PATHOPHYSIOLOGY
OF HEART DISEASE

*A Collaborative Project
of Medical Students and Faculty*

SECOND EDITION

PATHOPHYSIOLOGY
OF HEART DISEASE

*A Collaborative Project
of Medical Students and Faculty*

SECOND EDITION

EDITOR

Leonard S. Lilly, M.D.

*Associate Professor of Medicine
Harvard Medical School
Cardiologist
Brigham and Women's Hospital
Boston, Massachusetts*

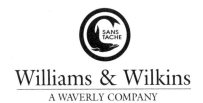

Williams & Wilkins

A WAVERLY COMPANY

BALTIMORE • PHILADELPHIA • LONDON • PARIS • BANGKOK
BUENOS AIRES • HONG KONG • MUNICH • SYDNEY • TOKYO • WROCLAW

Editor: Paul J. Kelly
Managing Editor: Crystal Taylor
Marketing Manager: Rebecca Himmelheber
Production Coordinator: Carol Eckhart
Project Editor: Karen M. Ruppert
Designer: Paul Fry
Illustration Planner: Lorraine Wrzosek
Cover Designer: Artech Graphics II
Typesetter: Peirce Graphic Services
Printer and Binder: Mack Printing Group

351 West Camden Street
Baltimore, Maryland 21201-2436 USA

Rose Tree Corporate Center
1400 North Providence Road
Building II, Suite 5025
Media, Pennsylvania 19063-2043 USA

Accurate indications, adverse reactions and dosage schedules for drugs are provided in this book, but it is possible that they may change. The reader is urged to review the package information data of the manufacturers of the medications mentioned.

Printed in the United States of America

First Edition, 1993

Library of Congress Cataloging-in-Publication Data

Pathophysiology of heart disease : a collaborative project of medical students and
    faculty / editor, Leonard S. Lilly. — 2nd ed.
        p.   cm.
    Developed by the medical students and cardiology faculty of Harvard Medical
    School.
    Includes bibliographical references and index.
    ISBN 0-683-30220-5
    1. Heart—Pathophysiology.   I. Lilly, Leonard S.   II. Harvard Medical School.
    [DNLM: 1. Heart Diseases—physiopathology. WG 200 P2973 1997]
    RC682.9.P255 1997
    616. 1' 207—dc21
    DNLM/DLC
    for Library of Congress   97-25006
                                                                                                                          CIP

The publishers have made every effort to trace the copyright holders for borrowed material. If they have inadvertently overlooked any, they will be pleased to make the necessary arrangements at the first opportunity.

To purchase additional copies of this book, call our customer service department at **(800) 638–0672** or fax orders to **(800) 447–8438.** For other book services, including chapter reprints and large quantity sales, ask for the Special Sales department.

Canadian customers should call **(800) 665–1148**, or fax **(800) 665–0103.** For all other calls originating outside of the United States, please call **(410) 528–4223** or fax us at **(410) 528–8850.**

Visit Williams & Wilkins on the Internet: http://www.wwilkins.com or contact our customer service department at **custserv@wwilkins.com.** Williams & Wilkins customer service representatives are available from 8:30 am to 6:00 pm, EST, Monday through Friday, for telephone access.

98 99 00 01
2 3 4 5 6 7 8 9 10

To Carolyn,

To Jonathan and

To Norma and David Lilly

Foreword

It is axiomatic that when designing any new product or service, the needs of the prospective user must receive primary consideration. Regrettably, this is rarely the case with medical textbooks, which play such a vital role in the education of students, residents, fellows, practicing physicians, and paramedical professionals. A large majority of books are written for anyone who will read—or preferably buy—them. As a consequence they often provide a little for everyone but not enough for anyone. Many medical textbooks are reminiscent of the one-room schoolhouse, which included pupils ranging from the first to the twelfth grade. The need to deal with subject matter at enormously disparate levels of sophistication interfered with the educational process.

Medical educators appreciate that the needs of medical students exposed to a subject for the first time differ importantly from those of practicing physicians who wish to review an area learned previously or to be updated on new developments in a field with which they already have some familiarity. The lack of textbooks designed specifically for students leads faculty at schools around the country to spend countless hours preparing and duplicating voluminous lecture notes, and providing students with custom-designed "camels" (a camel is a cow created by a committee).

Pathophysiology of Heart Disease, a collaborative project of Harvard Medical Students and Faculty, represents a refreshing and innovative departure in the preparation of a medical text. Students, i.e., potential consumers, dissatisfied with currently available textbooks of cardiology made their needs clear. Fortunately, their pleas fell on receptive ears. Dr. Leonard Lilly, who joined our faculty after completing his clinical training at the Brigham and Women's Hospital and Harvard Medical School, has played a catalytic role in this project. He has brought together a group of talented students and faculty to produce this fine introductory text on the pathophysiology of heart disease *specifically* designed to meet the needs of medical students during their initial encounters with patients with heart disease. The text, tables, and illustrations are readily comprehensible to students. While *Pathophysiology of Heart Disease* is not meant to be encyclopedic or all-inclusive, it is remarkably thorough.

Quite appropriately, the first edition of this book has been received enthusiastically and is a recommended text in many medical schools. It has been translated into other languages, has received two awards of excellence from the American Medical Writers Association, and it has triggered at least two other student–faculty collaborative book projects.

Dr. Lilly and his colleagues—both faculty and students—have made a significant and unique contribution in preparing this important book. This second edition is not only an expanded but also an updated version of the first edition. As such, it will prove to be even more valuable.

EUGENE BRAUNWALD, M.D.
Distinguished Hersey Professor of Medicine,
Harvard Medical School;
Faculty Dean for Academic Programs,
Brigham and Women's Hospital
and Massachusetts General Hospital,
Boston, Massachusetts

Preface

This textbook is a comprehensive introduction to diseases of the cardiovascular system. Although excellent reference books of cardiology are available, their encyclopedic content can overwhelm the beginning student. Therefore, this text was written to serve as a simplified bridge between courses in basic physiology and the care of patients on the hospital wards and in the clinics. It is intended to help medical students and physicians-in-training form a solid foundation of knowledge of diseases of the heart and circulation, and is designed so that it can be read in its entirety during the one-month period usually allocated to courses in cardiovascular pathophysiology. Emphasis has been placed on the basic mechanisms by which cardiac illnesses develop, in order to facilitate the later in-depth study of clinical diagnosis and therapy.

The original motivation for writing this book was the need for such a text voiced by our medical students, as well as their desire to participate in its creation and direction. Consequently, the book's development is unusual in that it represents a close collaboration between Harvard medical students and cardiology faculty, who shared in the writing and editing of the manuscript. The goal of this pairing was to focus the subject matter on the needs of the student, while providing the expertise of our faculty members. One of the most important aims of student participation was to ensure that sufficient attention is provided to those concepts that they had found most difficult to learn during their own pathophysiology course work. In this updated second edition of *Pathophysiology of Heart Disease*, the collaborative effort has continued, between a new generation of medical students and our cardiovascular faculty.

The introductory chapters of the book review basic cardiac anatomy and physiology, and describe the tools needed for understanding the clinical aspects of subsequent material. These tools include interpretation of heart sounds and murmurs, imaging and catheterization techniques, and the electrocardiogram. The main body of the book addresses the major groups of cardiovascular diseases. The chapters are designed and edited to be read in sequence, but are sufficiently cross-referenced so that they can also be used out of order. The final chapter discusses the major classes of cardiovascular drugs and explains the physiologic rationale for their uses.

The diagrams and tables were devised to present information in a clear, straightforward manner. After an initial reading of the text, subsequent glances at the figures and tables should quickly prompt recall of the described pathophysiology.

It has been a great privilege for me to collaborate with the 56 talented, creative, and energetic students who contributed to the first and second editions of this book. Their enthusiasm and dedication have significantly facilitated the completion of this project. I am also indebted to my faculty colleague coauthors for their time, their expertise, and their encouragement.

Several individuals provided illustrative material for certain figures: we thank Eric Isselbacher, Krishna Kandarpa, Finn Mannting, Robert Pugatch, Helmutt Rennke, Stanley Robbins, and Frederick Schoen for their assistance. We also gratefully acknowledge constructive advice from H. Thomas Aretz, Dennis Claflin, Bruce Ewenstein, Daniel Federman, Gil Gross, and Robert Handin.

It has been a pleasure to work with the

editorial and production staffs of our publisher, Williams & Wilkins. In particular, we thank Crystal Taylor, Carol Eckhart, Paul Kelly, and their associates for their invaluable assistance and enthusiastic participation in bringing this edition to completion.

On behalf of the contributors, I hope that this book enhances your understanding of cardiovascular diseases, and that you find this learning path a beneficial and enjoyable one!

LEONARD S. LILLY, M.D.
BOSTON, MASSACHUSETTS

Contributors

Student Contributors

Gopa Bhattacharyya (M.D. '97)
Chapter 5

Price Kerfoot (M.D. '96)
Chapter 4

Oscar Benavidez (M.D. '98)
Chapter 2

Kyle Low (M.D. '97)
Chapter 4

Rahul Deshmukh (M.D. '97)
Chapter 13

C. Geoffrey McDonough (M.D. '97)
Chapter 15

Stephen K. Frankel (M.D. '95)
Chapters 8 & 9

Shona Pendse (M.D. '97)
Chapter 3

David Grayzel (M.D. '97)
Chapter 10

Thomas G. Roberts (M.D. '97)
Chapter 14

Douglas W. Green (M.D. '97)
Chapter 16

Marc S. Sabatine (M.D. '95)
Chapters 6, 7, 11 & 12

Kirsten Greineder (M.D. '98)
Chapter 1

David Sloane (M.D. '97)
Chapter 17

Sharon Horesh (M.D. '97)
Chapter 3

Allison Smith (M.D. '97)
Chapter 13

Steven N. Kalkanis (M.D. '97)
Chapter 17

Raymond Tabibiazar (M.D. '98)
Chapter 16

Faculty Contributors

Elliott M. Antman, M.D.
Associate Professor of Medicine
Harvard Medical School
Director, Levine Cardiac Unit
Brigham and Women's Hospital
Boston, Massachusetts

John A. Bittl, M.D.
Associate Professor of Medicine
Harvard Medical School
Director of Interventional Cardiology
Brigham and Women's Hospital
Boston, Massachusetts

Eugene Braunwald, M.D. *(Foreword)*
Distinguished Hersey Professor of Medicine
Harvard Medical School
Faculty Dean for Academic Programs at
Brigham and Women's Hospital and
Massachusetts General Hospital
Boston, Massachusetts

Patricia Challender Come, M.D.
Associate Professor of Medicine
Harvard Medical School
Cardiologist, Harvard Pilgram Health Care
Senior Physician, Beth Israel Deaconess
Hospital and Associate Physician
Brigham and Women's Hospital
Boston, Massachusetts

Mark A. Creager, M.D.
Associate Professor of Medicine
Harvard Medical School
Clinical Director, Vascular Medicine and
Atherosclerosis Unit, Cardiovascular Division
Brigham and Women's Hospital
Boston, Massachusetts

G. William Dec, M.D.
Associate Professor of Medicine
Harvard Medical School
Medical Director
Cardiac Transplantation Program
Massachusetts General Hospital
Boston, Massachusetts

Michael A. Fifer, M.D.
Associate Professor of Medicine
Harvard Medical School
Director, Coronary Care Unit
Massachusetts General Hospital
Boston, Massachusetts

Michael D. Freed, M.D.
Associate Professor of Pediatrics
Harvard Medical School
Senior Associate in Cardiology and Chief
Inpatient and Outpatient Cardiology Services
Children's Hospital
Boston, Massachusetts

Leonard I. Ganz, M.D.
Assistant Professor of Medicine
Medical College of Pennsylvania-Hahnemann
School of Medicine
Electrophysiology Section
Cardiovascular Division
Allegheny General Hospital
Pittsburgh, Pennsylvania

Allan Goldblatt, M.D.
Associate Professor of Pediatrics
Harvard Medical School
Emeritus Chief of Pediatric Cardiology
Massachusetts General Hospital
Boston, Massachusetts

Peter Libby, M.D.
Professor of Medicine
Harvard Medical School
Director, Vascular Medicine
and Atherosclerosis Unit
Brigham and Women's Hospital
Boston, Massachusetts

Leonard S. Lilly, M.D.
Associate Professor of Medicine
Harvard Medical School
Cardiologist, Brigham and Women's Hospital
Boston, Massachusetts

Patrick T. O'Gara, M.D.
Assistant Professor of Medicine
Harvard Medical School
Director of Clinical Cardiology
Vice Chairman for Clinical Affairs
Department of Medicine
Brigham and Women's Hospital
Boston, Massachusetts

Gary R. Strichartz, Ph.D.
Professor of Anaesthesia (Pharmacology)
Harvard Medical School
Director, Anesthesia Research Labs
Brigham and Women's Hospital
Boston, Massachusetts

Contents

Basic Cardiac Structure and Function

Kirsten Greineder,
Gary R. Strichartz,
and Leonard S. Lilly

A knowledge of normal cardiac structure and function is crucial to the understanding of diseases that afflict the heart. This chapter reviews basic cardiac anatomy, electrophysiology, and the events that lead to cardiac contraction.

CARDIAC ANATOMY AND HISTOLOGY

Although the study of cardiac anatomy dates back to ancient times, interest in this field has gained recent momentum. The development of sophisticated cardiac imaging procedures such as coronary angiography, echocardiography, computed tomography, and magnetic resonance imaging has made essential an intimate knowledge of the spatial relationships of cardiac structures. Such information also proves helpful in understanding the pathophysiology of heart disease. This section emphasizes the aspects of cardiac anatomy that are important to the clinician; that is, the "functional" anatomy.

Pericardium

The heart and roots of the great vessels are enclosed by a fibroserous sac called the pericardium (Fig. 1.1). This structure consists of two layers: a strong outer fibrous layer and an inner serosal layer. The inner serosal layer adheres to the external wall of the heart and is called the **visceral pericardium.** The visceral pericardium reflects back on itself and lines the outer fibrous layer, forming the **parietal pericardium.** The space between the visceral and parietal layers contains a thin film of pericardial fluid that allows the heart to beat in a minimal-friction environment.

The pericardium is attached to the sternum and the mediastinal portions of the right and left pleurae. Its many connections to surrounding structures keep the pericardial sac firmly anchored within the thorax and therefore help to maintain the heart in its normal position.

Emanating from the pericardium in a superior direction are the aorta, the pulmonary artery and the superior vena cava (Fig. 1.1). The inferior vena cava projects through the pericardium inferiorly.

Surface Anatomy of the Heart

The heart is shaped roughly like a cone and consists of four muscular chambers.

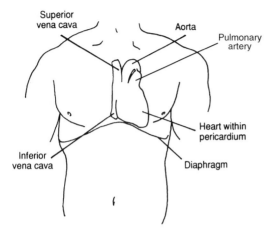

Figure 1.1. The position of the heart in the chest.
The superior vena cava, aorta, and pulmonary artery
exit superiorly, whereas the inferior vena cava
projects inferiorly.

The right and left ventricles are the main
pumping chambers. The less muscular right
and left atria deliver blood to their respective ventricles.

Several terms are used to describe the
heart's surfaces and borders (Fig. 1.2). The
apex is formed by the tip of the left ventricle, which points inferiorly, anteriorly, and
to the left. The **base** or posterior surface of
the heart is formed by the atria, mainly the
left, and lies between the lung hila. The **anterior** surface of the heart is shaped by the
right atrium and ventricle. Since the left
atrium and ventricle lie more posteriorly,
they form only a small strip of this anterior
surface. The **inferior** surface of the heart is
formed by both ventricles, primarily the
left. This surface of the heart lies along the
diaphragm, hence, it is also referred to as
the "diaphragmatic" surface.

Observing the chest from an anteropos-
terior view (such as on a chest radiograph,
as described in Chapter 3), four recognized
borders of the heart are apparent. The right
border is established by the right atrium
and is almost in line with the superior and
inferior vena cavae. The inferior border is
nearly horizontal and is formed mainly by
the right ventricle, with a slight contribution from the left ventricle near the apex.
The left ventricle and a portion of the left
atrium make up the left border of the heart,

whereas the superior border is shaped by
both atria. From this description of the surface of the heart emerge two basic "rules" of
normal cardiac anatomy: 1) right-sided
structures lie mostly anterior to their left-
sided counterparts, and 2) atrial chambers
are located mostly to the right of their corresponding ventricles.

Internal Structure of the Heart

Four major valves are present in the normal heart that direct blood flow in a forward direction and prevent backward leakage. The atrioventricular valves (tricuspid
and mitral) separate the atria and ventricles,
whereas the semilunar valves (pulmonic
and aortic) separate the ventricles from the
great arteries. All four heart valves are attached to the fibrous **cardiac skeleton** (Fig.
1.3). The cardiac skeleton is composed of
dense connective tissue and serves as a site
of attachment for the valves, and for the
ventricular and atrial muscles.

The surface of the heart valves and the
interior surface of the heart chambers are
lined by a single layer of endothelial cells,
termed the **endocardium.** The subendocardial tissue contains fibroblasts, elastic
and collagenous fibers, veins, nerves, and
branches of the conducting system and is
continuous with the connective tissue of the
heart muscle layer, the myocardium. The
myocardium is the thickest layer of the
heart and consists of bundles of cardiac
muscle cells, the histology of which is described below. External to the myocardium
is a layer of connective tissue and adipose
tissue through which pass the larger blood
vessels and nerves that supply the heart
muscle. The **epicardium** is the outermost
layer of the heart and is identical to, and just
another term, for the visceral pericardium
described above.

Right Atrium and Ventricle

Opening into the **right atrium** are the superior and inferior vena cavae and the coronary sinus (Fig. 1.4). The vena cavae return

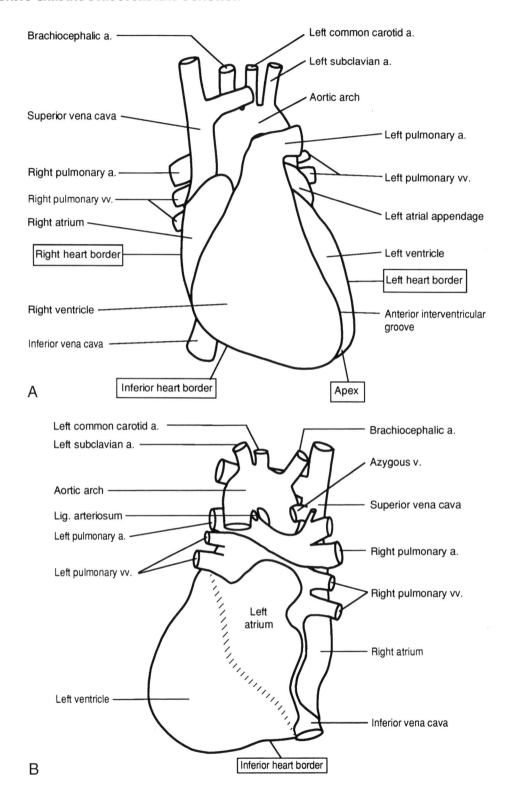

Figure 1.2.   A. The anterior view of the heart and great vessels. **B.** The posterior aspect (or base) of the heart and great vessels, as viewed from the back. a, artery; vv, veins.

Anterior

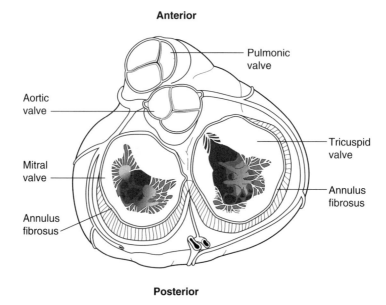

Posterior

Figure 1.3.   The four heart valves viewed from above with atria removed. The figure depicts the period of ventricular filling (diastole) during which the tricuspid and mitral valves are open and the semilunar valves (pulmonic and aortic) are closed. Each annulus fibrosus surrounding the mitral and tricuspid valves is thicker than those surrounding the pulmonic and aortic valves.

deoxygenated blood from the systemic veins into the right atrium, whereas the coronary sinus caries venous return from the coronary arteries. The interatrial septum forms the posteromedial wall of the right atrium and separates it from the left atrium. The **tricuspid valve** is located in the floor of the atrium and opens into the right ventricle.

The **right ventricle** (Fig. 1.4) is roughly triangular in shape, and its superior aspect forms a cone-shaped outflow tract, which leads to the pulmonary artery. Although the inner wall of the outflow tract is smooth, the rest of the ventricle is covered by a number of irregular bridges (termed **trabeculae carneae**) that give the right ventricular wall

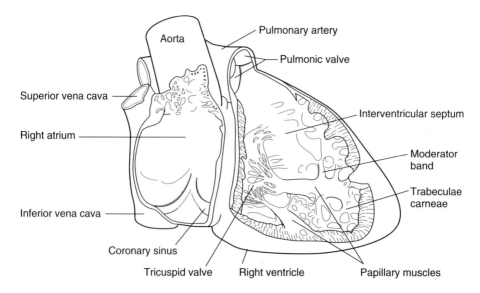

Figure 1.4.   Interior structures of the right atrium and right ventricle. (Modified from Goss CM. Gray's Anatomy. 29th ed. Philadelphia: Lea and Febiger, 1973:547).

a spongelike appearance. A large trabecula that crosses the ventricular cavity is called the **moderator band.** It carries a component of the right bundle branch of the conducting system to the ventricular muscle.

The right ventricle contains three **papillary muscles,** which project into the chamber and via their thin, stringlike **chordae tendineae** attach to the edges of the tricuspid valve leaflets. The leaflets, in turn, are attached to the fibrous ring that supports the valve between the right atrium and ventricle. Contraction of the papillary muscles prior to other regions of the ventricle tightens the chordae tendineae, drawing the leaflets of the tricuspid valve together. This action prevents blood from regurgitating into the right atrium during ventricular contraction.

At the apex of the right ventricular outflow tract is the **pulmonic valve,** which leads to the pulmonary artery. This valve consists of three cusps attached to a fibrous ring. During relaxation of the ventricle, elastic recoil of the pulmonary arteries forces blood back toward the heart, distending the valve cusps toward one another. This action closes the pulmonic valve and prevents regurgitation of blood back into the right ventricle.

Left Atrium and Ventricle

Entering the posterior half of the **left atrium** are the four pulmonary veins (Fig. 1.5A). The wall of the left atrium is about 2 mm thick, being slightly greater than that of the right atrium. The mitral valve opens into the left ventricle through the inferior wall of the left atrium.

The cavity of the **left ventricle** is approximately cone-shaped and longer than that of the right ventricle. In healthy adult hearts, the wall thickness is 9 to 11 mm, roughly three times that of right. The aortic vestibule is a smooth-walled part of the left ventricular cavity located just inferior to the aortic valve. Inferior to this region, most of the ventricle is covered by trabeculae carneae, which are finer and more numerous than in the right ventricle.

The left ventricular chamber (Fig. 1.5B) contains two large papillary muscles. These are larger than their counterparts in the right ventricle, and their chordae tendineae are thicker, but less numerous. The chordae tendineae of each papillary muscle distribute to both leaflets of the **mitral valve.** Similar to the case in the right ventricle, tensing of the chordae tendineae during left ventricular contraction helps the mitral leaflets close properly to prevent the backward leakage of blood.

The **aortic valve** separates the left ventricle from the aorta. Surrounding the aortic valve opening is a fibrous ring to which is attached the three cusps of the valve. Just above the right and left aortic valve cusps in the aortic wall are the origins of the right and left coronary arteries (Fig. 1.5B).

Interventricular Septum

The interventricular septum is the thick wall between the left and right ventricles. It is composed of a muscular and a membranous part (Fig. 1.5B). The margins of this septum can be traced on the surface of the heart by following the anterior and posterior interventricular grooves. Owing to the greater hydrostatic pressure within the left ventricle, the large muscular portion of the septum bulges toward the right ventricle. The small, oval-shaped membranous part of the septum is thin and located just inferior to the cusps of the aortic valve.

To summarize the functional anatomic points presented in this section, we now review the path of blood flow through the heart. Deoxygenated blood is delivered to the heart through the inferior and superior vena cavae, which enter into the right atrium. Flow continues through the tricuspid valve orifice into the right ventricle. Contraction of the right ventricle propels the blood across the pulmonic valve to the pulmonary artery and lungs, where carbon dioxide is released and oxygen is taken up. The oxygen-rich blood returns to the heart through the pulmonary veins to the left atrium, then passes across the mitral valve into the left ventricle. Contraction of the left

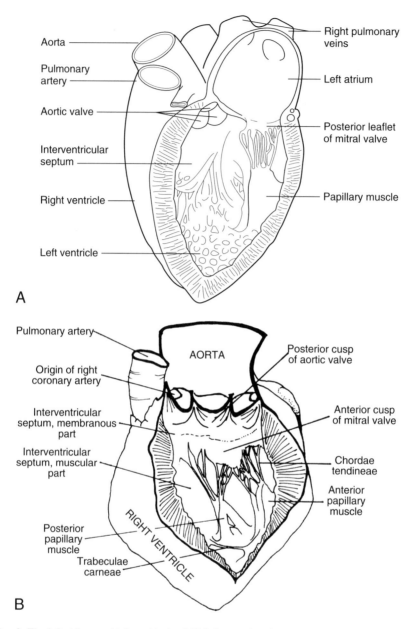

Figure 1.5. **A.** The left atrium and left ventricular (LV) inflow and outflow regions. **B.** Interior structures of the LV cavity. (Modified from Agur AMR, Lee MJ. Grant's Atlas of Anatomy. 9th ed. Baltimore: Williams & Wilkins, 1991:59.)

ventricle pumps the oxygenated blood across the aortic valve into the aorta, whereupon it is distributed to all other tissues of the body.

Impulse Conducting System

The impulse conducting system (Fig. 1.6) consists of specialized cells that initiate the

heartbeat and electrically coordinate contractions of the heart chambers. The **sinoatrial (SA) node** is a small mass of specialized cardiac muscle fibers in the wall of the right atrium. It is located to the right of the superior vena cava entrance and normally initiates the electrical impulse for contraction. The **atrioventricular (AV) node** lies beneath the endocardium in the inferoposterior part of the interatrial septum.

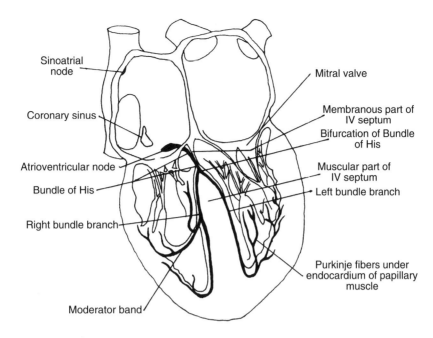

Figure 1.6. Main components of the cardiac conduction system include the sinoatrial node, atrioventricular node, bundle of His, right and left bundle branches, and the Purkinje fibers. The moderator band carries a large portion of the right bundle.

Distal to the AV node is the **bundle of His,** which perforates the interventricular septum posteriorly. Within the septum, the bundle of His bifurcates into a broad sheet of fibers that continues over the left side of the septum, known as the **left bundle branch,** and a compact, cablelike structure on the right side, the **right bundle branch.**

The right bundle branch is thick and deeply buried in the muscle of the interventricular septum, and continues towards the apex. Near the junction of the interventricular septum and the anterior wall of the right ventricle, the right bundle branch becomes subendocardial and bifurcates. One branch travels across the right ventricular cavity in the moderator band, whereas the other continues toward the tip of the ventricle. These branches eventually arborize into a finely divided anastomosing plexus that travels throughout the right ventricle.

Functionally, the left bundle branch is divided into an anterior and a posterior fascicle and a small branch to the septum. The anterior fascicle runs anteriorly toward the apex, forming a subendocardial plexus in the area of the anterior papillary muscle. The posterior fascicle travels to the area of

the posterior papillary muscle, then divides into a subendocardial plexus and spreads to the rest of the left ventricle.

The subendocardial plexuses of both ventricles send distributing **Purkinje fibers** to the ventricular muscle. Impulses within the His-Purkinje system are transmitted first to the papillary muscles and then throughout the walls of the ventricles, allowing papillary muscle contraction to precede that of the ventricles. This coordination prevents regurgitation of blood flow through the atrioventricular valves, as discussed above.

Cardiac Innervation

The heart is innervated by both parasympathetic and sympathetic afferent and efferent nerves. Preganglionic *sympathetic* neurons located within the upper five to six thoracic levels of the spinal cord synapse with second-order neurons in the cervical sympathetic ganglia. Traveling within the cardiac nerves, these fibers terminate in the heart and great vessels. Preganglionic *parasympathetic* fibers originate in the dorsal motor nucleus of the medulla and pass as branches of the vagus nerve to the heart and great vessels. Here the fibers synapse with second-order neurons located in ganglia within these structures. A rich supply of vagal afferents from the inferior and posterior aspects of the ventricles mediate important cardiac reflexes, whereas the abundant vagal efferent fibers to the SA and AV nodes are active in modulating electrical impulse initiation and conduction.

Cardiac Vessels

The cardiac vessels consist of the coronary arteries and veins and the lymphatic vessels. The largest components of these systems lie within the loose connective tissue in the epicardial fat.

Coronary Arteries

The heart muscle is supplied with oxygen and nutrients by the right and left coronary arteries, which arise from the root of the aorta just above the aortic valve cusps (Figs. 1.5B, 1.7). After their origin, these vessels pass anteriorly, one on each side of the pulmonary artery (Fig. 1.7).

The large **left main coronary artery** passes between the left atrium and the pulmonary trunk to reach the atrioventricular groove. Here, it divides into the **left anterior descending (LAD) coronary artery** and the circumflex artery. The LAD travels within the anterior interventricular groove toward the cardiac apex. During its descent on the anterior surface, the LAD gives off septal branches that supply the anterior two-thirds of the interventricular septum and the apical portion of the anterior papillary muscle. The LAD also gives off diagonal branches that supply the anterior surface of the left ventricle. The **circumflex artery** continues within the left atrioventricular groove and passes around the left border of the heart to reach the posterior surface. It gives off large obtuse marginal branches that supply the lateral and posterior wall of the left ventricle.

The **right coronary artery (RCA)** travels in the right atrioventricular groove, passing posteriorly between the right atrium and ventricle. It supplies blood to the right ventricle via acute marginal branches. In most individuals, the distal RCA gives rise to a large branch, the **posterior descending artery** (Fig. 1.7C). This vessel travels from the inferoposterior aspect of the heart to the apex and supplies blood to the inferior and posterior walls of the ventricles and the posterior one-third of the interventricular septum. Just prior to giving off the posterior descending branch, the RCA usually gives off the **AV nodal artery.**

The posterior descending and AV nodal arteries arise from the RCA in 85% of the population. In approximately 8% of individuals, the posterior descending artery arises from the circumflex artery instead. In the remaining population, the heart's posterior blood supply is contributed to from branches of both the RCA and the circumflex.

The blood supply to the sinoatrial node is also most often (70% of the time) derived from the RCA. However, in 25% of normal hearts, the **SA nodal artery** arises from the circumflex artery, and in 5% of cases, both the RCA and the circumflex contribute to this vessel.

From their epicardial locations, the coronary arteries send perforating branches into the ventricular muscle, which form a richly branching and anastomosing vasculature in the walls of all of the cardiac chambers. From this plexus arise a massive number of capillaries that form an elaborate network surrounding each cardiac muscle fiber. The muscle fibers located just beneath the endocardium, particularly those of the papillary muscles and the thick left ventricle, are supplied either by the terminal branches of the coronary arteries or directly from the ventricular cavity through tiny vascular channels, known as **thebesian veins.**

Collateral connections, usually < 200 μm in diameter, exist at the subarteriolar level between the coronary arteries. In the normal heart, few of these collateral vessels are visible. However, they may become larger and functional when atherosclerotic disease obstructs a coronary artery, thereby providing flow to distal portions of the vessel from a nonobstructed neighbor.

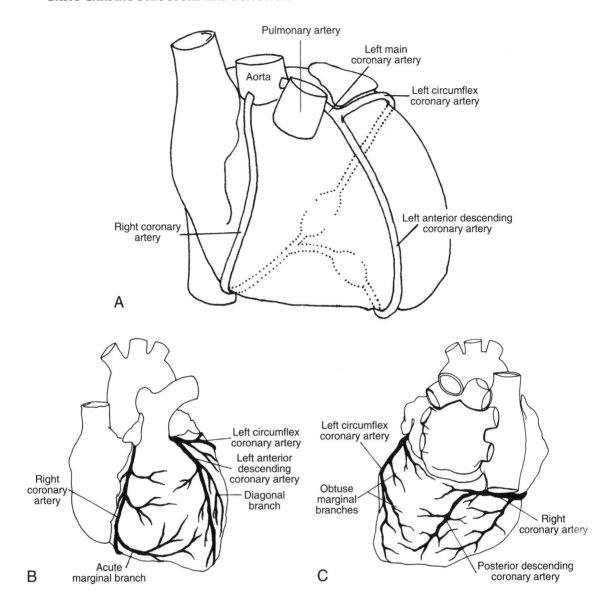

Figure 1.7. Coronary artery anatomy. A. Schematic representation of the right and left coronary arteries demonstrates their orientation to one another; the left main artery bifurcates into the circumflex artery, which perfuses the lateral and posterior aspects of the left ventricle (LV), and the anterior descending artery, which perfuses the LV anterior wall, anterior portion of the intraventricular septum, and a portion of the anterior right ventricular (RV) wall. The right coronary artery (RCA) perfuses the right ventricle and variable portions of the posterior left ventricle through its terminal branches. The posterior descending artery most often arises from the RCA. **B.** Anterior view of the heart demonstrating the coronary arteries and their major branches. **C.** Posterior view of the heart demonstrating the terminal portions of the right and circumflex coronary arteries and their branches.

Coronary Veins

The coronary veins follow a distribution similar to that of the major coronary arteries. These vessels return blood from the myocardial capillaries to the right atrium predominantly via the coronary sinus. The major veins lie in the epicardial fat, usually superficial to the coronary arteries. The thebesian veins, mentioned above, provide an additional potential route for a small amount of direct blood return to the cardiac chambers.

Lymphatic Vessels

The heart lymph is drained by an extensive plexus of valved vessels located in the subendocardial connective tissue of all four chambers. This lymph drains to the epicardial plexus of lymphatic vessels in the interstitial connective tissue. These smaller vessels anastomose to form several large lymphatic vessels that follow the distribution of the coronary arteries and veins. Each of these large vessels then combines in the atrioventricular groove to form a single large lymphatic vessel, which eventually exits the heart to reach the mediastinal lymphatic plexus and ultimately the thoracic duct.

Histology of Ventricular Myocardial Cells

The mature myocardial cell (also termed **myocyte**) measures up to 25 μm in diameter and 100 μm in length. The cell shows a cross-striated banding pattern similar to that of skeletal muscle. However, unlike the multinucleated skeletal myofibers, myocardial cells contain only one or two centrally located nuclei. Surrounding each myocardial cell is connective tissue with a rich capillary network.

Each myocardial cell contains numerous **myofibrils,** which are long chains of individual **sarcomeres,** the fundamental contractile units of the cell (Fig. 1.8). Each sarcomere is made up of two groups of overlapping filaments of contractile proteins. Biochemical and biophysical interactions occurring between these myofilaments produce muscle contraction. Their structure and function are described later in this chapter.

Within each myocardial cell the neighboring sarcomeres are all in register, producing the characteristic cross-striated banding pattern seen by light microscopy.

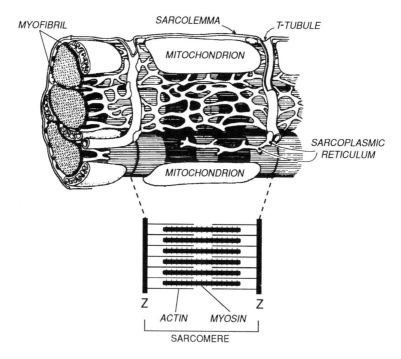

Figure 1.8.   Top. Schematic representation of the ultrastructure of the myocardial cell. The cell consists of multiple parallel myofibrils surrounded by mitochondria. The T tubules are invaginations of the cell membrane (the sarcolemma) that increase the surface area for ion transport and transmission of electrical impulses. The intracellular sarcoplasmic reticulum houses the majority of intracellular calcium and abuts the T tubules. (Modified from Katz AM. Physiology of the Heart. 2nd ed. New York: Raven Press, 1992:21.) **Bottom.** Expanded view of a sarcomere, the basic unit of contraction. Each myofibril consists of serially connected sarcomeres, that extend from one Z line to the next. The sarcomere is composed of alternating thin (actin) and thick (myosin) myofilaments.

The relative densities of the cross bands identify the location of the contractile proteins within the sarcomere. Under physiologic conditions the overall sarcomere length (Z to Z distance) varies between 2.2 and 1.5 μm during the cardiac cycle. The larger dimension reflects the degree of fiber stretch during ventricular filling, whereas the smaller one represents the extent of fiber shortening during contraction.

The myocardial cell membrane is termed the **sarcolemma.** A specialized region of the membrane is the **intercalated disk,** a distinct characteristic of cardiac muscle tissue. Intercalated disks are seen on light microscopy as darkly staining transverse lines that cross chains of cardiac cells at irregular intervals. They represent the gap junction complexes at the interface of adjacent cardiac fibers and establish structural and electrical continuity between the myocardial cells.

Another functional feature of the cell membrane is the **transverse tubular system (or T tubules).** This complex system is characterized by deep, fingerlike invaginations of the sarcolemma (Figs. 1.8, 1.9). Similar to the intercalated disks, transverse tubular membranes establish pathways for rapid transmission of the excitatory electrical impulses that initiate contraction. The T tubule system increases the surface area of the sarcolemma in contact with the extracellular environment, allowing the transmembrane ion transport accompanying excitation and relaxation to occur quickly and synchronously.

The **sarcoplasmic reticulum** is an extensive intracellular tubular membrane network that complements the T tubule system both structurally and functionally. The sarcoplasmic reticulum abuts the T tubules at right angles in lateral sacs, called the terminal cisternae (Fig. 1.9). These sacs house the majority of the intracellular calcium stores, the release of which is important in linking membrane excitation with activation of the contractile apparatus. The lateral sacs also abut the intercalated disks and the sarcolemma, providing each with a complete system for excitation-contraction coupling.

To serve the tremendous metabolic demand placed on the heart and the need for a constant supply of high energy phosphates, the myocardial cell has an abundant concentration of mitochondria. These organelles are located between the individual myofibrils and constitute approximately 35% of the cell volume (Fig. 1.8).

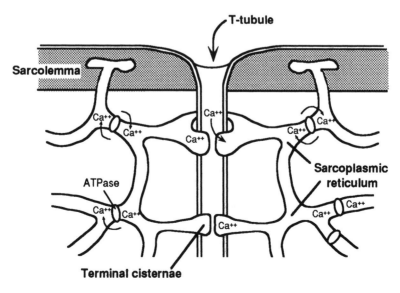

Figure 1.9. Schematic view of the tubular systems of the myocardial cell. The T tubules, invaginations of the sarcolemma, abut the sarcoplasmic reticulum at right angles at the terminal cisternae sacs. This relationship is important in linking membrane excitation with intracellular release of calcium from the sarcoplasmic reticulum.

BASIC ELECTROPHYSIOLOGY

Rhythmic contraction of the heart relies on the organized propagation of electrical impulses along its conduction pathway. The marker of electrical stimulation, the **action potential,** is created by a sequence of ion fluxes through specific channels in the sarcolemma. To provide a basis for understanding how electrical impulses lead to cardiac contraction, we now review the process of cellular depolarization and repolarization. This material serves as an important foundation for topics addressed later in this book, including electrocardiography (Chapter 4) and cardiac arrhythmias (Chapters 11 and 12).

Cardiac cells capable of electrical excitation are of three electrophysiologic types, the properties of which have been studied by intracellular microelectrode and patch-clamp recordings:

1. Pacemaker cells (e.g., SA node, AV node)
2. Specialized rapidly conducting tissues (e.g., Purkinje fibers)
3. Ventricular and atrial muscle cells

The sarcolemma of each of these cardiac cell types is a phospholipid bilayer that is largely impermeable to ions. There are specialized proteins interspersed throughout the membrane that serve as ion channels, cotransporters, and active transporters (Fig. 1.10). These transporters help maintain ionic concentration gradients and charge differentials between the inside and the outside of the cardiac cells. Normally, Na^+ and Ca^{++} concentrations are much higher outside of the cell, and K^+ concentrations much higher inside.

Ion Channels

Ion channels are specialized proteins that span the cell membrane and contain hydrophilic pores through which certain charged atoms can pass. There are several types of cardiac ion channels, which vary by two functional properties: selectivity and gating.

Each type of channel is **selective** for a specific ion, which is a manifestation of the size and structure of its pore. For example, in cardiac calls, some channels permit the passage of sodium ions, some are specific for potassium, whereas others allow only calcium to pass through.

An ion can pass through its specific channel only at certain times. That is, the ion channel is **gated:** at any given moment, the channel is in either an open or closed state. The more time that a channel is in its open state, the larger the number of ions that pass through it and therefore, the greater the transmembrane current. For cardiac ion channels involved in the generation of the action potential, it is the voltage across the membrane that determines whether the channel is open or closed. Therefore, the gating of such channels is **voltage-sensitive.** As the membrane voltage changes during depolarization and repolarization of the cell, specific channels open and close, with corresponding alterations in the ion fluxes across the sarcolemma.

As an example of voltage-sensitive gating, let's consider the cardiac channel known as the **fast sodium channel.** The transmembrane protein that forms this channel assumes different conformations depending on the cell's membrane potential (Fig. 1.11). At a potential of -90 mV (the typical "resting voltage" of a ventricular muscle cell), the channels are primarily in a closed, *resting state,* such that Na^+ ions cannot pass through. In this resting state, the channels are available for conversion to the open configuration.

A rapid wave of depolarization (which causes the membrane potential to become less negative) "activates" the resting channels to the *open state,* through which Na^+ ions readily permeate; thus, an inward Na^+ current ensues. However, the activated channels remain open for only a brief time, a few thousandths of a second, and then spontaneously close, to an *inactive state* (Fig. 1.11C). Channels in this closed, inactivated conformation cannot be directly converted back to the open state; the "gating" portions of the channel protein are largely immobilized by the inactivation process.

The inactivated state persists until the

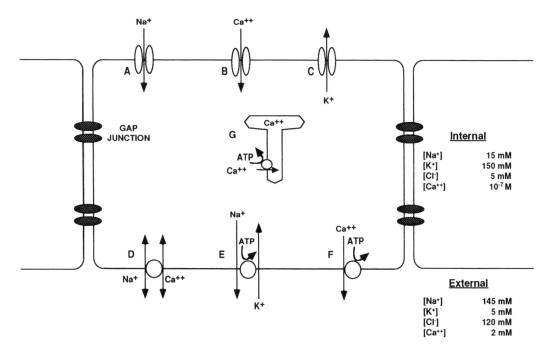

Figure 1.10.   Ion channels, cotransporters, and active transporters of the myocyte. A. Sodium entry through the "fast" sodium channel is responsible for the rapid upstroke (phase 0) of the action potential (AP) in nonpacemaker cells. **B.** Calcium enters the cell through the "slow" calcium channel during phase 2 of the Purkinje and muscle cell AP, and is the main channel responsible for depolarization of pacemaker cells. **C.** Potassium exits through the potassium channel to repolarize the cell during phase 3 of the AP, and open potassium channels help maintain the resting potential (phase 4) of nonpacemaker cells. **D.** Sodium/calcium exchanger helps maintain the low intracellular calcium concentration. **E.** Sodium/potassium ATPase pump maintains concentration gradients for these ions. **F, G.** Active calcium pumps aid removal of calcium to the external environment and sarcoplasmic reticulum, respectively.

membrane voltage has repolarized nearly back to its original resting level. Until it does so, the closed, inactivated channel prevents any flow of sodium ions. Therefore, during normal cellular depolarization, the voltage-dependent fast sodium channels conduct for a short period of time, then close and are unable to reopen until the cell membrane has nearly fully repolarized.

Another important attribute of cardiac fast sodium channels should be noted. If the transmembrane voltage of a cardiac cell is *slowly* depolarized and maintained *chronically* at levels less negative than the usual resting potential, inactivation of channels occurs *without* initial opening (Fig. 1.11). Furthermore, as long as the less negative potential exists, the closed, inactive state *never* returns to the resting state, such that the fast sodium channels in such a cell are continuously unable to conduct Na$^+$ ions. This is the typical case in cardiac pacemaker

cells (e.g., SA and AV node) in which the membrane voltage is generally less negative than -70 mV throughout the cardiac cycle. As a result, the fast sodium channels in pacemaker cells are persistently inactivated, and do not play a role in the generation of the action potential in these cells.

Calcium and potassium channels in cardiac cells also act in voltage-dependent fashions, but they behave differently than the sodium channels, as will be described in the following sections.

Resting Potential

In cardiac cells at rest, prior to excitation, the electrical charge differential between the inside and outside of a cell is known as the **resting potential.** The magnitude of the resting potential depends upon two main properties: 1) the concentration gradient of ions

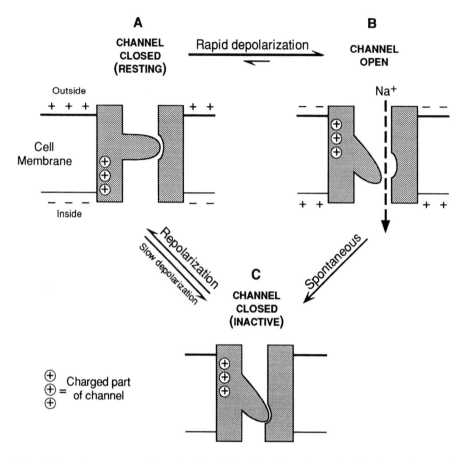

Figure 1.11. Schematic representation of gating of "fast" sodium channels. A. In the resting membrane, most channels are in the closed, resting state. **B.** Rapid, large depolarizations force the charged parts of the channel to translocate, activating the channel to the open conformation, and Na+ ions permeate into the cell. **C.** From the open state, the channels spontaneously close to the inactivated state, from which reopening cannot directly occur. This closed, inactive state persists until repolarization returns the channel to the resting state. Note that when cells are *slowly* depolarized, they may enter the closed, inactive state directly from the resting state, without channel opening.

between the inside and outside of the cell, and 2) which ion channels are open at rest.

Similar to other tissues such as nerve cells and skeletal muscle, the potassium concentration is much greater inside cardiac cells compared to outside. This is attributed to cell membrane transporters, the most important of which is the ATP-dependent Na+/K+ pump, which exchanges Na+ ions in an outward direction for K+ movement inward.

Cardiac myocytes contain potassium channels that are open in the resting state, at a time when other ionic channels (i.e., sodium and calcium) are closed. Therefore, *the resting cell membrane is much more permeable to potassium than to other ions.* As a result

of its open channels at rest, K+ fluxes in an outward direction down its concentration gradient, removing positive charges from the cell. The predominant counterions for potassium within the cell are large negatively charged proteins that are unable to diffuse out of the cell along with K+. Thus as potassium ions exit the cell, the anions that are left behind cause the interior of the cell to become electrically negative with respect to the outside.

However, as the interior of the cell becomes more and more *negatively* charged by the outward flux of potassium, the *positively* charged K+ ions are attracted back toward the cellular interior, an effect that slows their net exit from the cell. Thus, there are two opposing forces directing the flux of potassium ions across their open channels in the resting state (Fig. 1.12): 1) the concentration gradient favors outward passage of potassium, whereas 2) the electrostatic force attracts potassium back into the cell. At steady state, the balance between these chemical and electrical forces determine the resting potential, which is approximately −90 mV in ventricular muscle cells. This electrical potential at rest can be predicted by the Nernst equation for potassium, as shown in the figure.

In the resting state, the permeability of the cardiac muscle cellular membrane for sodium is minimal because the sodium channels are essentially closed. Nonetheless, there is a slight leak of sodium ions through their channels into the cell. This tiny inward current of positively charged sodium ions explains why the actual resting potential is slightly less negative than would be predicted if the cell membrane were truly only permeable to potassium ions.

The sodium ions that slowly leak into the myocyte at rest (and the much larger amount that enters during the action potential as described below) are continuously removed from the cell and returned to the extracellular environment. This is accomplished by the ATP-dependent Na^+/K^+ pump, which extrudes sodium from the cell in exchange for potassium. In this process, three Na^+ ions are moved in an outward direction for each two K^+ ions inward, creating a net outward flow of positive charges. This net outward movement of cations also contributes to maintaining the cell interior more negatively charged than the outside.

Action Potential

When the cell membrane voltage is altered, its permeability to specific ions changes. The changes in ion permeability are a reflection of the voltage-gating of the ion channels, and each type of channel has a characteristic pattern of activation and inactivation that determines the progression of the electrical signal. This discussion be-

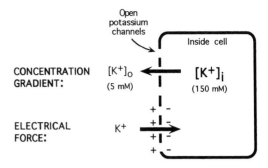

$$\text{Equilibrium potential} = -61.5 \log ([K^+]_i / [K^+]_o)$$

Figure 1.12. The resting potential of a cardiac muscle cell is determined by the balance between the concentration gradient and electrostatic forces for potassium, because only potassium channels are open at rest. The concentration gradient favors outward movement of K^+, whereas the electrical force attracts the positively charged K^+ ions inward. The equilibrium (resting) potential can be approximated by the Nernst equation for potassium, as shown in the figure.

gins by following the development of the action potential in a typical cardiac muscle cell (Fig. 1.13). The unique characteristics of action potentials in cardiac pacemaker cells will be described later.

Cardiac Muscle Cell

Until otherwise provoked, the resting potential of the cardiac muscle cell remains stable, at approximately −90 mV. This resting state prior to depolarization is known as **phase 4** of the action potential. Following phase 4, four additional phases characterize depolarization and repolarization of the cell (Fig. 1.13):

Phase 0. At the resting membrane voltage, sodium and calcium channels are closed. Any process that makes the membrane potential less negative than the resting value causes some sodium channels to open. As Na^+ channels open, sodium ions rapidly enter the cell, flowing down their concentration gradient (the sodium concentration is greater outside of the cell), because these positively charged ions are attracted to the negatively charged cellular interior. The entry of Na^+ ions into the cell causes the transmembrane potential to become progressively less negative, which in

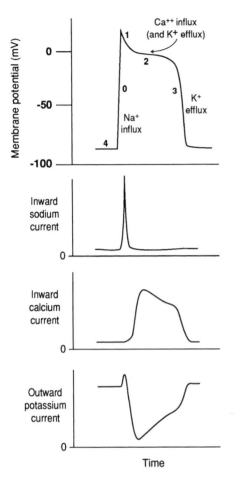

Figure 1.13. Schematic representation of a myocyte action potential (AP), and relative net ion currents for Na$^+$, Ca^{++}, and K$^+$. The resting potential is represented by phase 4 of the AP. Following depolarization, Na$^+$ influx results in the rapid upstroke of phase 0; a transient outward potassium current is responsible for partial repolarization during phase 1; slow Ca^{++} influx (and relatively low K$^+$ efflux) results in the plateau of phase 2; final rapid repolarization is largely due to K$^+$ efflux during phase 3.

turn causes more sodium channels to open and promotes further sodium entry into the cell. When the membrane voltage approaches the **threshold potential** (approximately −70 mV in cardiac muscle cells), enough of these "fast" Na$^+$ channels have opened to generate a self-sustaining inward Na$^+$ current. The magnitude of entry of positively charged Na$^+$ ions, driven by their concentration gradient, neutralizes the membrane potential to zero, and transiently into the positive range.

This prominent influx of sodium ions is responsible for the rapid upstroke, or phase

0, of the action potential. However, the Na$^+$ channels remain open for only a few thousandths of a second and are then quickly inactivated, preventing further influx (Fig. 1.13). Thus, while activation of these fast Na$^+$ channels causes the rapid early depolarization of the cell, the rapid inactivation makes their major contribution to the action potential short-lived.

Phase 1. Following rapid phase 0 depolarization, a transient current of repolarization returns the membrane potential to approximately 0 mV. The responsible current appears to be due primarily to an outward flow of K$^+$ ions through a type of transiently activated potassium channel.

Phase 2. This relatively long phase of the action potential is mediated by a balance of persistent outward K$^+$ current opposed by an inward Ca^{++} current through calcium channels (termed "L-type" calcium channels), which begin to open during phase 0 (when the membrane voltage reaches approximately −40 mV). When these channels open, Ca^{++} flows down its concentration gradient into the cell. Ca^{++} entry proceeds in a more gradual fashion than the initial influx of sodium, because the activation of calcium channels is slower and the channel remains open much longer than the fast Na$^+$ channel (Fig. 1.13). During this phase, the Ca^{++} influx, and the relatively low permeability to K$^+$ efflux, maintains a voltage of approximately 0 mV for a prolonged period, known as the **plateau.** Calcium ions that enter the cell during this phase play an important role in triggering additional internal calcium release from the sarcoplasmic reticulum ("calcium-induced calcium release"), which is important in initiating myocyte contraction, as discussed below.

As the Ca^{++} channels gradually inactivate, and the efflux of K$^+$ begins to exceed the influx of calcium, phase 3 begins.

Phase 3. This is the final period of repolarization that returns the transmembrane voltage back to the resting potential of approximately −90 mV. An outward potassium current, and low membrane permeability for other cations are responsible for this rapid repolarization. This phase completes the action potential cycle, with a return to resting phase 4, preparing the cell for the next stimulus for depolarization.

In order to preserve normal transmembrane ionic concentration gradients, the sodium and calcium that enter the cell during depolarization must be returned to the extracellular environment. Similarly, potassium ions must return to the cell interior. The exchange of Na^+ and K^+ across the cell membrane is mediated via the ATP-dependent Na^+/K^+ pump. Excess Ca^{++} in the cell is eliminated primarily by Na^+/Ca^{++} exchange, and a lesser amount by the ATP-consuming calcium pump.

Specialized Conduction System

The previous section applies to the action potential of cardiac muscle cells. The cells of the specialized conduction system (e.g., Purkinje fibers) behave similarly, although the resting potential is slightly more negative, and the upstroke of phase 0 is even more rapid.

Pacemaker Cells

The upstroke of the action potential of cardiac muscle cells described in the previous sections does not normally occur spontaneously. Rather, when a wave of depolarization reaches the myocyte from neighboring cells, its membrane potential becomes less negative and an action potential is triggered.

Certain heart cells do not require external provocation to initiate their action potential. Rather, they are capable of self-initiated depolarization in a rhythmic fashion and are known as **pacemaker cells.** They are endowed with the property of **automaticity,** by which the cells undergo *spontaneous* depolarization during phase 4. When the threshold voltage is reached in such cells, the upstroke of an action potential is triggered (Fig. 1.14).

Cells that display pacemaker behavior include the sinoatrial node (the "natural pacemaker" of the heart) and the atrioventricular node. Although atrial and ventricular muscle cells do not normally display au-

tomaticity, they may do so under disease conditions such as ischemia.

The shape of the action potential of a pacemaker cell is different from that of a ventricular muscle cell in three ways:

1. The maximum negative voltage of pacemaker cells is approximately -60 mV, substantially less negative than the resting potential of ventricular muscle cells (-90 mV). *The persistently less negative membrane voltage of pacemaker cells causes the fast sodium channels within these cells to remain inactivated.*

2. Unlike cardiac muscle cells, phase 4 of the pacemaker cell action potential is not flat, but has an upward slope, representing spontaneous gradual depolarization. This spontaneous depolarization is due to an ionic flux known as the **pacemaker current** (termed I_f). Current evidence indicates that the pacemaker current is carried predominently by Na^+ ions. The ion channel through which the pacemaker current passes is different from the fast sodium channel responsible for phase 0 of cardiac muscle cell depolarization. Rather, this pacemaker channel opens during *repolarization* of the cell, as the membrane potential approaches its most negative values. The inward flow of pos-

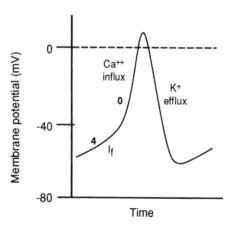

Figure 1.14. Action potential of a pacemaker cell. Phase 4 is characterized by gradual, spontaneous depolarization, owing to the pacemaker current (I_f). When the threshold potential is reached, at about -40 mV, the upstroke of the action potential follows. The upstroke of phase 0 is less rapid than in nonpacemaker cells, because the current represents Ca^{++} influx through the relatively slow calcium channels.

itively charged Na^+ ions through the pacemaker channel causes the membrane potential to become progressively less negative during phase 4, ultimately depolarizing the cell to its threshold voltage (Fig 1.14), and gradually deactivating the pacemaker channels.

3. The phase 0 upstroke of the pacemaker cell action potential is much less rapid and reaches a lower amplitude than that of a cardiac muscle cell. This is so because the fast sodium channels of the pacemaker cells are inactivated, and the upstroke of the action potential relies solely on Ca^{++} influx through the relatively slow calcium channels.

Repolarization of pacemaker cells occurs in a fashion similar to ventricular muscle cells, and is due to 1) inactivation of the calcium channels, and 2) increased activation of potassium channels with enhanced K^+ efflux from the cell.

Refractory Periods

Compared with electrical impulses in nerves and skeletal muscle, the cardiac action potential is much longer in duration. This results in a prolonged refractory period during which the muscle cannot be restimu-

lated. These long periods are physiologically necessary, because they allow the ventricles sufficient time to empty their contents and refill prior to the next cardiac contraction.

There are different levels of refractoriness during the action potential, as illustrated in Figure 1.15. The degree of refractoriness primarily reflects the number of fast Na^+ channels that have recovered from their inactive state, and are capable of reopening. As phase 3 of the action potential progresses, an increasing number of Na^+ channels recover and can respond to the next depolarization. This, in turn, corresponds to an increasing probability that a stimulus will trigger an action potential and result in a propagated impulse.

The *absolute* refractory period refers to the time during which the cell is completely unexcitable to a new stimulation. The *effective* refractory period includes the absolute refractory period but extends beyond it to include a short interval of phase 3, during which stimulation produces a localized action potential that is not strong enough to propagate further. The *relative* refractory period is the interval during which stimulation triggers an action potential that is conducted, but because the cell is stimulated from a voltage less negative than the resting potential, its upstroke is less steep and of lower amplitude and its conduction veloc-

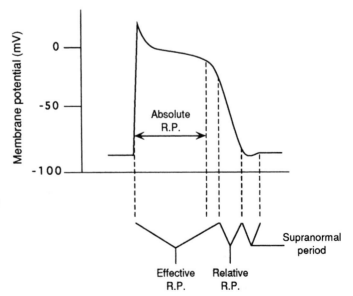

Figure 1.15. Refractory periods (RP) of the myocyte. During the absolute refractory period (ARP), the cell is unexcitable to stimulation. The effective refractory period includes a brief period beyond the ARP during which stimulation produces a localized depolarization that doesn't propagate. During the relative refractory period, stimulation produces a weak action potential (AP) that propagates, but more slowly than usual. During the supranormal period, a weaker-than-normal stimulus can trigger an AP.

ity slower than normal (see section on Impulse Conduction below). Following the relative refractory period, a short "supranormal" period is present, in which a less-than-normal stimulus can trigger an action potential.

The refractory period of atrial cells is shorter than that of ventricular muscle cells, so that atrial rates can generally exceed ventricular rates during rapid arrhythmias, as we will explore in Chapter 11.

Impulse Conduction

During depolarization, the electrical impulse spreads along each cardiac cell, and rapidly from cell to cell, because each myocyte is connected to its neighbors through low-resistance gap junctions. The speed of tissue depolarization (phase 0) and the conduction velocity along the cell depend on the number of sodium channels and on the magnitude of the resting potential. Tissues with a high concentration of Na^+ channels, such as Purkinje fibers, have a large fast inward current, which spreads rapidly within and between cells to support rapid conduction. In contrast, the less negative the resting potential, the greater the number of inactivated fast sodium channels, and therefore the less rapid the upstroke velocity will be (Fig. 1.16). Thus, alterations in the resting potential greatly affect the upstroke and conduction velocity of the action potential.

Normal Sequence of Cardiac Depolarization

Electrical activation of each heart beat is normally initiated at the sinoatrial node (Fig. 1.6). The impulse spreads to the surrounding atrial muscle through intercellular gap junctions that provide electrical continuity between the cells. Ordinary atrial muscle fibers participate in the propagation of the impulse from the SA to the AV node, although in certain regions the fibers are more densely arranged, facilitating conduction.

Fibrous tissue surrounds the atrioventricular valves, such that there is no direct electrical connection between the atrial and ventricular chambers other than through the AV node. As the electrical impulse reaches the AV node, a delay in conduction (approximately 0.1 sec) is encountered. This delay occurs because the small-diameter fibers in this region conduct slowly, and the action potential is of the "slow" pacemaker type (recall that in pacemaker tissue, the fast sodium channels are permanently inactivated, and the upstroke velocity relies on the slower calcium channels). The pause in conduction at the AV node is beneficial because it allows the atria time to contract and fully empty their contents prior to ventricular stimulation. In addition, the delay allows the AV node to serve as a "gatekeeper" of conduction from atria to ventricles, which is critical for limiting the rate of ventricular stimulation during abnormally rapid atrial rhythms.

After traversing the AV node, the cardiac

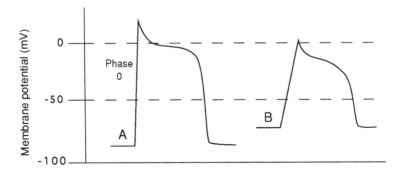

Figure 1.16. Dependence of speed of depolarization on resting potential. A. Normal resting potential (RP) and normal rapid rise of phase 0. **B.** Less negative RP results in slower rise of phase 0, and lower maximum amplitude of the action potential.

action potential spreads into the rapidly conducting bundle of His and Purkinje fibers, which distribute the electrical impulses to the bulk of the ventricular muscle cells. This allows for precisely timed stimulation and smooth contraction of the ventricular myocytes.

EXCITATION-CONTRACTION COUPLING

We now review how the action potential leads to physical contraction of cardiac muscle cells, a process known as excitation-contraction coupling. During this process, chemical energy in the form of high energy phosphate compounds is translated into the mechanical energy of myocyte contraction.

There are several distinct proteins responsible for cardiac muscle cell contraction (Fig. 1.17). Two of the proteins, actin and myosin, are the chief contractile elements. Two other proteins, tropomyosin and troponin, serve regulatory functions.

Myosin is arranged in thick filaments, each composed of lengthwise stacks of approximately 300 molecules. The myosin filament exhibits globular heads that are evenly spaced along its length, and contain myosin ATPase, an enzyme that is necessary for contraction to occur. **Actin,** a smaller molecule, is arranged in thin filaments as an alpha-helix consisting of two strands that interdigitate between the thick myosin filaments (Fig. 1.8). **Titin** (also termed connectin) is a recently discovered protein that helps tether myosin to the Z-line of the sarcomere and also provides elasticity to the contractile process.

Tropomyosin is a double helix that lies in the grooves between the actin filaments and, in the resting state, inhibits the interaction between myosin heads and actin, thus preventing contraction. **Troponin** sits at regular intervals along the actin strands and is composed of three subunits. The troponin C (TN-C) subunit is responsible for binding calcium ions that regulate the contractile process. The troponin I (TN-I) subunit inhibits the ATPase activity of the actin-myosin interaction. The troponin T (TN-T) subunit links the troponin complex to the actin and tropomyosin molecules.

During phase 2 of the action potential, Ca^{++} enters the myocyte through the calcium channels in the sarcolemma and T tubules. The relatively small amount of calcium that enters the cell in this fashion is not sufficient to cause contraction of the myofibrils, but it acts as a trigger for much greater Ca^{++} release from the sarcoplasmic reticulum (Fig. 1.18). As a result, the concentration of calcium in the cytosol increases tenfold.

As calcium ions bind to TN-C, the activity of TN-I is inhibited, which induces a conformational change in tropomyosin. The latter event unblocks the active site between actin and myosin, enabling contraction to proceed.

Contraction ensues as myosin heads bind to actin filaments and "flex," thus causing the interdigitating thick and thin filaments to move past each other in an ATP-dependent reaction (Fig. 1.19). The first step in this process is activation of the myosin head by hydrolysis of ATP, following which the myosin head binds to actin and forms a cross bridge. The interaction

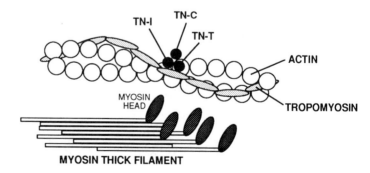

Figure 1.17. Schematic diagram of the main contractile proteins of the myocyte, actin and myosin. Tropomyosin and troponin (components TN-I, TN-C, TN-T) are regulatory proteins.

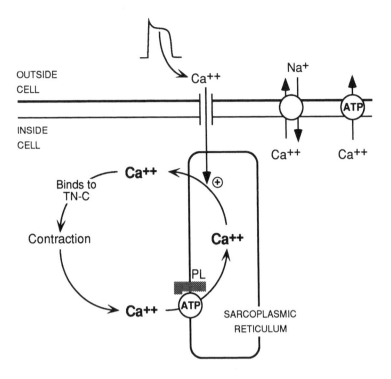

Figure 1.18.   Calcium ion movements during excitation and contraction in cardiac muscle cells. Ca^{++} **enters the cell through calcium channels during phase 2 of the action potential, triggering a much larger calcium release from the sarcoplasmic reticulum (SR).** The binding of cytosolic Ca^{++} to troponin-C (TN-C) results in contraction. Relaxation occurs as Ca^{++} returns to the SR by the ATP-dependent calcium pump. Phospholamban (PL) is a major regulator of this pump, inhibiting Ca^{++} uptake in its dephosphorylated state. Excess intracellular calcium is returned to the extracellular environment by sodium-calcium exchange and to a smaller degree by the sarcolemmal ATP-dependent Ca^{++} pump.

between the myosin head and actin results in a conformational change in the head, causing it to flex. This flexing motion exerts force on the actin filament and pulls it inward.

Next, while the myosin head and actin are still attached, an additional ATP molecule binds to the myosin head and displaces the ADP that had resulted from the previous ATP hydrolysis. The binding of new ATP causes the myosin head to release the actin filament, and hydrolysis of the new ATP returns the myosin head to its unflexed position, preparing it for the next cycle. Progressive coupling and uncoupling of actin and myosin cause the muscle fiber to shorten by increasing the overlap between the myofilaments within each sarcomere. In the presence of ATP, this process continues for as long as the calcium concentration remains sufficient to

inhibit the troponin-tropomyosin blocking action.

At the conclusion of phase 2 of the action potential, the Ca^{++} channels close so that there is no further influx into the sarcoplasm. Meanwhile, calcium is continuously pumped back into the sarcoplasmic reticulum and out of the cell (Fig. 1.18). As calcium ions are dissociated from troponin C, tropomyosin once again inhibits the actin-myosin interaction, leading to relaxation of the contracted cell. The contraction-relaxation cycle can then be repeated with the next action potential.

There is substantial evidence that the concentration of Ca^{++} within the cytosol is the major determinant of the force of cardiac contraction with each heart beat. Mechanisms that raise the intracellular Ca^{++} enhance force development, whereas factors that lower Ca^{++} reduce the contractile force.

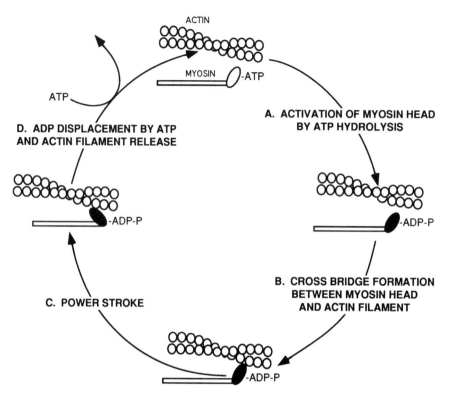

Figure 1.19. The contractile process. A. Myosin head is activated by hydrolysis of ATP. **B.** During cellular depolarization, cytoplasmic calcium concentration increases and removes the troponin-tropomyosin inhibition, such that a crossbridge is formed between actin and myosin. **C.** The myosin head flexes, drawing the actin filament inward. **D.** ADP is released and replaced by ATP, releasing the myosin head from the actin filament. The head extends to bind further down the actin filament, and the process repeats, causing the muscle fiber to shorten. The cycle continues until calcium concentration decreases at the end of phase 2 of the action potential.

Beta-adrenergic Stimulation and Cellular Signaling

Beta-adrenergic stimulation is one mechanism that enhances calcium fluxes in the myocyte and thereby strengthens the force of ventricular contraction (Fig. 1.20). When catecholamines (e.g., norepinephrine) bind to the myocyte β_1-adrenergic receptor, the transmembrane guanine nucleotide regulatory protein system (G proteins) stimulates membrane-bound adenylate cyclase. The latter enzyme enhances production of cyclic AMP (cAMP). cAMP activates intracellular protein kinases, which phosphorylate cellular proteins, including L-type calcium channels within the cell membrane. Phosphorylation of the calcium channel increases Ca^{++} influx, triggering a corresponding increase in Ca^{++} release from the sarcoplasmic reticulum and enhancing the force of contraction.

Beta-adrenergic stimulation of the myocyte also enhances myocyte *relaxation*. The return of Ca^{++} from the cytosol to the sarcoplasmic reticulum (SR) is regulated by **phospholamban** (PL), a low molecular weight protein in the SR membrane. In its dephosphorylated state, PL inhibits Ca^{++} uptake by the SR calcium ATPase pump (Fig. 1.18). However, beta-adrenergic activation of protein kinases (Fig. 1.20) causes PL to become phosphorylated, an action that blunts PL's inhibitory effect. The subsequently greater uptake of calcium ions by the SR hastens Ca^{++} removal from the cytosol and therefore promotes myocyte relaxation. The increased cAMP activity also results in phosphorylation of TN-I, an action that inhibits actin-myosin interactions, and therefore further enhances relaxation of the cell.

Thus, physiologic or pharmacologic catecholamine stimulation of the myocyte β_1

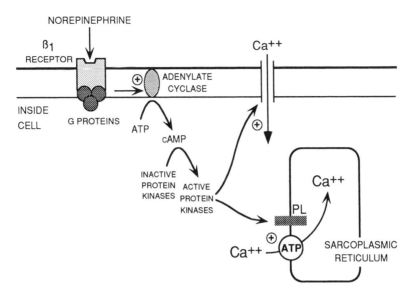

Figure 1.20. The effect of beta-adrenergic stimulation on cellular signaling and calcium ion movement. The binding of a ligand (e.g., norepinephrine) to the β_1-receptor causes G-protein-mediated stimulation of adenylate cyclase and formation of cyclic AMP (cAMP). The latter activates protein kinases, which phosphorylate cellular proteins, including ion channels. Phosphorylation of the slow Ca^{++} channel enhances calcium movement into the cell, and therefore strengthens the force of contraction. Protein kinase also phosphorylates phospholamban (PL), reducing the latter's inhibition of Ca^{++} uptake by the sarcoplasmic reticulum. The enhanced removal of Ca^{++} from the cytosol facilitates relaxation of the myocyte.

adrenergic receptor enhances both contraction and relaxation of the cell. We will refer back to these important properties in later chapters.

SUMMARY

The anatomic structure, cellular composition, and conduction pathways of the heart form an efficient system for repetitive, organized contractions. As such, the heart is capable of purposeful stimulation billions of times during the lifespan of a normal individual. With each contraction cycle, the heart receives and propagates blood through the circulation, to provide nutrients to and remove waste products from the body's tissues.

In the chapters that follow, we will explore what can go wrong with this extraordinary system.

Acknowledgments   The previous edition of this chapter was written by Stephanie Harper, MD, Scott Hyver, MD, Paul Kim, MD, Laurence Rhines, MD, James D. Marsh, MD, and Leonard S. Lilly, MD.

ADDITIONAL READING

Braunwald E, et al. Mechanisms of Contraction of the Normal and Failing Heart. Boston: Little, Brown & Co., 1976.

Di Francesco D. Pacemaker mechanisms in cardiac tissue. Ann Rev Physiol 1993;55:455–472.

Grupp IL, et al. The contribution of phospholamban, a sarcoplasmic reticulum phosphoprotein, to myocardial contractility in health and disease. Heart Failure 1995;11:48–61.

Hille B. Ionic Channels of Excitable Membranes. 2nd ed. Sunderland, MA: Sinauer Assoc., 1992.

Katz AM. Physiology of the Heart. 2nd ed. New York: Raven Press, 1992.

Katz AM. Cardiac ion channels. N Engl J Med 1993;328:1244–1251.

Linder ME, Gilman AG. G proteins. Scientific American, 1992;267(1):36–43.

Roberts R. Molecular Basis of Cardiology. Boston: Blackwell Scientific Publications, 1993.

Trautwein W, Hescheler J. Regulation of cardiac L-type calcium current by phosphorylation and G proteins. Ann Rev Physiol 1990;52:257–274.

Heart Sounds and Murmurs

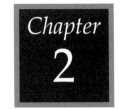

Oscar Benavidez, Allan Goldblatt, and Leonard S. Lilly

Diseases of the heart often manifest themselves as abnormalities of the physical examination, including pathologic heart sounds and murmurs. These findings are clues to the underlying disease pathophysiology, and proper interpretation is necessary for successful diagnosis and management. This chapter describes heart sounds of the normal cardiac cycle, then focuses on the origins of pathologic heart sounds and cardiac murmurs.

In this chapter, many cardiac diseases are briefly mentioned as examples of abnormal heart sounds and murmurs. Each of these conditions is described in greater detail later in this book, so it is not necessary to memorize the examples presented here. Rather, it is preferable to understand the mechanisms by which the abnormal sounds are produced, so that their descriptions will make sense in later chapters.

CARDIAC CYCLE

The cardiac cycle consists of precisely timed electrical and mechanical events that result in the rhythmic atrial and ventricular contractions that propel blood into the pulmonary and systemic circulations. Mechanical **systole** refers to ventricular contraction, and **diastole** to ventricular relaxation and filling (Fig. 2.1). Throughout the cycle, the right and left atria continuously accept blood returning to the heart from the systemic veins and from the pulmonary veins, respectively. During diastole, blood passes from the atria into the ventricles across the open tricuspid and mitral valves. In late diastole, atrial contraction propels a final bolus of blood into the ventricles, which produces a slight pressure rise, termed the "a" wave.

Contraction of the ventricles follows, signaling the onset of mechanical systole. As the ventricles start to contract, pressure within them rapidly exceeds atrial pressures, resulting in the forced closure of the tricuspid and mitral valves, which produces the first heart sound, termed S_1 (Fig. 2.1). S_1 has two nearly superimposed components: the mitral component slightly precedes the tricuspid component because of the earlier electrical stimulation and onset of left ventricular contraction.

As the ventricular pressures rapidly rise, they exceed the diastolic pressures within the pulmonary artery and aorta, thus opening the pulmonic and aortic valves, and blood is ejected into the pulmonary and systemic circulations. At the conclusion of the ventricular ejection phase, the ventricular pressures fall below those of the pulmonary artery and aorta, such that the pulmonic and aortic valves are forced to close, producing the second heart sound, termed S_2. S_2 also consists of two components: The aortic component (A_2) normally precedes the

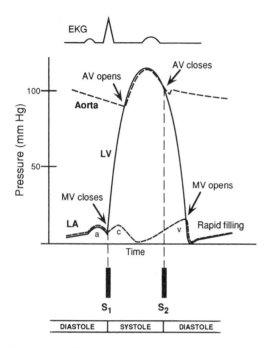

Figure 2.1. The normal cardiac cycle, showing pressure relationships between the left-sided heart chambers. During diastole, the mitral valve (MV) is open, so that the left atrial (LA) and left ventricular (LV) pressures are equal. In late diastole, LA contraction causes a small rise in pressure in both the LA and LV (the "a" wave). During systolic contraction, the LV pressure rises, and when it exceeds the LA pressure, the MV closes, contributing to the first heart sound (S_1). As LV pressure rises above the aortic pressure, the aortic valve (AV) opens, which is a silent event. As the ventricle begins to relax and its pressure falls below that of the aorta, the AV closes, contributing to the second heart sound (S_2). As LV pressure falls further, below that of the LA, the MV opens, which is silent in the normal heart. In addition to the "a" wave, the LA pressure curve displays two additional positive deflections: the "c" wave represents a small rise in LA pressure as the MV closes and bulges toward the atrium, and the "v" wave is due to passive filling of the LA from the pulmonary veins during systole, when the MV is closed.

the duration of systole remains constant, the length of diastole varies with the heart rate: the faster the heart rate, the shorter the diastolic phase. The main heart sounds, S_1 and S_2, provide a framework from which all other heart sounds and murmurs can be timed.

Most modern stethoscopes have two chest pieces with which to auscultate the heart. The "bell" chest piece is meant to be applied lightly to the skin, whereby it accentuates low frequency sounds. The "diaphragm" chest piece is pressed firmly against the skin, which eliminates low frequencies and therefore accentuates high frequency sounds and murmurs.

HEART SOUNDS

First Heart Sound (S_1)

S_1 is produced by closure of the mitral and tricuspid valves in early systole, and is loudest near the apex of the heart (Fig. 2.2). It is a high-frequency sound, best heard with the diaphragm of the stethoscope. Although mitral closure usually precedes tricuspid closure, they are separated by only approximately 0.01 sec, such that the human ear appreciates only a single sound through the stethoscope. An exception occurs in patients with right bundle branch block (see Chapter 4), in whom these components *may* be audibly split, because of delayed closure of the tricuspid valve.

pulmonic component (P_2) because the diastolic pressure gradient between the aorta and left ventricle is higher than that between the pulmonary artery and right ventricle. The ventricular pressures continue to fall during the relaxation phase, and as they drop below the pressures in the right and left atria, the tricuspid and mitral valves open, followed by diastolic ventricular filling and repetition of the cycle.

At the bedside, therefore, systole can be approximated by the period from S_1 to S_2, and diastole from S_2 to the next S_1. Although

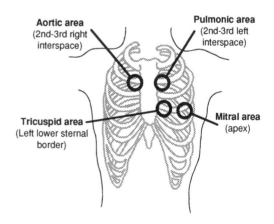

Figure 2.2. Standard positions of stethoscope placement for cardiac auscultation.

Three factors determine the intensity of S_1: 1) the distance between the open valve leaflets at the onset of ventricular systole, 2) the mobility of the leaflets (normal, or rigid because of stenosis), and 3) the rate of ventricular pressure elevation (Table 2.1).

The distance between the open valve leaflets at the onset of systole is affected by the PR interval on the electrocardiogram, the period between the onset of atrial and ventricular activation. Normal atrial contraction initiated by the P wave forces the tricuspid and mitral valve leaflets apart. As they start to drift back together, ventricular contraction forces them shut, from whatever position they are at, as soon as ventricular pressure exceeds that in the atrium. An *accentuated* S_1 results when the PR interval is shorter than normal because the valve leaflets have not had sufficient time to drift back together, and are forced shut from a relatively wide apart distance at the onset of ventricular contraction.

Similarly, in mild mitral stenosis a prolonged diastolic pressure gradient exists between the left atrium and ventricle, keeping the bodies of the mitral leaflets farther apart than normal during diastole. Since the leaflets are relatively wide apart at the onset of systole, they are forced shut loudly when the left ventricle contracts.

S_1 also may be accentuated when the heart rate is more rapid than normal (i.e., tachycardia), because diastole is shortened and therefore ventricular contraction forces together the tricuspid and mitral leaflets from relatively wide apart positions, because they have had insufficient time to drift together.

Conditions that *reduce* the intensity of S_1 are also listed in Table 2.1. In first-degree AV nodal block, a diminished S_1 results from a prolonged PR interval, which delays the onset of ventricular contraction: following atrial contraction, the mitral and tricuspid valves have *additional* time to float back together so that the leaflets are forced closed from only a small distance apart.

In patients with mitral regurgitation (see Chapter 8), S_1 is often diminished in intensity, because the mitral leaflets may not

TABLE 2.1. Causes of Altered Intensity of S_1

Accentuated S_1
1. Shortened PR interval
2. Mild mitral stenosis
3. High cardiac output states or tachycardia (e.g., exercise or anemia)

Diminished S_1
1. Lengthened PR interval: first-degree AV nodal block
2. Mitral regurgitation
3. Severe mitral stenosis
4. "Stiff" left ventricle (e.g., systemic hypertension)

come into full contact with one another as they close. In *severe* mitral stenosis, the leaflets are nearly fixed in position throughout the cardiac cycle, and that reduced movement can also lessen the intensity of S_1.

In patients with "stiffened" ventricles (e.g., a hypertrophied or scarred left ventricle), atrial contraction results in a higher than normal left ventricular diastolic pressure. This higher pressure accelerates the drifting together of the mitral leaflets in diastole, so that when ventricular contraction commences, the leaflets are forced together from a smaller than normal distance apart, and therefore S_1 may be reduced in intensity.

Second Heart Sound (S_2)

The second heart sound results from the closure of the aortic and pulmonic valves, and therefore has aortic (A_2) and pulmonic (P_2) components. Unlike S_1, which is usually auscultated as a single sound, the components of S_2 vary with the respiratory cycle: they are normally fused as one sound during expiration, but become audibly separated during inspiration, a situation termed "normal splitting of S_2" (Fig. 2.3).

One explanation for normal splitting of S_2 is as follows: expansion of the chest during inspiration causes the intrathoracic pressure to become more negative. The negative pressure transiently increases the capacitance (and reduces the impedance) of the intrathoracic pulmonary vessels. As a result, there is a temporary delay in the diastolic "back pressure" of the pulmonary artery responsible for closure of the pulmonic valve. Thus, P_2 is delayed—i.e., it oc-

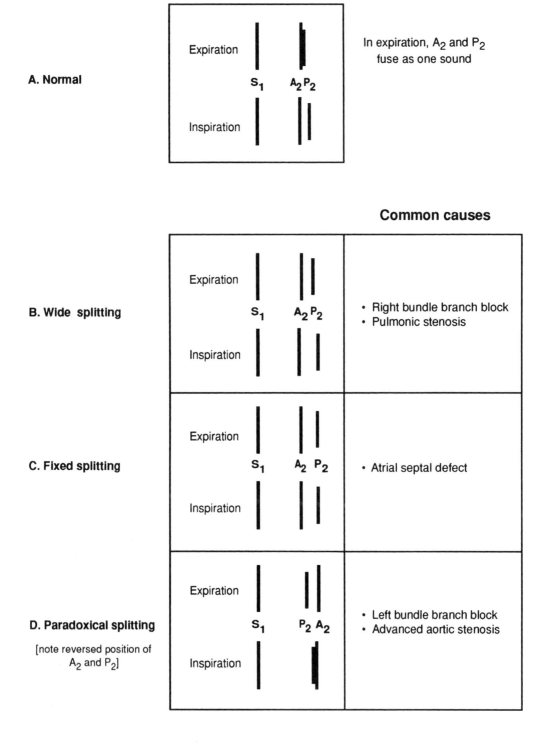

Figure 2.3.   Splitting patterns of the second heart sound (S$_2$). S$_1$, first heart sound; A$_2$, aortic component; P$_2$, pulmonic component of S$_2$.

curs *later* during inspiration than during expiration.

Inspiration has the *opposite* effect on A_2. Since the capacity of the intrathoracic pulmonary veins is increased by the negative pressure during inspiration, the venous return to the left atrium and ventricle temporarily decreases. Reduced filling of the LV translates to a reduced stroke volume during the next systolic contraction, and therefore shortens the time required for LV emptying. Therefore, aortic valve closure (A_2) occurs earlier in inspiration than during expiration. The combination of an earlier A_2 and delayed P_2 during inspiration causes audible separation of these two components of the second heart sound. Since the components of S_2 are high-frequency sounds, they are best heard with the diaphragm of the stethoscope, and splitting of the sounds is usually most easily appreciated near the second left intercostal space next to the sternum (the "pulmonic" area).

Abnormalities of S_2 include alterations in its intensity and changes in the pattern of splitting. The intensity of S_2 depends on the velocity of blood coursing back toward the valves from the aorta and pulmonary artery after the completion of ventricular contraction, and the suddenness with which that motion is arrested by the closing valves. In systemic or pulmonary arterial hypertension, the diastolic pressure in the respective great artery is higher than normal, such that the velocity of the blood surging toward the valve is elevated, and S_2 is accentuated. Conversely, in severe aortic or pulmonic valve stenosis the valve commissures are nearly fixed in position, such that the contribution of the stenotic valve to S_2 is diminished.

Widened splitting of S_2 refers to an increase in the time interval between A_2 and P_2, such that the two components are audibly separated even during expiration, and become more widely separated in inspiration (Fig. 2.3). This pattern is usually the result of delayed closure of the pulmonic valve, which occurs in right bundle branch block (RBBB) and pulmonic valve stenosis.

Fixed splitting of S_2 is defined as a widened interval of splitting between A_2 and P_2 that persists unchanged through the respiratory cycle (Fig. 2.3). The most common abnormality that causes fixed splitting of S_2 is an atrial septal defect (see Chapter 16). In that condition, a chronic volume overload of the right-sided circulation results in a high-capacitance, low-resistance pulmonary vascular system. This alteration in pulmonary artery hemodynamics delays the "back pressure" responsible for closure of the pulmonic valve. Thus, P_2 occurs later than normal, even during expiration, such that there is wider than normal separation of A_2 and P_2. The pattern of splitting doesn't change (i.e., it is fixed) during the respiratory cycle, because inspiration does not substantially further increase the already elevated pulmonary vascular capacitance.

Paradoxical splitting (or "reversed" splitting) refers to audible separation of A_2 and P_2 during *expiration* that disappears on *inspiration,* the opposite of the normal situation. It reflects a delay in the closure of the aortic valve, such that P_2 *precedes* A_2. In adults, the most common cause is left bundle branch block (LBBB). In LBBB, the spread of electrical activity through the left ventricle is impaired, resulting in delayed ventricular contraction and late closure of the aortic valve such that it *follows* P_2. During inspiration, as in the normal case, the pulmonic valve closure sound is delayed and the aortic valve closure sound moves earlier. This results in superimposition of the two sounds, and therefore, there is no apparent split at the height of inspiration (Fig. 2.3). In addition to LBBB, paradoxical splitting may be observed under circumstances in which left ventricular ejection is prolonged, such as aortic stenosis.

Extra Systolic Heart Sounds

Extra systolic heart sounds may occur in early, mid, or late systole.

Early Extra Systolic Heart Sounds

Abnormal early systolic sounds, or "ejection clicks," occur shortly after S_1, and coincide with the opening of the aortic or pulmonic valves (Fig. 2.4). These sounds have a sharp, high-pitched quality so that they are heard best with the diaphragm of the stethoscope placed over the aortic and pulmonic areas. Ejection clicks indicate the presence of aortic or pulmonic valve stenosis or dilatation of the pulmonary artery or aorta. In stenosis of the aortic or pulmonic valve, the sound occurs as the valve leaflets reach their maximal level of ascent into the great artery, just prior to blood ejection. At that moment, the rapidly ascending valve reaches its elastic limit and decelerates abruptly, an action thought to result in the sound generation. In dilatation of the root

of the aorta or pulmonary artery, the sound is associated with sudden tensing of the aortic or pulmonic root with the onset of blood flow into the vessel. The aortic ejection click is heard at both the base and the apex of the heart, and does not vary with respiration. In distinction, a pulmonic ejection click is heard only at the base and its intensity diminishes during inspiration.

Mid or Late Extra Systolic Heart Sounds

Clicks occurring in mid or late systole are usually because of systolic prolapse of the mitral or tricuspid valves, in which the leaflets bulge abnormally from the ventricular side of the atrioventricular junction to the atrial side during ventricular contraction, often accompanied by valvular regurgitation. They are loudest over the mitral or tricuspid auscultatory regions, respectively (Fig. 2.2).

Extra Diastolic Heart Sounds

Extra heart sounds may also be heard in diastole. These include the opening snap (OS), the third heart sound (S_3), the fourth heart sound (S_4), and the pericardial knock.

Opening Snap

Opening of the mitral and tricuspid valves is normally silent, but valvular stenosis, usually the result of rheumatic heart disease, produces an opening sound, termed a "snap," shortly after S_2. It is a sharp, high-pitched sound, and its timing does not vary significantly with respiration. In mitral stenosis (which is much more common than tricuspid valve stenosis), the OS is heard best between the apex and the left sternal border, just after the aortic closure sound (A_2), when the left ventricular pressure falls below that of the left atrium (Fig. 2.4). Because of its proximity to A_2, the A_2-OS sequence can be confused with a widely split second heart sound, but careful auscultation at the pulmonic area during inspiration reveals *three* sounds occurring in rapid succession (Fig. 2.5), which corre-

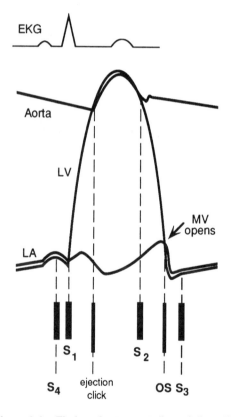

Figure 2.4. Timing of extra systolic and diastolic heart sounds. S_4 is produced by atrial contraction into a "stiff" left ventricle (LV). An ejection click follows the opening of the aortic or pulmonic valve in cases of valve stenosis or dilatation of the corresponding great artery. An S_3 occurs during the period of rapid ventricular filling; it is normal in young individuals, but its presence in adults implies LV contractile dysfunction. The timing of an opening snap (OS) is placed for comparison, but it is not likely that all of these sounds would appear in the same individual. LA, left atrium.

spond to aortic closure (A_2), pulmonic clo-sure (P_2), then the opening snap (OS). The three sounds become two on expiration, as A_2 and P_2 fuse.

The more severe the stenosis, the shorter is the interval between A_2 and the opening snap. This occurs because the degree of left atrial pressure elevation corresponds to the severity of mitral stenosis. Thus, when the ventricle relaxes, the greater the left atrial pressure, the earlier the mitral valve opens. Compared with severe stenosis, in mild dis-ease, left atrial pressure is less elevated, so that it takes longer for the left ventricular pressure to fall below that of the atrium. Therefore, in mild mitral stenosis, the open-ing snap is widely separated from A_2, whereas in more severe stenosis, the A_2-OS internal is narrower.

Third Heart Sound (S_3)

When present, an S_3 occurs in early dias-tole, following the opening of the atrioven-tricular valves, during the ventricular rapid filling phase (Fig. 2.4). It is a dull, low-pitched sound best heard with the bell of the stethoscope placed over the cardiac apex while the patient lies in the left lateral decubitus position. Production of the S_3 sound appears to result from tensing of the chordae tendinae as rapid filling of the ven-tricle causes expansion of the chamber.

The third heart sound is a normal finding in children and young adults. In these groups, an S_3 implies the presence of a sup-ple ventricle that can undergo normal rapid expansion in early diastole. Conversely, when heard in a middle-aged or older adult, an S_3 is often a sign of disease, indicating volume overload owing to congestive heart failure, or the increased transvalvular flow that accompanies advanced mitral or tricus-pid regurgitation. A pathologic S_3 is often referred to as a **ventricular "gallop."**

Fourth Heart Sound (S_4)

When an S_4 is present, it occurs in late di-astole and coincides with contraction of the atria (Fig. 2.4). This sound is generated by

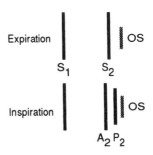

Figure 2.5. Timing of the opening snap (OS) in mitral stenosis does not change with respiration. Upon inspiration, normal splitting of the second heart sound (S_2) is observed so that three sounds are heard. A_2, aortic component; P_2, pulmonic component of S_2.

the left (or right) atrium vigorously con-tracting against a *stiffened* ventricle. Thus, an S_4 usually indicates the presence of car-diac disease, specifically a decrease in ven-tricular compliance, usually due to ven-tricular hypertrophy or myocardial ischemia. Like an S_3, the S_4 is a dull, low-pitched sound, and is heard best with the bell of the stethoscope. In the case of the left-sided S_4, the sound is loudest at the apex, with the patient lying in the left lateral de-cubitus position. An S_4 is sometimes re-ferred to as an **atrial "gallop."**

Quadruple Rhythm or Summation Gallop

In a patient with both an S_3 and S_4, those sounds, in conjunction with S_1 and S_2, pro-duce a quadruple beat. If a patient with such a quadruple rhythm develops tachy-cardia, diastole becomes shorter in dura-tion, the S_3 and S_4 sounds coalesce, and a **"summation gallop"** results. The summa-tion of S_3 and S_4 is heard as a long middias-tolic, low-pitched sound, often louder than S_1 and S_2.

Pericardial Knock

A pericardial knock is an uncommon, high-pitched sound that occurs in patients with severe constrictive pericarditis (see Chapter 14). It appears early in diastole soon after S_2, and can be confused with an opening snap or an S_3. However, the knock appears slightly later in diastole than the timing of an opening snap and is louder and occurs earlier than the ventricular gallop. It results from the abrupt cessation of ventricular filling in early diastole, which is the hallmark of constrictive pericarditis.

MURMURS

A murmur is the sound generated by turbulent blood flow. Under normal conditions, the flow of blood is laminar through the vascular bed and is therefore silent. However, as a result of hemodynamic and/or structural changes in the vasculature, laminar flow can become disturbed and produce an audible noise. Murmurs result from the following mechanisms:

1. Flow across a partial obstruction (e.g., aortic stenosis)
2. Increased flow through normal structures (e.g., aortic systolic murmur associated with a high output state, such as anemia)
3. Ejection into a dilated chamber (e.g., aortic systolic murmur associated with aneurysmal dilatation of the aorta)
4. Regurgitant flow across an incompetent valve (e.g., mitral regurgitation)
5. Abnormal shunting of blood from a high-pressure to a lower-pressure vascular chamber (e.g., ventricular septal defect)

Murmurs are described by their timing, intensity, pitch, shape, location, radiation, and response to maneuvers. *Timing* refers to whether the murmur occurs during systole, diastole, or is continuous (i.e., begins in systole and continues into diastole). The *intensity* of the murmur can be quantified by the following grading system:

Systolic Murmurs

Grade 1/6: Barely audible (i.e., medical students cannot hear it!)
Grade 2/6: Faint, but immediately audible
Grade 3/6: Easily heard
Grade 4/6: Easily heard and associated with a palpable thrill
Grade 5/6: Very loud; heard with stethoscope lightly on chest

Grade 6/6: Audible without the stethoscope directly on the chest wall

Diastolic Murmurs

Grade 1/4: Barely audible
Grade 2/4: Faint, but immediately audible
Grade 3/4: Easily heard
Grade 4/4: Very loud

Pitch refers to the frequency of the murmur, ranging from high to low. High-frequency murmurs are caused by large pressure gradients between chambers (e.g., aortic stenosis), and are best appreciated using the diaphragm chest piece of the stethoscope. Low-frequency murmurs imply less of a pressure gradient between chambers (e.g., mitral stenosis), and are best heard using the stethoscope's bell piece.

Shape describes how the murmur changes in intensity from its onset to its completion. For example, a "crescendo-decrescendo" (or "diamond-shaped") murmur first rises, then falls off in intensity. Other shapes include "decrescendo" (i.e., the murmur begins at its maximum intensity and grows softer) and "uniform" (the intensity of the murmur doesn't change).

Location refers to the murmur's region of maximum intensity, and is usually described in terms of specific auscultatory areas (Fig. 2.2):

- "aortic" area (2nd–3rd right intercostal space, next to sternum)
- "pulmonic" area (2nd–3rd left intercostal space, next to sternum)
- "tricuspid" area (lower left sternal border)
- "mitral" area (cardiac apex).

From their primary locations, murmurs may be heard to *radiate* to various areas of the chest, and such patterns of transmission relate to the direction of the turbulent flow. Finally, similar types of murmurs can be distinguished from one another by simple bedside *maneuvers*, such as standing upright, Valsalva (forceful expiration against a closed airway) or clenching of the fists, each of which alter the heart's loading conditions, and can affect the intensity of many murmurs.

When describing a murmur, some or all

of these descriptors are listed. For example, a physician might describe a patient's murmur of aortic stenosis as follows: "a grade III/VI high-pitched, crescendo-decrescendo systolic murmur, heard best at the upper right sternal border, radiating towards the neck."

Systolic Murmurs

Systolic murmurs are subdivided into systolic ejection murmurs, pansystolic murmurs, and late systolic murmurs (Fig. 2.6).

A **systolic ejection murmur** is typical of aortic or pulmonic valve stenosis. It begins after the first heart sound, and terminates before or during S_2, depending on its severity and whether the obstruction is of the aortic or pulmonic valve. The murmur is of the crescendo-decrescendo type (i.e., its intensity rises and then falls).

The ejection murmur of *aortic stenosis* begins in systole after S_1, from which it is separated by a short audible gap (Fig. 2.7). This gap corresponds to the period of isovolumetric contraction of the left ventricle (the period after the mitral valve has closed, but the aortic valve has not yet opened). The murmur becomes more intense as flow increases across the aortic valve during the rise in left ventricular pressure (crescendo). Then, as the ventricle relaxes, forward flow

decreases, and the murmur lessens in intensity (decrescendo), and finally ends prior to the aortic component of S_2. The murmur may be immediately preceded by an ejection click, especially in mild forms of aortic stenosis.

Although the intensity of the murmur does not correlate well with the severity of aortic stenosis, other features do. For example, the more severe the stenosis, the longer it takes to force blood across the valve, and the later the murmur peaks in systole (Fig. 2.8). Also note in the figure that as the severity of stenosis increases, the aortic component of S_2 softens, as the leaflets become more rigidly fixed in place.

Aortic stenosis causes a high-frequency murmur, reflecting the sizable pressure gradient across the valve. It is best heard in the "aortic area" in the second and third right interspaces close to the sternum. The murmur typically radiates towards the neck (the direction of turbulent blood flow), but often can be heard in a wide distribution, including the cardiac apex.

When a systolic ejection murmur is due to *pulmonic stenosis*, it also begins after S_1, may also be preceded by an ejection click, but may extend beyond A_2. That is, if the stenosis is severe, it will result in a very prolonged right ventricular ejection time, elongating the murmur, which will continue beyond A_2 and end just prior to closure of the

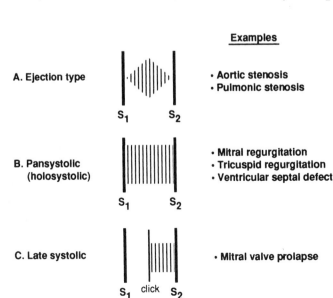

Examples

A. Ejection type

S_1 S_2

• Aortic stenosis
• Pulmonic stenosis

B. Pansystolic (holosystolic)

S_1 S_2

• Mitral regurgitation
• Tricuspid regurgitation
• Ventricular septal defect

C. Late systolic

S_1 click S_2

• Mitral valve prolapse

Figure 2.6. Classification of systolic murmurs. Ejection murmurs are crescendo-decrescendo in configuration, whereas pansystolic murmurs are uniform throughout systole. A late systolic murmur often follows a midsystolic click, and suggests mitral (or tricuspid) valve prolapse.

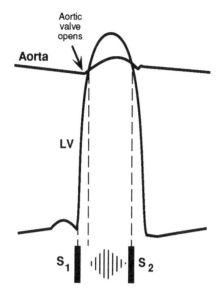

Figure 2.7.   Systolic ejection murmur of aortic stenosis. There is a short delay between the first heart sound (S_1) and the onset of the murmur. S_2, second heart sound; LV, left ventricle.

pulmonic valve (P_2). Pulmonic stenosis is usually loudest at the 2nd–3rd left interspaces close to the sternum. It does not radiate as widely as aortic stenosis, but sometimes it is transmitted towards the neck or left shoulder.

Young adults often have *benign systolic ejection murmurs* owing to increased systolic flow across normal aortic and pulmonic valves. This type of murmur often becomes softer, or disappears when the patient sits upright.

Pansystolic (also termed **holosystolic**) murmurs are caused by regurgitation of blood across an incompetent mitral or tricuspid valve or through a ventricular septal defect (VSD) (Fig. 2.6). These murmurs are characterized by a uniform intensity throughout systole. In mitral and tricuspid valve regurgitation, as soon as ventricular pressure exceeds atrial pressure (i.e., when S_1 occurs), there is immediate retrograde flow across the regurgitant valve. Thus, there is no gap between S_1 and the onset of these pansystolic murmurs, in distinction to the systolic ejection murmurs discussed above. Similarly, there is no significant gap between S_1 and the onset of the systolic murmur of a VSD, since left ventricular sys-

tolic pressure exceeds right ventricular systolic pressure (and flow occurs) quickly after the onset of contraction.

The pansystolic murmur of advanced *mitral regurgitation* continues through the aortic closure sound because left ventricular pressure remains greater than that in the left atrium, at the time of aortic closure. The murmur is heard best at the apex, is high-pitched and "blowing" in quality, often radiates toward the left axilla, and its intensity does not change with respiration.

Tricuspid valve regurgitation is best heard along the left lower sternal border. It generally radiates to the right of the sternum and is high-pitched and "blowing" in quality. The intensity of the murmur *increases* with inspiration, because the negative intrathoracic pressure induced during inspiration

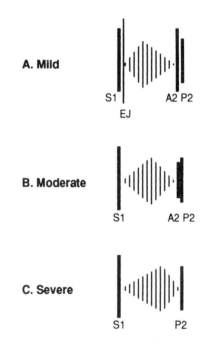

Figure 2.8.   The severity of aortic stenosis affects the shape of the systolic murmur and the heart sounds. A. In mild stenosis, an ejection click (EJ) is often present, followed by an early peaking crescendo-decrescendo murmur, and a normal A_2. **B.** As the stenosis becomes more severe, the peak of the murmur becomes more delayed in systole and the intensity of A_2 lessens. The prolonged ventricular ejection time delays A_2 so that it merges with or occurs after P_2; the ejection click may not be heard. **C.** In severe stenosis, the murmur peaks very late in systole, and A_2 is usually absent, because of immobility of the valve leaflets.

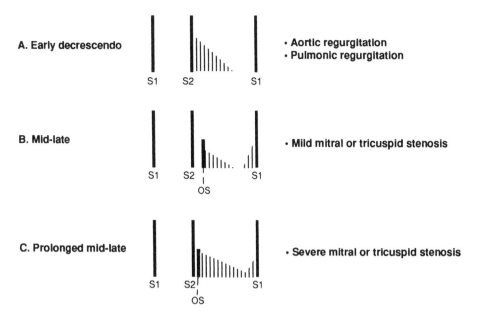

A. Early decrescendo

S1   S2   S1

• **Aortic regurgitation**
• **Pulmonic regurgitation**

B. Mid-late

S1   S2   S1
         OS

• **Mild mitral or tricuspid stenosis**

C. Prolonged mid-late

S1   S2   S1
         OS

• **Severe mitral or tricuspid stenosis**

Figure 2.9. Classification of the diastolic murmurs. A. An early diastolic decrescendo murmur is typical of aortic or pulmonic valve regurgitation. **B.** Mid to late low-frequency rumbling murmurs are usually the result of mitral or tricuspid valve stenosis, which follow a sharp opening snap (OS). Presystolic accentuation of the murmur occurs in patients in normal sinus rhythm because of the transient rise in atrial pressure during atrial contraction. **C.** In more severe mitral or tricuspid valve stenosis, the opening snap and diastolic murmur occur earlier, and the murmur is prolonged.

enhances venous return to the heart. The latter augments right ventricular stroke volume, thereby increasing the amount of regurgitated blood.

The murmur of a *ventricular septal defect* is heard best at the fourth to sixth left intercostal spaces, is high-pitched, and may be associated with a palpable thrill. The intensity of the murmur does not increase with inspiration and does not radiate to the axilla, which helps distinguish it from tricuspid and mitral regurgitation, respectively. Of note, the *smaller* the VSD, the greater the turbulence of blood flow between the left and right ventricles, and the *louder* the murmur. Some of the loudest murmurs you will ever hear are those of small VSDs.

Late systolic murmurs begin in mid to late systole and continue to A_2. They most often reflect mitral regurgitation due to prolapse of the valve leaflets into the left atrium during ventricular contraction (Fig. 2.6). This murmur is usually preceded by a midsystolic click, and is described further in Chapter 8.

Diastolic Murmurs

Diastolic murmurs are divided into early decrescendo murmurs and mid to late rumbling murmurs (Fig. 2.9). **Early diastolic murmurs** result from regurgitant flow through either the aortic or pulmonic valve, with the former being much more common in adults. If produced by *aortic valve regurgitation*, the murmur begins at A_2, has a decrescendo shape, and terminates prior to the next S_1. Because relaxation of the left ventricle is rapid, a significant pressure gradient develops immediately between the aorta and left ventricle in aortic regurgitation, and the murmur therefore displays its maximum intensity at its onset. Thereafter, as the aortic diastolic pressure and the gradient between the two chambers fall, the murmur decreases. Aortic regurgitation is a high-pitched murmur, best heard using the diaphragm of the stethoscope along the left sternal border with the patient sitting, leaning forward and exhaling.

Pulmonic regurgitation, usually due to pulmonary hypertension in adults, has a similar early diastolic decrescendo profile. It is best heard in the "pulmonic" area, and its intensity may increase with inspiration.

Mid to late diastolic murmurs result from either turbulent flow across a *stenotic mitral or tricuspid valve* or less commonly from increased flow across a normal mitral or tricuspid valve (Fig. 2.9). If because of stenosis, the murmur begins after S_2 and is preceded by an opening snap. The shape of this murmur is unique. In early diastole, following the opening snap, the murmur is at its loudest because the pressure gradient between the atrium and ventricle is at its maximum. The murmur then decrescendos or disappears totally during diastole as the transvalvular gradient decreases. The degree to which the murmur fades depends on whether the stenosis is severe, in which case the murmur will be prolonged, or mild, such that the murmur disappears in mid to late diastole. Whether the stenosis is mild or severe, the murmur intensifies at the end of diastole (in patients in normal sinus rhythm), when atrial contraction accelerates flow across the valve (Fig. 2.9). The murmur of mitral stenosis is low-pitched and is heard best with the bell of the stethoscope at the apex, while the patient lies in the left lateral decubitus position. The much less common murmur of tricuspid stenosis is heard best near the xiphoid process.

Hyperdynamic states such as fever, anemia, hyperthyroidism, and exercise cause increased flow across the normal tricuspid and mitral valves, and can therefore occasionally result in a diastolic murmur. In patients with mitral regurgitation or a ventricular septal defect, the expected systolic murmurs can be accompanied by a diastolic murmur across the mitral valve because of the increased volume of blood flow. Similarly, patients with either tricuspid regurgitation or an atrial septal defect (see Chapter 16) may have an additional soft diastolic flow murmur across the tricuspid valve.

Continuous Murmurs

Continuous murmurs are heard throughout the cardiac cycle without an audible hiatus between systole and diastole. Such murmurs result from conditions in which a persistent pressure gradient exists between two structures during both systole and diastole. An example is the murmur of patent ductus arteriosus, in which there is an abnormal communication between the aorta and pulmonary artery (see Chapter 16). During systole, blood flows from the high-pressure ascending aorta through the ductus into the lower-pressure pulmonary artery. During diastole, the aortic pressure remains greater than that in the pulmonary artery and flow continues across the ductus. This murmur begins in early systole, crescendos to its maximum at S_2, and decrescendos to the next S_1 (Fig. 2.10). The maximal intensity of the murmur occurs at S_2 because that is approximately when the gradient between the aorta and pulmonary artery is the greatest.

The "to-and-fro" combined murmur in a patient with *both* aortic stenosis and aortic regurgitation could be mistaken for a continuous murmur (Fig. 2.10): During systole there is a diamond-shaped ejection murmur, and during diastole a decrescendo

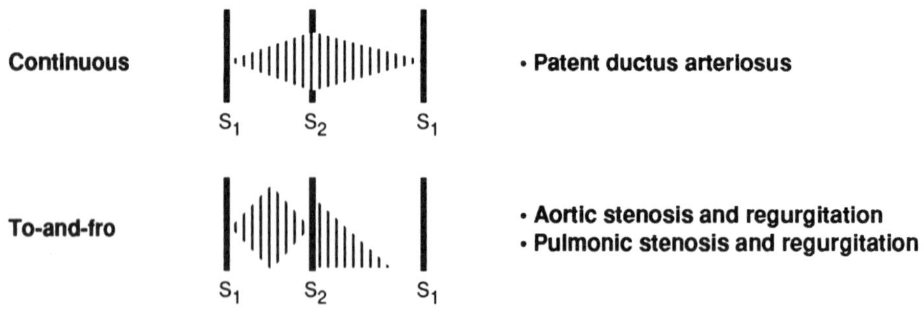

Figure 2.10.   A continuous murmur peaks at, and extends through, the second heart sound (S_2). A "to-and-fro" murmur is not continuous; rather, there is a systolic component and a distinct diastolic component, separated by S_2.

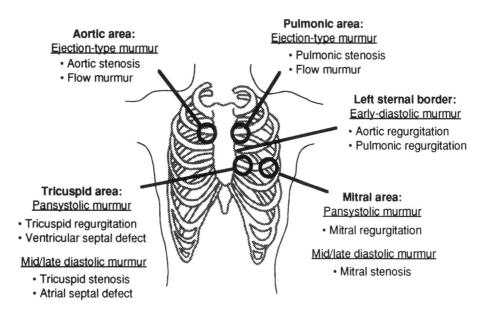

Aortic area:
Ejection-type murmur
• Aortic stenosis
• Flow murmur

Pulmonic area:
Ejection-type murmur
• Pulmonic stenosis
• Flow murmur

Left sternal border:
Early-diastolic murmur
• Aortic regurgitation
• Pulmonic regurgitation

Tricuspid area:
Pansystolic murmur
• Tricuspid regurgitation
• Ventricular septal defect

Mid/late diastolic murmur
• Tricuspid stenosis
• Atrial septal defect

Mitral area:
Pansystolic murmur
• Mitral regurgitation

Mid/late diastolic murmur
• Mitral stenosis

Figure 2.11. Locations where the murmurs presented in this chapter demonstrate their maximum intensities.

murmur. However, in the case of such a to-and-fro murmur, the sound does not extend through S2, as it has discrete systolic and diastolic components.

SUMMARY

Abnormal heart sounds and murmurs are common in acquired and congenital heart disease. Although it may seem diffi-cult to remember even the basic features presented here, it will become easier as you learn more about the pathophysiology of these conditions, and as your physical diagnosis experience grows. For now, just remember that the information is here, and refer to it as needed. Tables 2.2 and 2.3, and Figure 2.11 summarize features of the most common heart sounds and murmurs described in this chapter.

TABLE 2.2. Common Heart Sounds

Sound	Location (& Pitch)	Significance
S_1	Apex (high-pitched)	Normal closure of mitral and tricuspid valves
S_2	Base (high-pitched)	Normal closure of aortic (A_2) and pulmonic (P_2) valves
Extra Systolic Sounds		
Ejection clicks	*Aortic:* apex & base *Pulmonic:* base (both are high-pitched)	Aortic or pulmonic stenosis, or dilatation of aortic root or pulmonary artery
Mid/late click	*Mitral:* apex *Tricuspid:* left lower sternal border (both are high-pitched)	Mitral or tricupid valve prolapse
Extra Diastolic Sounds		
Opening snap	Apex (high-pitched)	Mitral stenosis
S_3	(*left-sided*): Apex (low-pitched)	Normal in children Abnormal in adults: indicates heart failure or volume overload state
S_4	(*left-sided*): Apex (low-pitched)	Reduced ventricular compliance

TABLE 2.3. Common Murmurs

Murmur Type		Examples	Location & Radiation
Systolic ejection	S_1 S_2	Aortic stenosis	2nd right interspace → neck (but may radiate widely)
		Pulmonic stenosis	2nd–3rd left interspace
Pansystolic	S_1 S_2	Mitral regurgitation	Apex → axilla
		Tricuspid regurgitation	Left lower sternal border → right lower sternal border
Late systolic	S_1 S_2	Mitral valve prolapse	Apex → axilla
Early diastolic	S_2 S_1	Aortic regurgitation	Along left side of sternum
		Pulmonic regurgitation	Upper left side of sternum
Mid/late diastolic	S_2 S_1	Mitral stenosis	Apex

ADDITIONAL READING

Bates B. A Guide to Physical Examination and History Taking. Philadelphia: JB Lippincott, 1995.

Constant J. Bedside Cardiology. 4th ed. Boston: Little, Brown, 1993.

DeGowin RL, DeGowin EL. Bedside Diagnostic Examination. New York: Macmillan, 1994.

Leon DL, Shaver JA. Physiologic Principles of Heart Sounds and Murmurs. American Heart Association Monograph Number 46. New York: American Heart Association, 1975.

Marriott HJL. Bedside Cardiac Diagnosis. Philadelphia: JB Lippincott, 1993.

Perloff JK, Braunwald E. Physical examination of the heart and circulation. In: Braunwald E, ed. Heart Disease: a Textbook of Cardiovascular Medicine. 5th ed. Philadelphia: WB Saunders, 1997:15–52.

Sapira JD. The Art and Science of Bedside Diagnosis. Baltimore: Williams & Wilkins, 1990:283–330.

Acknowledgments   The previous edition of this chapter was written by Bradley S. Marino, MD, and Allan Goldblatt, MD.

Diagnostic Imaging and Catheterization Techniques

*Sharon Horesh, Shona Pendse,
and Patricia Challender Come*

Diagnostic imaging plays an essential role in the assessment of cardiac function and pathology. The most commonly used techniques are chest radiography, echocardiography, cardiac catheterization with cineangiography, and nuclear imaging. The cardiovascular applications of computed tomography (CT) scanning and magnetic resonance imaging (MRI) are currently being defined.

This chapter presents an introductory overview of these techniques as they are used to assess the cardiovascular disorders described in this book. It would be beneficial to familiarize yourself with the information now, but not to memorize the details. The chapter is meant as a reference, so that you can look back to it while reading subsequent material.

CARDIAC RADIOGRAPHY

The penetration of x-rays through the body is inversely proportional to tissue density. Air-filled tissues, such as the lung, absorb few x-rays and expose the underlying film, causing it to appear black. In contrast, dense materials, such as bone, absorb more radiation and appear white, or radiopaque. For a boundary to show between two structures, they must differ in density. Myocardium, valves, and other intracardiac structures have densities similar to adjacent blood; consequently, radiography cannot delineate these structures unless they happen to be calcified. However, heart borders adjacent to lung are depicted clearly because heart and air-filled lung have different densities. If the lung adjacent to the heart is diseased, however, as in pulmonary edema, consolidation, or collapse, the lung density will match that of the heart, and the cardiac border will be ill-defined.

Frontal and lateral radiographs are routinely used to assess the heart and lungs (Fig. 3.1). The *frontal* view is usually a posterior-anterior (PA) image in which the x-rays are transmitted from behind (i.e., posterior to) the patient, travel through the body, and then expose a sheet of film placed against the chest on the anterior side. In the standard *lateral* view, the patient's left side is placed against the film plate and the x-

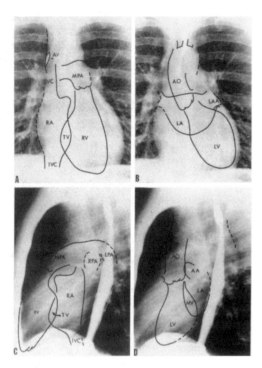

Figure 3.1. Posteroanterior (**A** and **B**) and lateral (**C** and **D**) chest radiographs from an individual without cardiopulmonary disease illustrating cardiac chambers and valves. AV, azygos vein; SVC, superior vena cava; RA, right atrium; IVC, inferior vena cava; TV, tricuspid valve; RV, right ventricle; MPA, main pulmonary artery; AO, aorta; LA, left atrium; LAA, left atrial appendage; LV, left ventricle; RPA, right pulmonary artery; LPA, left pulmonary artery; MV, mitral valve. (Reprinted with permission from Come PC, ed. Diagnostic Cardiology: Noninvasive Imaging Techniques. Philadelphia: JB Lippincott, 1985.)

rays pass through the body from right to left. The frontal radiograph is particularly good for assessing the size of the left ventricle, left atrial appendage, pulmonary artery, aorta, and superior vena cava; the lateral view evaluates right ventricular size, posterior borders of the left atrium and ventricle, and PA diameter of the thorax. In some cases, optimal evaluation of the heart requires right and left anterior oblique views as well.

Cardiac Silhouette

Chest radiographs are used to evaluate the size of heart chambers and the pulmonary consequences of heart disease. Alterations in chamber size are reflected by changes in the cardiac silhouette. In the frontal view of adults, the heart shadow should occupy 50% or less of the maximal width of the thorax, measured between the inner margins of the ribs. In children, normal cardiac diameter may be up to 60% of thoracic width. The cardio/thoracic ratio is used instead of absolute measurements, in order to account for differences in body habitus.

There are several situations in which the cardiac silhouette inaccurately reflects heart size. An elevated diaphragm or narrow chest PA diameter, for example, may cause the heart to appear to spread out transversely. Consequently, the silhouette on a PA chest film may be greater than 50% of the thorax even though the *actual* heart size is normal. Therefore, the chest PA diameter should be assessed on the lateral view before one concludes that a frontal image truly represents an enlarged heart. The presence of a pericardial effusion can also cause enlargement of the cardiac silhouette, because fluid and myocardium affect x-ray penetration similarly.

Radiographs reflect changes due to dilatation of cardiac chambers and great vessels. Hypertrophy alone *may not* result in radiographic abnormalities, because it generally occurs at the expense of the cavity's internal volume and produces little or no change in overall cardiac size. Hypertrophy is more readily suspected from changes in electrocardiographic QRS voltage, and wall thickness can be accurately quantitated by other techniques, such as echocardiography. Major causes of chamber and great vessel dilatation include heart failure, valvular lesions, abnormal intracardiac and extracardiac communications (shunts), and certain pulmonary disorders. Because dilatation takes time to develop, recent lesions, such as *acute* mitral insufficiency, may present without apparent cardiomegaly.

The pattern of chamber enlargement may suggest specific disease entities. For example, dilatation of the left atrium and right ventricle, accompanied by signs of pulmonary hypertension, suggests mitral stenosis (Fig. 3.2). In contrast, dilatation of

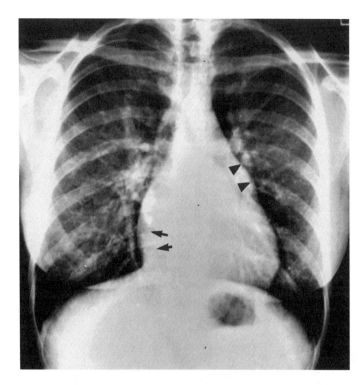

Figure 3.2.   Posteroanterior chest radiograph from a patient with severe mitral stenosis and secondary pulmonary vascular congestion. The radiograph shows a prominent left atrial appendage (arrowheads) with consequent straightening of the left heart border and suggestion of a double density right cardiac border (arrows) produced by the enlarged left atrium. The aortic silhouette is small, which suggests chronic low cardiac output. Radiographic signs of pulmonary vascular congestion include increased caliber of upper zone pulmonary vessel markings and decreased caliber of lower zone vessels.

the pulmonary artery and right heart chambers, but without enlargement of the left-sided heart dimensions, suggests pulmonary vascular obstruction or increased pulmonary artery blood flow (e.g., due to an atrial septal defect; see Fig. 3.3).

The shape of the dilated chamber may also provide etiologic clues. For instance, in left ventricular volume overload due to valvular insufficiency, the ventricle tends to enlarge primarily in its long axis, displacing the apex downward and to the left. In contrast, when left ventricular dilation results from primary myocardial dysfunction, left ventricular length and width are generally both increased, causing the heart to appear globular.

Dilatation of the aorta and pulmonary artery can also be detected by chest radiographs. Causes of aortic dilatation include aneurysm, dissection, and aortic valve disease (Fig. 3.4). The pulmonary artery may

be enlarged in patients with left-to-right shunts, which cause increased pulmonary blood flow (Fig. 3.3), and in those with pulmonary hypertension of diverse causes. Isolated enlargement of the proximal left pulmonary artery is seen in some patients with pulmonic stenosis.

Pulmonary Manifestations

The appearance of the pulmonary vasculature on chest radiographs reflects changes in pulmonary arterial pressure, pulmonary venous pressure, and pulmonary blood flow. Increased pulmonary venous pressure, as occurs in left heart failure, causes increased vascular markings, redistribution of blood flow from the bases to the apices of the lungs, pulmonary edema, the presence of abnormal septal lines, and pleural effusions (Fig. 3.5). Blood flow redistribution

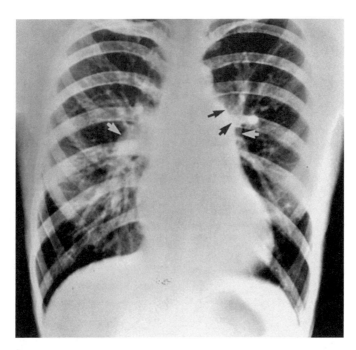

Figure 3.3.   Posteroanterior chest radiograph of a patient with pulmonary hypertension secondary to an atrial septal defect. Radiographic signs of pulmonary hypertension include pulmonary artery dilatation (black arrows) (compare with the appearance of left atrial appendage dilatation in Figure 3.2) and large central pulmonary arteries (white arrows) associated with small peripheral vessels (a pattern known as "peripheral pruning").

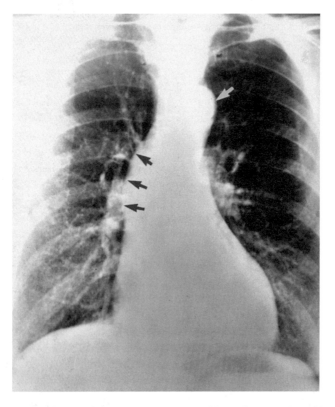

Figure 3.4.   Posteroanterior chest radiograph from a patient with aortic stenosis and insufficiency secondary to a bicuspid aortic valve. In addition to poststenotic dilatation of the ascending aorta (black arrows), the transverse aorta (white arrow) is prominent, which suggests aortic insufficiency in addition to stenosis.

appears as an increase in the number or width of vascular markings at the apex. (Compare Figure 3.5 with healthy lungs in Figure 3.1.) Interstitial and alveolar pulmonary edema produce opacity radiating from the hilar region bilaterally (known as a "butterfly pattern") and air bronchograms, respectively. Septal lines (or Kerley lines), which depict fluid in interlobular spaces, result from interstitial edema. Pleural effusions cause blunting of the costodiaphragmatic angles.

Changes in pulmonary blood flow may also cause alterations in the appearance of the pulmonary vessels. Focal oligemia (decreased flow) may result from pulmonary embolism or replacement of functioning lung tissue by emphysematous bullae. Large central pulmonary arteries, in association with small peripheral vessels ("peripheral pruning"), suggest pulmonary hypertension (Fig. 3.3).

Table 3.1 summarizes the major radiographic findings in common forms of cardiac disease.

ECHOCARDIOGRAPHY

Echocardiography plays an important role in the diagnosis and serial evaluation of many cardiac disorders. It is safe, noninvasive, relatively inexpensive, and capable of accurately depicting a wide array of heart diseases. High-frequency (ultrasonic) waves, generated by a piezoelectric transducer, travel through body tissue and are reflected at interfaces where there are differences in the acoustic impedance of adjacent tissues. The reflected waves return to the transducer and cause mechanical deformation of the piezoelectric ceramic. The distance between the transducer and each anatomic reflecting surface is calculated automatically

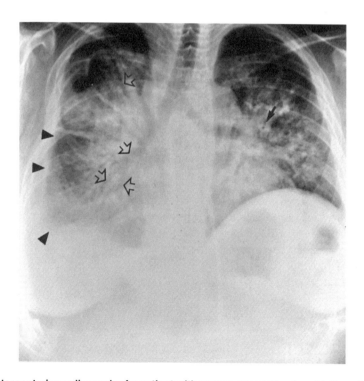

Figure 3.5. Posteroanterior radiograph of a patient with severe congestive heart failure. Pulmonary vascular congestion is indicated by vascular redistribution from the bases to the apices of the lungs (although in severe CHF there is increased pulmonary vascular markings throughout the lung fields), peribronchiolar cuffing (black arrow), and pleural effusion, which is indicated by blunting of the costodiaphragmatic angle and tracking up the right lateral hemithorax (black arrowheads). The presence of interstitial and alveolar edema produces perihilar haziness and air bronchograms (open arrows), which occur when the radiolucent bronchial tree is contrasted with opaque edematous lung tissue. (Courtesy of Robert Pugatch, MD, Brigham and Women's Hospital, Boston, MA)

TABLE 3.1. Chest Radiography of Common Cardiac Disorders

Congestive heart failure	• Vascular redistribution from bases to apices of the lungs • Perivascular haziness • Peribronchiolar cuffing • Air bronchograms • Pleural effusions
Pulmonic valve stenosis	• Poststenotic dilatation of pulmonary artery • Normal cardiac chamber sizes • Clear lung fields
Aortic valve stenosis	• Poststenotic dilatation of ascending aorta • Normal cardiac chamber sizes (until heart fails) • Normal pulmonary vasculature
Aortic regurgitation	• Left ventricular enlargement • Dilated aorta
Mitral stenosis	• Enlarged left atrium • Small aorta (if chronic low cardiac output) • Signs of pulmonary venous congestion

Mitral regurgitation	• Left atrial dilatation
	• Left ventricular dilatation
	• If severe:
	    • Right ventricular dilatation
	    • Signs of congestive heart failure

by the machine from the time elapsed between the initiation and reception of the sound waves, and images are constructed.

Three types of echocardiographic studies are generally performed: 1) M-mode, 2) two-dimensional (2-D), and 3) Doppler Imaging. Each type of imaging can be performed from a variety of locations. Most commonly, *transthoracic* studies are performed, in which images are obtained by placing the transducer on the surface of the chest. When greater structural detail is required, *transesophageal* imaging is performed, as described below.

M-mode echocardiography was the first cardiac application of ultrasonography. It is now used rarely by itself, because it provides only limited data from one narrow ultrasonic beam—images along a single line are displayed. M-mode techniques are used today for measurement of wall thicknesses, chamber diameters, and accurate temporal resolution of valve motion (Fig. 3.6).

In **2-D echocardiography,** multiple ultrasonic beams are transmitted through a wide arc. The returning signals are integrated to produce two-dimensional images of the heart on a video monitor. Thus, this technique depicts anatomic relationships and defines the movement of cardiac structures relative to one another. The wide fields of view enhance the ability of 2-D echocardiograms to detect and display wall and valve motion, abnormal shunts, and intracardiac masses such as vegetations, thrombi, and tumors.

Each two-dimensional plane (Fig. 3.7) delineates only part of a given cardiac structure. Optimal evaluation of the entire heart is achieved by using combinations of views. These include the standard parasternal long axis, parasternal short axis, apical four-chamber, apical two-chamber, and subcostal views. The *parasternal long axis* view is recorded with the transducer in the third or fourth intercostal space to the left of the sternum. This view is particularly useful for evaluation of the left atrium, mitral valve, left ventricle, and left ventricular outflow tract, which includes the aortic valve and adjacent interventricular septum. To obtain the *parasternal short axis* views, the transducer is rotated 90° from its position for the parasternal long axis view. The short axis images depict transverse planes of the heart. Several different levels are imaged to assess the aortic valve, mitral valve, and left ventricular wall motion. *Apical views* are produced when the transducer is placed at the point of maximal cardiac impulse. The apical four-chamber view evaluates the mi-

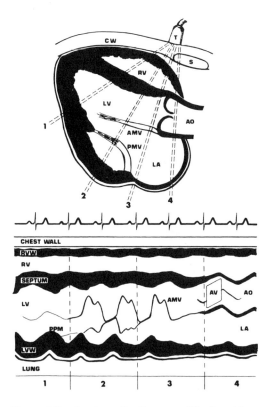

Figure 3.6. A schematic diagram of the heart in a parasternal long axis view is illustrated in the upper drawing. Below it is an electrocardiogram and an M-mode echocardiogram generated by changes in the direction of the transducer from position 1 to position 4. Chamber sizes and wall thicknesses can be measured along the vertical axis. Wall thickening and wall thinning with ventricular contraction and relaxation are evident, as is movement of the aortic and mitral valves. CW, chest wall; T, echocardiographic transducer; S, sternum; RV, right ventricle; LV, left ventricle; AO, aortic root; AMV, anterior mitral valve leaflet; LA, left atrium; RVW, right ventricular wall; AV, aortic valve; PPM, posterior papillary muscle region; LVW, left ventricular wall. (Reprinted with permission from Come PC. Echocardiography in diagnosis and management of cardiovascular disease. Compr Ther 1980;6:7–17. By permission of International Publishing Group, Cleveland, OH.)

tral and tricuspid valves, and the atrial and ventricular chambers, including the motion of the lateral, septal, and apical left ventricular walls. The apical two-chamber view shows only the left side of the heart, and it depicts movement of the anterior, inferior, and apical walls. In some patients, such as those with obstructive airways disease or obesity, the above views do not provide adequate depiction of cardiac structures because of signal attenuation caused by the in-

creased air or adipose tissue. In such patients the *subcostal view*, in which the transducer is placed inferior to the rib cage, may provide a better ultrasonic window, allowing visualization of all four cardiac chambers.

Doppler ultrasonography evaluates blood flow direction, turbulence, and velocity, and it permits estimation of pressure gradients within the heart and great vessels. Doppler studies are based on the physical principle that waves reflected from a moving object undergo a frequency shift according to the moving object's velocity relative to the source of the waves. Color flow mapping converts the Doppler signals to an arbitrarily chosen scale of colors that represent direction, velocity, and turbulence of blood flow in a semiquantitative way. The colors are superimposed on 2-D echocardiographic images and show the location of stenotic and regurgitant valvular lesions and of abnormal communications within the heart and great vessels. For example, Doppler echocardiography in a patient with mitral regurgitation shows a jet of retrograde flow into the left atrium during systole (Fig. 3.8).

Modern echocardiography machines automatically convert sound frequency shifts into blood flow velocity measurements. The components of that calculation are:

$$v = \frac{fs \cdot c}{2 \cdot f_o \cdot (\cos \theta)}$$

where v equals blood flow velocity (m/sec); fs, Doppler frequency shift (kHz); c, velocity of sound in body tissue (m/sec); θ, angle between the transmitted sound pulse and the mean axis of blood flow; f_o, frequency of the sound pulse emitted from the transducer (MHz).

Transesophageal echocardiography (TEE) uses a miniaturized transducer mounted at the end of a modified endoscope to transmit and receive ultrasound waves from within the esophagus, thus producing very clear images of the neighboring cardiac structures (Fig. 3.9) and much of the thoracic aorta. Progressive refinements in technology have created small probes with biplanar or multiplanar capabilities, as well as Doppler

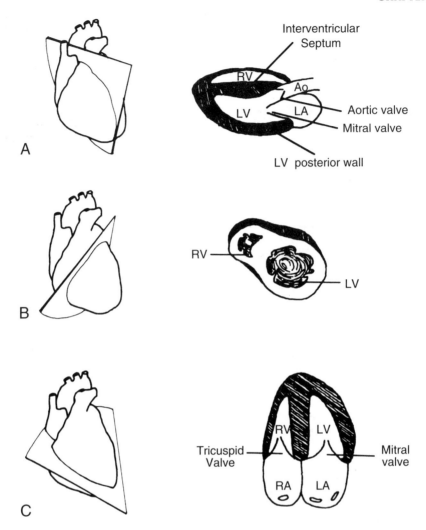

Figure 3.7.   Transthoracic two-dimensional echocardiographic views. A. Parasternal long axis view. **B.** Parasternal short axis view. **C.** Apical 4-chamber view. LA, left atrium; RA, right atrium; LV, left ventricle; RV, right ventricle; Ao, aorta.

as Doppler imaging. Transesophageal echocardiography is particularly helpful in the assessment of aortic and atrial abnormalities, conditions that are less well-visualized by conventional transthoracic echo imaging. For example, TEE is more sensitive than transthoracic echo for the detection of thrombus within the left atrial appendage (Fig. 3.10). The proximity of the esophagus to the heart makes TEE imaging particularly advantageous in patients in whom transthoracic echo images are unsatisfactory (e.g., patients with chronic obstructive lung disease).

TEE is also advantageous in the evaluation of patients with prosthetic heart valves. During standard transthoracic imaging, ar-

tificial mechanical valves reflect a large portion of ultrasound waves, thus masking visualization of more posterior structures. TEE aids visualization of the posterior chambers in such patients, and is therefore the most sensitive noninvasive technique for evaluating perivalvular leaks.

TEE is commonly used to evaluate patients with cerebral ischemia of unexplained etiology, since it can identify cardiovascular causes for emboli with a high sensitivity. These etiologies include intracardiac thrombi or tumors, atherosclerotic debris within the aorta, and valvular vegetations. TEE is also sensitive and specific for the detection of aortic dissection.

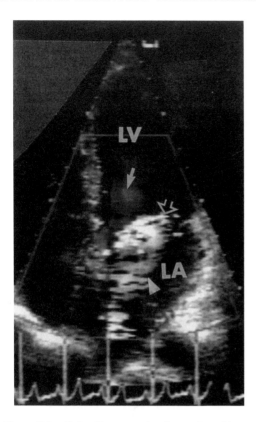

Figure 3.8. Color-flow mapping (reproduced in gray tones) of Doppler ultrasonography superimposed on an apical four-chamber two-dimensional echocardiogram from a patient with mitral regurgitation. The break in the EKG tracing at the peak of the T wave shows that the image represents systole. Forward systolic flow is visualized heading from the left ventricle toward the aortic root (arrow), and retrograde systolic flow (mitral regurgitation) is seen projecting into the left atrium (arrowhead). The mitral valve (open arrow) separates the left ventricle and atrium. LV, left ventricle; LA, left atrium. (Courtesy of Marilyn Riley, BS, Beth Israel Deaconess Hospital, Boston, MA)

Transesophageal echocardiography is often used in the operating room during surgical procedures. It permits intraoperative monitoring to determine the success of repair of congenital and valvular lesions. In addition, imaging of ventricular wall motion can identify periods of myocardial ischemia during high-risk surgeries.

Contrast echocardiography is frequently used in the evaluation of congenital heart disease, as it is highly sensitive for the detection of abnormal intracardiac shunts. In this technique, an echocardiographic contrast agent (e.g., agitated saline) is rapidly injected into a peripheral (usually a bra-

chial) vein. Using standard echocardiographic imaging, the "contrast" can be visualized passing through the cardiac chambers. Normally, there is rapid opacification of the right-sided chambers, but since the contrast is filtered out (harmlessly) in the lungs, it does not reach the left-sided chambers. However, in the presence of an intracardiac or intrapulmonary shunt with abnormal right-to-left heart blood flow, contrast will appear in the left sided chambers as well.

Intravascular ultrasound is presently a research tool used to investigate the coronary arteries and cardiac chambers. Advances in this technique, in conjunction with angioplasty procedures, have enhanced the understanding of coronary anatomy and pathology.

Echocardiography can identify and often quantify the severity of valvular lesions, complications of coronary artery disease, septal defects, intracardiac masses, cardiomyopathy, ventricular hypertrophy, pericardial disease, aortic disease, and congenital heart disease. Echocardiographic evaluation includes assessment of cardiac chamber sizes, wall thicknesses, wall motion, valvular function, and blood flow and intracardiac hemodynamics. A few of these topics are highlighted below.

Ventricular Assessment

Two-dimensional echocardiography measures left ventricular systolic function by computing fractional changes between end-diastolic and end-systolic measurements. Left ventricular width, area, and volume in diastole and systole can be measured to permit assessment of contractile function. Two-dimensional echocardiography can also depict regional ventricular wall motion abnormalities, a sign of coronary artery disease. Right ventricular (RV) function is generally assessed qualitatively, because the RV does not lend itself as easily to geometric modeling as does the left ventricle. Two-dimensional echocardiography is also useful in evaluating ventricular wall thickness and mass, which is important in

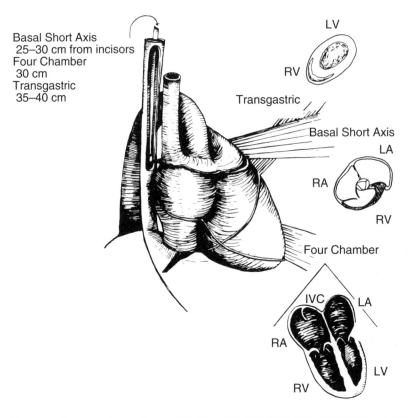

Basal Short Axis
 25–30 cm from incisors
Four Chamber
 30 cm
Transgastric
 35–40 cm

LV

RV

Transgastric

Basal Short Axis
LA

RA

RV

Four Chamber

IVC   LA

RA

LV

RV

Figure 3.9.   Transesophageal echocardiographic views. LA, left atrium; RA, right atrium; LV, left ventricle; RV, right ventricle; IVC, inferior vena cava; Ao, aorta. (Courtesy of Jane Freedman, MD, Boston University Medical Center, Boston, MA)

patients with hypertension, aortic stenosis, or hypertrophic cardiomyopathy (Fig. 3.11).

Valvular Lesions

Echocardiography is of great benefit in the assessment of valvular heart disease. The underlying causes of valvular abnormalities can often be identified and the severity of certain lesions (e.g., mitral stenosis or aortic stenosis) can be quantitated. For example, pressure gradients across stenotic valves can be calculated from the maximal blood flow velocity (v) measured distal to the valve, using the simplified Bernoulli equation:

$$\text{Pressure gradient} = 4 \times v^2$$

For example, if the peak velocity recorded distal to a stenotic aortic valve is 4 m/sec, then the calculated peak pressure gradient across the valve = $4 \times 4^2 = 64$ mm Hg. Other calculations (beyond the scope of

this book) yield fairly accurate noninvasive measurements of aortic, mitral and tricuspid valve areas.

Coronary Artery Disease (CAD)

Two-dimensional echocardiography can visualize ventricular wall motion abnormalities associated with infarcted or transiently ischemic myocardium. By evaluating the amount of abnormal systolic contraction and decreased systolic wall thickening, one can estimate the extent of an infarction and implicate the responsible coronary artery. Infarct size measured by 2-D echocardiography correlates well with other methods of quantification such as thallium perfusion defects, peak serum creatine kinase measurements and pathologic examination.

Echocardiography is also used to detect complications of acute myocardial infarction,

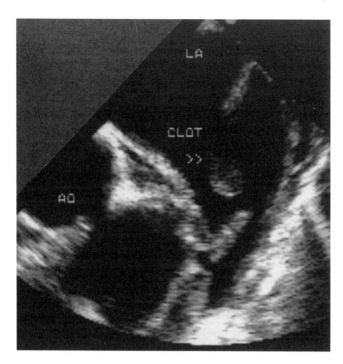

Figure 3.10. Transesophageal echocardiographic basal short-axis image from a patient with mitral stenosis illustrating a clot within the left atrial appendage. Transesophageal echocardiography is much more sensitive than transthoracic in imaging intra-atrial masses. LA, left atrium; AO, aorta. (Courtesy of Marilyn Riley, BS, Beth Israel Deaconess Hospital, Boston, MA)

including intraventricular thrombus formation, papillary muscle rupture, valvular dysfunction, ventricular septal rupture, aneurysm formation, and pericardial effusion.

Although echocardiography can depict these *consequences* of CAD, echo resolution is insufficient to directly image the coronary arteries themselves.

Stress echocardiography can be used to indirectly evaluate coronary artery disease, even in the absence of previous infarction. This technique assesses the development of left ventricular regional wall motion abnormalities induced by exercise or following infusion of specific pharmacologic agents, such as dobutamine and dipyridamole (see Chapter 6). Reversible myocardial ischemia is recognized by the development, during stress, of a wall motion abnormality in the region of reduced coronary blood supply.

Cardiomyopathy

Cardiomyopathies are heart muscle disorders that occur in three forms: dilated, hypertrophic, and restrictive (see Chapter 10). Echocardiography can often distinguish between these and permits assessment of the severity of myocardial dysfunction. For example, Figure 3.11 demonstrates the thickened ventricular walls typical of hypertrophic cardiomyopathy.

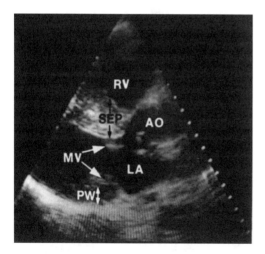

Figure 3.11. Diastolic parasternal long axis two-dimensional echocardiographic image from a patient with hypertrophic cardiomyopathy. A thickened septum (SEP), slight hypertrophy of the posterior ventricular wall (PW), and increased echogenicity of the septum are characteristic of hypertrophic cardiomyopathy. (Reprinted with permission from Come PC, ed. Diagnostic cardiology: noninvasive imaging techniques. Philadelphia: JB Lippincott, 1985.)

Pericardial Disease

Two-dimensional echocardiography can identify abnormal substances in the pericardial cavity (e.g., excessive pericardial fluid, fibrous material, tumor, clot). Tamponade and constrictive pericarditis, the main functional consequences of pericardial disease, may be associated with particular echocardiographic abnormalities. In tamponade, the increased pericardial pressure compresses the cardiac chambers, and results in cyclical "collapse" of the right atrium, right ventricle, and sometimes the left atrium (Fig. 3.12). Constrictive pericarditis is associated with increased thickness or reflectiveness of the pericardial echo and abnormal patterns of diastolic left ventricular wall motion.

Table 3.2 summarizes the salient echocardiographic features of common cardiac diseases.

CARDIAC CATHETERIZATION

In the diagnosis of many cardiovascular abnormalities, intravascular catheters are used to measure pressures in the heart chambers, to determine cardiac output and vascular resistances, and to inject radiopaque material to examine heart structures and blood flow. In 1929, Werner Forssmann performed the first cardiac

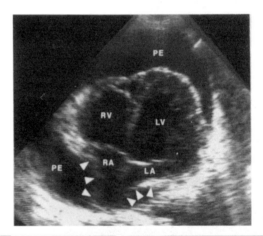

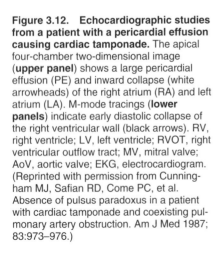
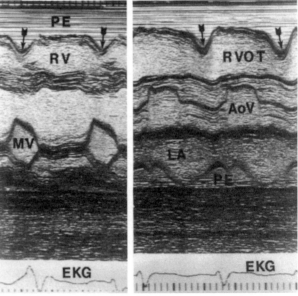

Figure 3.12. Echocardiographic studies from a patient with a pericardial effusion causing cardiac tamponade. The apical four-chamber two-dimensional image (**upper panel**) shows a large pericardial effusion (PE) and inward collapse (white arrowheads) of the right atrium (RA) and left atrium (LA). M-mode tracings (**lower panels**) indicate early diastolic collapse of the right ventricular wall (black arrows). RV, right ventricle; LV, left ventricle; RVOT, right ventricular outflow tract; MV, mitral valve; AoV, aortic valve; EKG, electrocardiogram. (Reprinted with permission from Cunningham MJ, Safian RD, Come PC, et al. Absence of pulsus paradoxus in a patient with cardiac tamponade and coexisting pulmonary artery obstruction. Am J Med 1987; 83:973–976.)

TABLE 3.2. Echocardiography in Common Cardiac Disorders

	Valvular Lesions
Mitral stenosis	• Enlarged left atrium • Thickened mitral valve leaflets • Decreased movement and separation of mitral valve leaflets • Decreased mitral valve orifice
Mitral regurgitation	• Enlarged left atrium (if chronic) • Enlarged left ventricle (if chronic) • Systolic flow from left ventricle into left atrium (by Doppler)
Aortic stenosis	• Thickened aortic valve cusps • Decreased valve orifice • Increased ventricular wall thickness
Aortic regurgitation	• Enlarged left ventricle • Abnormalities of aortic valve or aortic root
	Left Ventricular Function
Myocardial infarction and complications	• Hypokinetic, dyskinetic, or akinetic ventricular wall motion • Decreased ejection fraction • Thrombus within left ventricle • Aneurysm of ventricular wall • Septal rupture (abnormal Doppler flow) • Papillary muscle rupture • Pericardial effusion
Cardiomyopathies Dilated	• Enlarged ventricular chamber sizes • Normal ventricular wall thicknesses • Decreased systolic contraction
Hypertrophic	• Normal or decreased ventricular chamber sizes • Increased ventricular wall thickness • Diastolic dysfunction (assessed by Doppler)
Restrictive	• Normal or decreased ventricular chamber sizes • Enlarged atria • Increased ventricular wall thickness • Ventricular contractile function usually normal

catheterization, *on himself,* and humbly issued in the era of invasive cardiology. Much of what is known about the pathophysiology of valvular heart disease and congestive heart failure comes from decades of subsequent hemodynamic research in the cardiac catheterization laboratory.

Measurement of Pressure

Prior to catheterization of an artery or vein, the patient is mildly sedated, and a local anesthetic is used to numb the skin site of catheter entry. The catheter, attached to a pressure transducer outside of the body, is then introduced into the appropriate blood vessel. To measure pressures in the right atrium, right ventricle, and pulmonary artery, a catheter is usually inserted into a femoral, brachial or jugular *vein.* Pressures in the aorta and left ventricle are measured via catheters inserted into a brachial or femoral *artery.* Once in the blood vessel, the catheter is guided by fluoroscopy (x-ray images) to the area of study, where pressure measurements are made. Figure 3.13 depicts normal intracardiac pressures.

The measurement of pressures on the right side of the heart is usually performed with a specialized, balloon-tipped catheter that is advanced through the right side of the heart with the aid of normal blood flow. Typically, the catheter is inserted either percutaneously or via open incision into a peripheral vein and advanced toward the chest. When the catheter reaches a vein of suitable size (e.g., the inferior or superior vena cava), the balloon is inflated, which enables flotation of the catheter into the right heart and pulmonary artery.

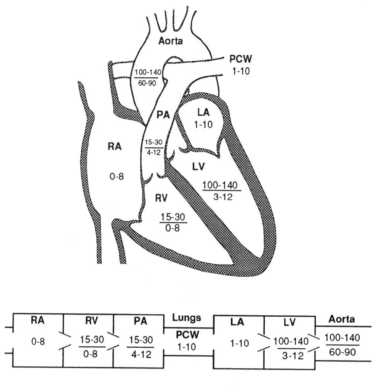

Figure 3.13. Diagrams indicating normal intracardiac chamber pressures. The top figure shows the normal anatomic relationship of the cardiac chambers, whereas the figure on the bottom shows a simplified schematic to clarify the pressure relationships. Numbers indicate pressures in mm Hg. RA, right atrial mean pressure; RV, right ventricular pressure; PA, pulmonary artery pressure; PCW, pulmonary capillary wedge mean pressure; LA, left atrial mean pressure; LV, left ventricular pressure.

Right Atrial Pressure

Right atrial pressure is equal to central venous pressure (estimated by the jugular venous pressure on physical exam), because no obstructing valves impede blood return into the right atrium. In addition, right atrial pressure normally equals right ventricular pressure in diastole, because the right heart functions as a common chamber when the tricuspid valve is open. The mean right atrial pressure is *reduced* when there is intravascular volume depletion. It is *elevated* in right ventricular failure, right-sided valvular disease, and cardiac tamponade (in which the cardiac chambers are surrounded by high-pressure pericardial fluid, as described in Chapter 14).

Certain abnormalities cause characteristic changes in individual components of the right atrial (and therefore jugular venous)

pressure (Table 3.3). For example, the two main causes of a prominent "a" wave are tricuspid stenosis and right ventricular hypertrophy. In these conditions, the right atrium contracts vigorously against either the obstructing tricuspid valve or a stiff right ventricle, generating a prominent pressure wave. A prominent "v" wave is observed in tricuspid regurgitation because normal right atrial filling is augmented by the regurgitated blood.

Right Ventricular Pressure

Right ventricular systolic pressure is increased by pulmonic valve stenosis or pulmonary hypertension. Right ventricular diastolic pressure increases when the right ventricle is subjected to pressure or volume overload, and may be a sign of right-heart failure.

TABLE 3.3. Causes of Increased Intracardiac Pressures

Chamber and Measurement	Causes
Right atrial pressure	• Right ventricular failure
	• Cardiac tamponade
a wave	• Tricuspid stenosis
	• Right ventricular hypertrophy
v wave	• Tricuspid regurgitation
	• Right ventricular failure
Right ventricular pressure	
Systolic	• Pulmonic stenosis
	• Right ventricular failure
	• Pulmonary hypertension
Diastolic	• Right ventricular failure
	• Cardiac tamponade
	• Right ventricular hypertrophy
Pulmonary artery pressure	
Systolic and diastolic	• Pulmonary hypertension
	• Left-sided CHF
	• Chronic lung disease
	• Pulmonary vascular
Systolic only	• Increased flow (L→R shunt)
Pulmonary artery wedge pressure	
	• Left-sided CHF
	• Mitral stenosis
	• Cardiac tamponade
a wave	• Mitral stenosis
v wave	• Mitral regurgitation
	• Ventricular septal defect
	• Decreased LV compliance

Pulmonary Artery Pressure

Elevation of systolic and diastolic pulmonary artery pressures occurs in three conditions: 1) *left*-sided heart failure, 2) parenchymal lung disease (e.g., chronic bronchitis or end-stage emphysema), and 3) pulmonary vascular disease (e.g., pulmonary embolism, primary pulmonary hypertension). Normally, the pulmonary artery diastolic pressure is equivalent to the left atrial pressure because of the low-resistance of the pulmonary vasculature that separates them. If the left atrial pressure rises because of left-sided heart failure, both systolic and diastolic pulmonary artery pressures increase in an obligatory manner to maintain forward flow through the lungs. This situation leads to "passive" pulmonary hypertension.

In certain conditions, however, pulmonary vascular resistance becomes abnormally high, which is manifest by an elevated pulmonary artery diastolic pressure compared with the left atrial pressure. In this setting, "reactive" pulmonary hypertension is said to exist. When pulmonary vascular obstructive disease develops as a complication of a chronic cardiac shunt (e.g., atrial or ventricular septal defect), it is called Eisenmenger's syndrome.

Pulmonary Artery Wedge Pressure

If a catheter is advanced into the right or left pulmonary artery, its tip will ultimately reach one of the small pulmonary artery branches and temporarily occlude forward blood flow beyond it. During that time, a column of stagnant blood stands between the catheter tip and the portions of the pulmonary capillary and pulmonary venous segments distal to it (Fig. 3.14). That column of blood acts as an "extension" of the catheter, and the pressure recorded through the catheter reflects that of the downstream chamber, namely the left atrium (LA). Such a pressure measurement is termed the "pulmonary artery wedge pressure" or "pulmonary capillary wedge pressure (PCW)" and it

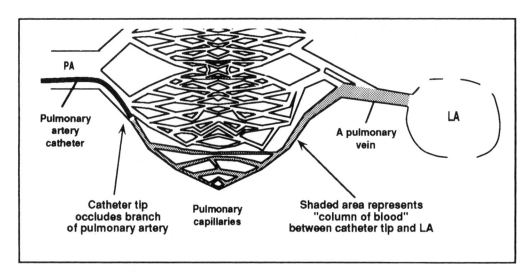

Figure 3.14. Diagram of pulmonary artery catheter inserted into a branch of the pulmonary artery (PA).
Flow is occluded in the arterial, arteriolar, and capillary vessels beyond the catheter; thus these vessels act as a conduit that transmits the left atrial (LA) pressure to the catheter.

closely matches the left atrial pressure in most individuals (and is therefore equivalent to the LA pressure tracing shown in Fig. 2.1). Furthermore, while the mitral valve is open during diastole, the pulmonary venous bed, left atrium, and left ventricle normally share equal pressures. Thus, the PCW is also used to estimate the left ventricular diastolic pressure, a measurement of ventricular preload (see Chapter 9). As a result of this important feature, the PCW measurement through a right-heart catheter is a key measurement while monitoring critically ill patients in the intensive care unit.

Elevation of the mean PCW is seen in left-sided heart failure and in mitral stenosis. The individual components of the PCW tracing may also become abnormally high. The "a" wave may be increased in conditions of decreased left ventricular compliance, such as left ventricular hypertrophy or acute myocardial ischemia (Table 3.3). The "v" wave is greater than normal when there is increased left atrial filling during ventricular contraction, such as in mitral regurgitation.

Measurement of Blood Flow

Cardiac output is measured by either the thermodilution method or the Fick tech-nique. In the thermodilution method, saline of a known temperature is injected rapidly into the right heart via a sidehole in a catheter 30 cm proximal to its tip. At the catheter tip, a thermistor registers the surrounding temperature in the pulmonary artery, which is transiently altered by the injected saline. The cardiac output is electronically calculated from the slope of the decay of the temperature change.

The commonly used Fick method is derived from the principle that consumption of oxygen by tissues is related to the O_2 content removed from blood as it flows through the capillary bed:

$$O_2 \text{ consumption} = O_2 \text{ content removed} \times \text{Flow}$$
$$\left(\frac{ml\,O_2}{min}\right) \qquad\qquad \left(\frac{ml\,O_2}{ml\,blood}\right)\left(\frac{ml\,blood}{min}\right)$$

Or, in other terms:

$$O_2 \text{ consumption} =$$
Arteriovenous O_2 difference $\times$ Cardiac output

in which arteriovenous O_2 difference equals the difference in oxygen content between the arterial and venous compartments. Total body oxygen consumption (normally $125 \pm 25\ ml\,O_2/min/m^2$) can be determined by analyzing expired air, and arterial and venous O_2 content is measured in blood samples. The cardiac output can then be calculated:

Cardiac output =

$$\frac{O_2 \text{ consumption}}{\text{Arteriovenous } O_2 \text{ difference}}$$

For example, if the arterial blood in a normal adult contains 190 ml O_2/L and the venous blood contains 150 ml O_2/L, the arteriovenous difference is 40 ml O_2/L. If this patient has a measured O_2 consumption of 200 ml/min, then the cardiac output is 5 L/min. In many forms of heart disease the cardiac output may be lower than normal. In that situation, the total body oxygen consumption does not change significantly; however, a greater percentage of O_2 is extracted per volume of circulating blood by the metabolizing tissues because of the decreased perfusion pressure. This leads to a lower than normal venous O_2 content and, therefore, an *increased* arteriovenous O_2 difference. So in the example described here, if the venous blood contains only 100 ml O_2/L, the arteriovenous O_2 difference is increased to 90 ml O_2/L, and the calculated cardiac output is reduced to 2.2 L/min.

Calculation of Vascular Resistances

Once pressures and cardiac output have been determined, pulmonary and systemic vascular resistances can be calculated from the following formulas:

$$PVR = \frac{MPAP - LAP}{CO} \times 80$$

PVR, pulmonary vascular resistance (dynes-sec-cm^{-5})
MPAP, mean pulmonary artery pressure (mm Hg)
LAP, mean left atrial pressure (mm Hg)
CO, cardiac output (L/min)

$$SVR = \frac{MAP - RAP}{CO} \times 80$$

SVR, systemic vascular resistance (dynes-sec-cm^{-5})
MAP, mean arterial pressure (mm Hg)
RAP, mean right atrial pressure (mm Hg)
CO, cardiac output (L/min)

Contrast Angiography

This technique, performed at the time of catheterization, uses radiopaque contrast material to visualize regions of the cardiovascular system. A catheter is introduced into an appropriate vessel and guided under fluoroscopy to the site where the contrast will be injected. Following administration of the contrast agent, x-rays are transmitted through the area of interest. A single exposure produces one film image, whereas a series of x-ray exposures are recorded to produce a "motion picture," termed a cineangiogram.

Selective injection of contrast material into the heart chambers is used to recognize valvular insufficiency, abnormal wall thickening, intracardiac shunts, thrombi within the heart, congenital malformations and to measure ventricular contractile function. To image the right heart chambers, injection is made through a catheter inserted into the inferior or superior vena cava, the right atrium, or the right ventricle. The left side of the heart can be imaged by contrast injection through a catheter advanced into the left ventricle (Fig. 3.15). Contrast injection into the coronary arteries is used to examine the location and severity of coronary atherosclerotic lesions (Figs. 3.16, 3.17).

A specialized type of contrast angiography, termed digital subtraction angiography (DSA), was developed to provide a clear image using less contrast material. In this technique, a computer processes the digitalized x-ray images and subtracts the background of soft tissue and bone, thus enhancing the image of the blood vessel or chamber into which contrast material was injected. DSA has certain advantages over conventional angiography: the techniques used to introduce contrast may be less invasive (e.g., use of smaller catheters) than those for conventional angiography, a lower concentration of contrast agent can be used, and greater image resolution may be achieved.

There is some risk associated with catheterization and contrast angiography. Complications are uncommon, but include myocardial perforation by the catheter, precipitation of arrhythmias and conduction

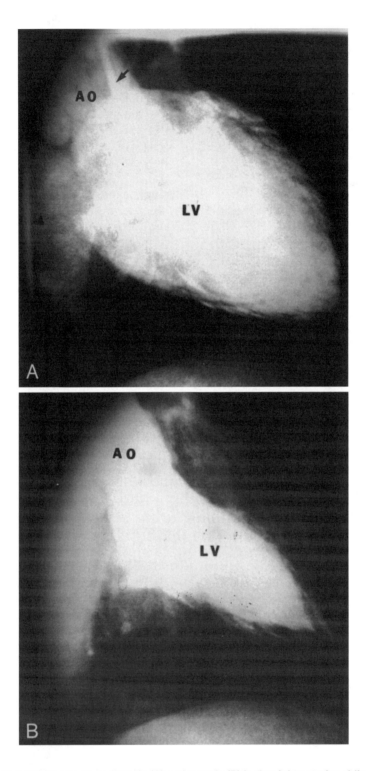

Figure 3.15.   Left ventriculograms in diastole (A) and systole (B) in the right anterior oblique projection from a patient with normal ventricular contractility. This view depicts movement of the anterior apical and inferior walls. A catheter (arrow) is used to inject contrast into the left ventricle (LV). The catheter can also be seen in the descending aorta (arrowhead). AO, aortic root. (Courtesy of John Bittl, MD, Brigham and Women's Hospital, Boston, MA)

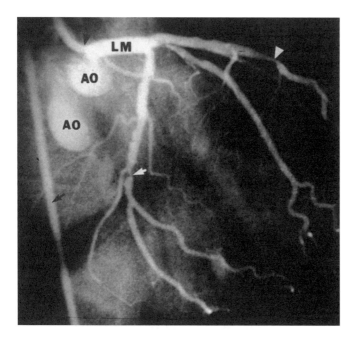

Figure 3.16. Left coronary artery angiogram in the right anterior oblique projection from a patient with diffuse coronary artery disease. The tip of the catheter (black arrowhead) is in the ostium of the left main (LM) coronary artery. The more distal catheter (black arrow) is seen within the descending aorta. The most critical stenoses are present in the left anterior descending (white arrowhead) and at the origin (white arrow) of the third obtuse marginal branch of the left circumflex coronary artery. Some contrast can also be visualized in two of the aortic sinuses (*AO*) just above the aortic valve. (Courtesy of John Bittl, MD, Brigham and Women's Hospital, Boston, MA)

blocks, damage to vessel walls, dislodgement of atherosclerotic plaques and infection. Complications resulting from the contrast medium itself include potential anaphylactic reactions or renal toxic effects.

Table 3.4 summarizes the catheterization findings in common cardiac abnormalities. Therapeutic interventional catheterization techniques, such as percutaneous translu-

minal coronary angioplasty, are discussed in Chapter 6.

NUCLEAR IMAGING

Heart function can be evaluated using injected radioactively labeled tracers and gamma-camera detectors. The resulting im-

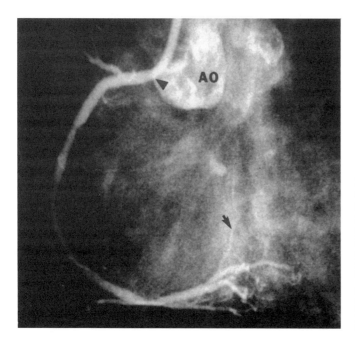

Figure 3.17. Right coronary artery angiogram in the left anterior oblique projection visualized with contrast injected by a catheter (arrowhead) positioned in the ostium of the dominant right coronary artery. Multiple areas of irregularities and stenosis can be seen. The AV nodal artery branches from the right coronary artery (arrow). AO, aorta. (Courtesy of John Bittl, MD, Brigham and Women's Hospital, Boston, MA)

TABLE 3.4. Cardiac Catheterization and Angiography in Cardiac Disorders

Coronary artery disease	• Identification of atherosclerotic lesions
Mitral regurgitation	• Large systolic v wave in left atrial pressure tracing
Mitral stenosis	• Abnormally high pressure gradient between left atrium and left ventricle in diastole
Tricuspid insufficiency	• Large systolic v wave in the right atrial pressure tracing
Aortic stenosis	• Systolic pressure gradient between left ventricle and aorta
Congestive heart failure	• Estimation of cardiac output
	• Calculation of systemic and pulmonary vascular resistances

ages reflect the distribution of the tracers within the cardiovascular system. Nuclear techniques are used to assess myocardial perfusion, to image blood passing through the heart and great vessels, to localize and quantify myocardial ischemia and infarction, and to assess myocardial metabolism.

Assessment of Myocardial Perfusion

Ischemia and infarction resulting from coronary artery disease can be detected by myocardial perfusion imaging using either of two radioisotopes: thallium-201 (Tl-201) or sestamibi (a synthetic complex of the isonitrile family that is abbreviated MIBI) labeled with technetium 99m (Tc-99m). These agents are equally sensitive in detecting areas of ischemic or scarred myocardium. However, each has certain advantages. For example, MIBI provides better image quality and is superior for detailed SPECT (single photon emission computed tomography) imaging. On the other hand, detection of myocardial cellular viability has been best documented by Tl-201 imaging.

In the case of thallium-201 imaging, the radioisotope is injected intravenously while a patient is exercising on a treadmill or stationary bicycle. Because thallium is a potassium analogue, it enters into normal myocytes, a process thought to be partially governed by the sodium-potassium ATPase pump. The intracellular concentration of thallium, estimated by the density of the image, depends on vascular supply (perfusion) and membrane function (tissue viability). In the normal heart, the radionuclide

scan shows a homogenous distribution of thallium in the myocardial tissue. Conversely, myocardial regions that are scarred (by previous infarction) or have transiently reduced perfusion with exercise (i.e., myocardial ischemia) do not accumulate as much thallium as normal tissue. Consequently, these areas will appear on the thallium scan as light, or "cold" spots.

When evaluating for myocardial ischemia, an initial set of images is taken right after exercise and thallium injection. Delayed images are acquired several hours later, because thallium accumulation does not remain fixed in myocytes. Rather, there is continuous redistribution of the isotope across the cell membrane. After 3 to 4 hours of redistribution, when additional images are obtained, all viable myocytes should have equal concentrations of thallium. Consequently, any defects due to myocardial *ischemia* on the initial postexercise scan will fill in on the delayed scan (and are therefore termed "reversible" defects), while those representing *infarcted* or scarred myocardium will persist as "cold" spots.

Of note, some myocardial segments that demonstrate persistent Tl-201 defects on both stress and redistribution imaging are falsely characterized as nonviable, scarred tissue. Sometimes, these areas represent ischemic, noncontractile but metabolically active areas that have the potential to regain function if blood flow is restored. For example, such areas may represent *hibernating* myocardium, segments that demonstrate diminished contractile function due to chronic reduction of coronary blood flow. This viable state can be differentiated from irreversibly scarred myocardium by repeat imaging after the injection of additional thallium-201 at rest, to enhance uptake by viable cells (Fig. 3.18).

MIBI, labeled with Tc-99m, is a large lipophilic molecule that, like thallium, is taken up in the myocardium in proportion to blood flow. The uptake mechanism differs in that the complex passes the myocyte membrane passively, driven by the negative membrane potential. Once intracellular, it further accumulates in the mitochondria, driven by the even more negative mitochondrial membrane potential. The myocardial distribution of MIBI reflects perfusion at the moment of injection and in distinction to thallium, it remains fixed intracellularly. Consequently, obtaining the MIBI imaging can be more convenient: Stress injection and imaging can be performed one day and rest injection and imaging the next. Alternatively, MIBI imaging can be undertaken as a one-day protocol in which an injection and imaging are performed at rest, using a small tracer dose, followed a couple of hours later by injection

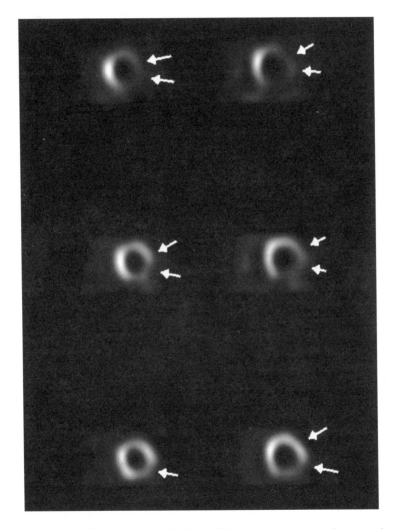

Figure 3.18. Myocardial viability study using Thallium-201. Images have been taken at peak stress (**upper panels**), early after re-injection of thallium (**middle panels**), and at four hours (delayed) after re-injection (**lower panels**). The left and right sided tomographic images are at the midventricular and basal ventricular levels, respectively. The stress images show decreased perfusion of the lateral wall (arrows). Both sets of re-injection images, which represent perfusion at rest, show improved (but not normal) uptake in the lateral wall. Note that the defect has filled in to a greater degree on the delayed, compared to the early re-injection images. This indicates that a portion of the lateral wall is irreversibly infarcted, but that there is also a component of reversible ischemia in the adjacent territory. (Courtesy of Finn Mannting, MD, Brigham and Women's Hospital, Boston, MA)

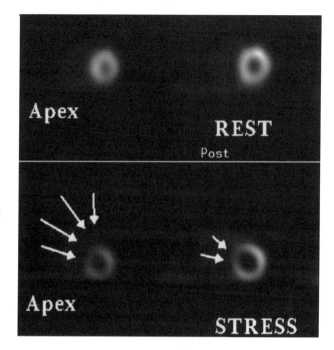

Figure 3.19. SPECT myocardial perfusion study using Tc-99m MIBI. Rest images (**upper panels**) and stress images (**lower panels**) are displayed for apical (**left panels**) and midventricular (**right panels**) tomographic views. There is uniform tracer uptake at rest. In the stress images, the arrows depict markedly reduced uptake in the apex, septum, and anterior wall. This study is consistent with moderately severe ischemia in the territory supplied by the left anterior descending coronary artery. (Courtesy of Finn Mannting, MD, Brigham and Women's Hospital, Boston, MA)

and imaging after exercise using a larger tracer dose (Fig. 3.19).

Exercise scintigraphic studies with either thallium-201 or Tc-99m MIBI have greater sensitivity and specificity (but are more expensive) than standard exercise electrocardiography for detecting ischemia due to coronary artery disease. Thus, nuclear exercise imaging is reserved for situations in which the exercise EKG results are either ambiguous or impossible to interpret because of an underlying EKG abnormality.

Blood Pool Imaging

Technetium-99m is an isotope used to image blood flow. To keep the radioactive tracer in the vascular system, it is usually first bound to red blood cells or to human serum albumin prior to injection. The technetium, administered as a bolus, is imaged at fixed times as the material passes through the heart and great vessels. Multiple images are displayed sequentially to produce a dynamic picture of blood flow.

Blood pool imaging is used to analyze right and left ventricular contractile function (Fig. 3.20). Calculations, such as determination of the ejection fraction, are based on the

difference between radioactive counts present in the ventricle at end-diastole and at end-systole. Therefore, measurements are largely independent of any assumptions of ventricular geometry. In addition, first-pass imaging and scans gated to the electrocardiogram permit recognition of abnormal cardiac and vascular shunts.

Assessment of Tissue Damage After Acute Myocardial Infarction

Technetium-99m bound to pyrophosphate preferentially binds to injured or necrotic myocardial cells, and areas of recent infarction will appear as bright or "hot" spots. Scans using this agent, to assist in the diagnosis of an acute MI, are best performed 24 to 72 hours after an infarction has occurred, because this is the time during which calcium, which binds pyrophosphate, is deposited in irreversibly damaged cells. After 4 to 5 days, the calcium is reabsorbed as scar tissue is formed; thereafter, no technetium will bind. This technique may be useful when detection of acute myocardial infarction using more traditional methods (EKG and cardiac enzymes, as described in Chapter 7) is inconclusive.

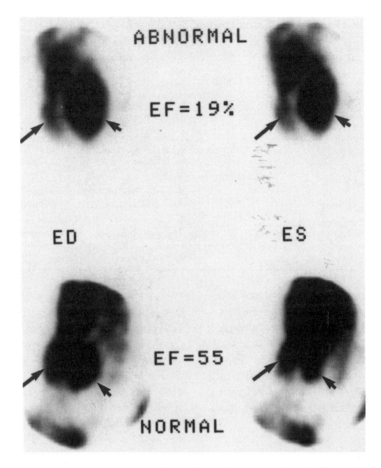

Figure 3.20.   Gated blood pool scans in the left anterior oblique projection in diastole (left panels) and systole (right panels) from a patient with ischemic cardiomyopathy (top panels) and from a normal individual (lower panels). The patient with ischemic cardiomyopathy has a dilated left ventricle (short black arrows) with globally reduced contraction. The right ventricle (long black arrows) is normal in size, but its contraction is also diminished. Normal contraction of the right ventricle (long black arrows) and the left ventricle (short black arrows) is evident in the normal subject. EF, ejection fraction; ED, end diastole; ES, end systole. (Courtesy of Jeff Kemp, Faulkner Hospital, Boston, MA)

Assessment of Myocardial Metabolism

Positron emission tomography (PET) is a technique used to measure cellular metabolism and regional myocardial blood flow *in vivo*. This technique involves incorporating positron-emitting isotopes (e.g., oxygen-15, carbon-11, nitrogen-13 or fluorine-18) into a metabolic tracer and using a sensitive positron camera to detect the tracer. To study glucose utilization in myocardial tissue, fluorine-18 is substituted for hydrogen in 2-deoxyglucose to produce fluoro-18 deoxyglucose, also known as [18]FDG. This substance competes with glucose both for transport into myocytes and for subsequent phosphorylation. Unlike glucose, however, [18]FDG is not metabolized further and becomes trapped within the cell. In normal myocardial metabolism, glucose is utilized for only 20% of energy production while free fatty acids provide the remaining 80%. In ischemic conditions, however, metabolism shifts toward glucose use, and the more ischemic the myocardial tissue, the stronger is the reliance on glucose. Thus, the amount of [18]FDG uptake provides a means of identifying ischemic, but viable, tissue.

To image blood flow, nitrogen 13-labeled ammonia, a potassium analogue, is used. By using both nitrogen 13-labeled ammonia and [18]FDG to evaluate regional blood flow and glucose uptake, respec-

TABLE 3.5. Nuclear Imaging in Cardiac Disorders

Myocardial Ischemia:
Stress-delayed-re-injection T1-201

- Low uptake during stress with complete or partial fill-in with delayed or re-injection images

Rest-stress sestamibi
- Normal uptake at rest with decreased uptake during stress

PET (N-13 ammonia/^{18}FDG)
- Decreased flow with normal or increased ^{18}FDG uptake during stress

Myocardial Infarction:
Stress-delayed-re-injection T1-201
- Low uptake during stress and low uptake after re-injection

Rest-stress sestamibi
- Low uptake in rest and stress images

PET (N-13 ammonia/^{18}FDG)
- Decreased flow and decreased ^{18}FDG uptake at rest

"Hibernating" Myocardium:
Rest-delayed T1-201
- Complete or partial fill-in of defects after re-injection

PET (N-13 ammonia/^{18}FDG)
- Decreased flow and increased ^{18}FDG uptake at rest

Assessment of Ventricular Function:
Tc-99m RBC gated blood pool imaging
- Assessment of global left and right ventricular function at rest or during exercise
- Regional wall motion and function

tively, PET scanning helps determine whether areas of decreased flow and contractile dysfunction represent scar tissue or whether the region is still viable (e.g., "hibernating" myocardium). In scar tissue, both blood flow to the affected area and ^{18}FDG uptake are decreased. Hibernating myocardium, in contrast, shows decreased blood flow but normal or elevated ^{18}FDG uptake. PET imaging is limited by the short half-life of the isotopes, necessitating production by a nearby linear accelerator, as well as by its expense.

Table 3.5 summarizes the findings of common cardiac conditions by nuclear imaging.

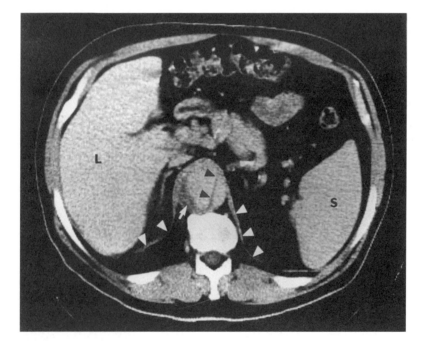

Figure 3.21. Abdominal CT scan from a patient with dissecting aortic aneurysm. Contrast has been injected into the vascular system and delineates the intimal flap (black arrowheads), which separates the opacified true and false lumens of the descending aorta. The nonopacified area in one lumen may represent a thrombus (white arrow). L, liver; S, spleen; white arrowheads, crura of the diaphragm.

COMPUTED TOMOGRAPHY

Computed tomography (CT) uses x-rays to produce a planar image of the heart. The standard CT technique is especially useful in assessing pericardial and aortic disease (Fig. 3.21). CT clearly delineates loculated pericardial effusions and pericardial thickening, which are often inadequately visualized by echocardiography. CT studies are useful in the diagnosis of aortic dissections and aneurysms and can be used to monitor patients who have had prior surgical treatment of these conditions. Newer modifications of cardiac CT include faster acquisition times, in an attempt to overcome the problem of cardiac motion that has limited the usefulness of this technique in imaging other cardiac structures.

MAGNETIC RESONANCE IMAGING (MRI)

This diagnostic tool uses a powerful magnetic field to obtain detailed images of internal structures. MRI provides extremely

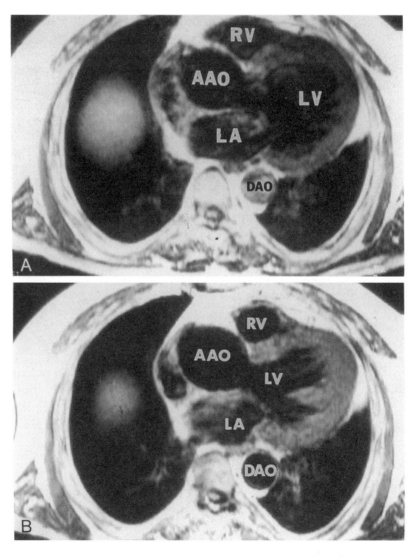

Figure 3.22. Transverse MRI images of the heart in diastole (A) and systole (B) from a normal individual. Clearly seen are the left ventricle (LV), right ventricle (RV), left atrium (LA), ascending aorta (AAO), and descending aorta (DAO). (Courtesy of Warren Manning, MD, Beth Israel Deaconess Hospital, Boston, MA)

detailed images of soft tissues and can be used to image a variety of cardiac abnormalities because vessels and heart chambers are clearly outlined (Fig. 3.22). Since MRI has the advantage of providing tomographic images in any plane without the use of ionized radiation, its use as a noninvasive technique is rapidly expanding. Cardiac MRI already has an established role in the assessment of congenital abnormalities and diseases of the aorta, including aneurysms and dissection. It is also used to assess intravascular thrombus, tumors and pericardial disease. Recent developments in MRI imaging include measurement of blood flow and of cardiac chamber volumes and ventricular mass. The clinical role of this technology in imaging the cardiovascular system is still relatively new and continues to be defined.

SUMMARY

This chapter has provided an overview of imaging and catheterization techniques that are available to assess cardiac structure and function. Many of these tools are expensive and yield similar information. However, when used in the appropriate settings, they provide a wealth of information to guide diagnosis and management of cardiovascular disorders. Tables 3.1 through 3.5 summarize the most common uses and findings.

ADDITIONAL READING

Baim D, Grossman W. Cardiac Catheterization, Angiography and Intervention. 5th ed. Baltimore: Williams & Wilkins, 1996.

Daniel WG, Mügge A. Medical progress: transesophageal echocardiography. New Engl J Med 1995;332:1268–1279.

Jain D, Zaret BL. Nuclear imaging techniques for the assessment of myocardial viability. Cardiology Clinics 1995;13:43–56.

Nishimura R, Miller FA, Callahan MJ, et al. Doppler echocardiography: theory, instrumentation, technique, and application. Mayo Clin Proc 1985;60:321–343.

Pennell DJ, Underwood R. Magnetic resonance imaging of the heart. Br J Hosp Med 1993;49:90–95, 98–102.

Popp R. Echocardiography. N Engl J Med 1990;323:101–109,165–172.

Ritchie JL, Bateman TM, Bonow RO, et al. Guidelines for clinical use of cardiac radionuclide imaging. Report of the American College of Cardiology/American Heart Association Task Force on Assessment of Diagnostic and Therapeutic Cardiovascular Procedures (Committee on Radionuclide Imaging). J Am Coll Cardiol 1995;25:521–547.

Seward JB, Khanderia BK, Freeman WK, et al. Multiplane transesophageal echocardiography: image orientation, examination technique, anatomic correlations, and clinical applications. Mayo Clinic Proceedings 1993;68: 523–551.

Skorton DJ, Schelbert HR, Wolf GL, Brundage BH, eds. Cardiac imaging: a companion to Braunwald's Heart Disease. 2nd ed. Philadelphia: WB Saunders, 1996.

Weyman AE. Principles and Practice of Echocardiography. 2nd ed. Baltimore: Williams & Wilkins, 1993.

Zaret BL, Wackers FJ. Medical progress: nuclear cardiology. N Eng J Med 1993;329:775–783,855–863.

Acknowledgments   The authors are grateful to Dr. Finn Mannting for his helpful suggestions during the preparation of this chapter. The previous edition of this chapter was written by Deborah Buccino, MD, Albert S. Tu, MD, and Patricia C. Come, MD.

The Electrocardiogram

Kyle Low, Price Kerfoot, and Leonard S. Lilly

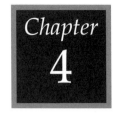

Chapter

4

Cardiac contraction relies on the organized flow of electrical impulses through the heart. The electrocardiogram (EKG or ECG) is an easily obtained recording of that activity, and provides a wealth of information about cardiac structure and function. This chapter presents the electrical basis of the EKG in health and disease, and will lead you through the basics of interpretation. To become fully adept at this technique, and to practice the principles described here, please also consult one of the complete electrocardiographic textbooks listed at the end of the chapter.

ELECTRICAL MEASUREMENT— SINGLE CELL MODEL

We begin by observing the propagation of an electrical impulse within a single cardiac muscle cell, illustrated in Figure 4.1. On the right side of the diagram, a voltmeter records the electrical potential across the cell, on graph paper. In the resting state, the cell is *polarized:* The entire outside of the cell is electrically positive with respect to the inside, because of the ionic distribution across the cell membrane. In this resting state, the voltmeter electrodes, which are placed on opposite *outside* surfaces of the cell, do not detect any electrical activity, because there is no electrical potential difference between them (the myocyte surface is homogeneously charged).

This equilibrium is disturbed, however,

by stimulation of the cell (Fig. 4.1B). During the action potential, as cations rush across the sarcolemma into the cell, the polarity at the stimulated region transiently reverses, such that the outside becomes negatively charged with respect to the inside; that is, the region **depolarizes.** At that moment, an electrical potential is created on the cell surface between the depolarized area (negatively charged surface), and the still polarized (positively charged surface) portions of the cell. An electrical current is therefore caused to flow between these two regions.

By convention, the direction of electrical current is said to flow *from* the negatively charged *to* the positively charged areas. Because the depolarization current in this example proceeds from left to right, that is, toward the (+) electrode of the voltmeter, an upward deflection is recorded. As the wave of depolarization spreads along the cell, additional electrical forces directed toward the (+) electrode record even a greater upward deflection (Fig. 4.1C). Once the cell has become fully depolarized (Fig. 4.1D), its outside is completely negatively charged with respect to the inside, the opposite of the initial resting condition. However, since the surface charge is homogeneous once again, the electrodes measure a potential difference of zero and the voltmeter records a neutral "flat line" during this period.

Note that in Figure 4.1E, if the electrode wires of the voltmeter had been reversed so that the (+) pole was placed to the *left* of the cell, then as the wave of depolarization pro-

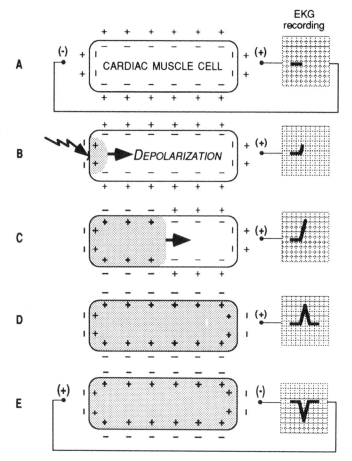

Figure 4.1. **Depolarization of a single cardiac muscle cell. A.** In the resting state, the surface of the cell is positively charged relative to the inside. Because the surface is homogeneously charged, the voltmeter electrodes outside of the cell do not record any electrical potential difference ("flat line" recording). **B.** Stimulation of the cell initiates depolarization (shaded area); the outside of the depolarized region becomes negatively charged relative to the inside. Because the current of depolarization is directed toward the (+) electrode of the voltmeter, an upward deflection is recorded. **C.** Depolarization spreads, creating a greater upward deflection by the recording electrode. **D.** The cell has become fully depolarized. The surface of the cell is now completely negatively charged compared with the inside. Because the surface is again homogeneously charged, a flat line is recorded by the voltmeter. **E.** Note that if the position of the voltmeter electrodes had been reversed, the wave of depolarization would have traveled away from the (+) electrode so that the EKG deflection would be downward.

ceeded toward the right, it would have headed *away* from the (+) electrode and the recorded deflection would have been *downward.* Please keep this relationship in mind when we discuss the polarity of EKG leads below.

Depolarization of the cell initiates cardiac muscle contraction, and is then followed by **repolarization,** the process by which the cellular charges return to the resting state (Fig. 4.2). As the left side of the cell begins to repolarize, its surface charge becomes positive once again. A current is therefore generated from the still negatively charged surface toward the positively charged area. Because this current is directed away from the voltmeter's (+) electrode, a downward deflection is recorded, opposite to that which was observed during the process of depolarization. Repolarization is a slower process than depolarization, so that the inscribed deflection of repolar-

ization is wider and of lower magnitude. Once the cell has returned to the resting state, the surface charges are once again homogeneous, and no further electrical potential is detected, resulting in a "flat line" on the voltmeter recording (Fig. 4.2C).

In the intact human heart, repolarization actually proceeds in the direction *opposite* that of depolarization, beginning at the *last* region to be depolarized (the reason for this is not known). Therefore, the deflection of repolarization is usually the inverse of what was presented in this example. That is, the current of repolarization (negative to positive flow) in Figure 4.2 would be directed *toward* the (+) electrode and would therefore inscribe an *upright* deflection on the recording. Thus, in a normal individual, the forces of depolarization and repolarization are usually oriented in the *same* direction on the EKG recording (Fig. 4–2D).

We have considered the depolarization

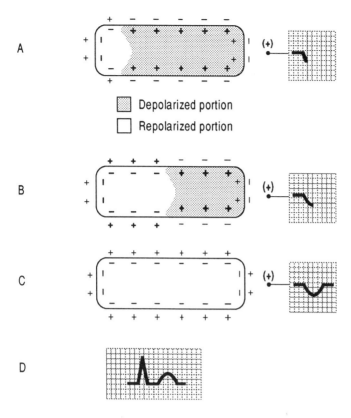

A
☒ Depolarized portion
☐ Repolarized portion

B

C

D

Figure 4.2. Sequence of repolarization of a single cardiac muscle cell.
A. As repolarization commences, positive charges re-emerge on the surface of the cell, and a current flows from the still negatively charged surface areas to the repolarized region. Because the current is directed away from the (+) electrode of the voltmeter, a downward deflection is recorded. **B.** Repolarization progresses. **C.** Repolarization has been completed and the outside surface of the cell is once again homogeneously charged, so that no further electrical potential is detected ("flat line" once again). **D.** In the human heart, repolarization proceeds in a direction *opposite* that of depolarization (would be from right to left in this example, and the wave of repolarization would be upright). Therefore, the *deflections of depolarization and repolarization of the normal intact heart are in the same direction,* as shown here. Note that the wave of repolarization is of lower amplitude, and more prolonged than that of depolarization.

and repolarization of a single cardiac muscle cell. As the wave of depolarization spreads rapidly through the heart, electrical forces are generated by each cell, and it is the sum of these forces, measured at the skin's surface, that is recorded by the EKG machine. The direction and magnitude of the deflections on the EKG recording depend on how the electrical forces are aligned to a set of specific reference axes, known as EKG leads.

EKG LEAD REFERENCE SYSTEM

When the EKG was first invented, the recording was made by dunking the patient's arms and legs into large buckets of electrolyte solution that were wired to the machine. As you can imagine, that was fairly messy, and fortunately is no longer necessary. Instead, wire electrodes are placed directly on the skin, in the arrangement shown in Figure 4.3. The right leg electrode is not used for measurement, but serves as an electrical ground.

The complete EKG tracing is formed by recording the electrical forces between standard positions of the skin electrodes. Figure 4.4 demonstrates the orientation of the six standard reference axes (termed EKG leads), which are electronically constructed by recording between the wire electrodes on the arms and left leg.

The EKG machine records lead aV_R by selecting the *r*ight arm electrode as the (+) pole with respect to the other electrodes. This is known as a **unipolar** lead, because there is no single (−) pole; rather, all of the other electrodes are averaged together to create a composite (−) reference. When the instantaneous electrical activity of the heart points in the direction of the right arm, an upward deflection is recorded in lead aV_R. However, when the electrical forces are heading away from the right arm, the EKG inscribes a downward deflection in aV_R.

Similarly, lead aV_F is recorded by setting the left leg as the (+) pole, such that a positive deflection is recorded when forces are directed toward the *f*eet. aV_L is selected when the *l*eft arm electrode is made the (+)

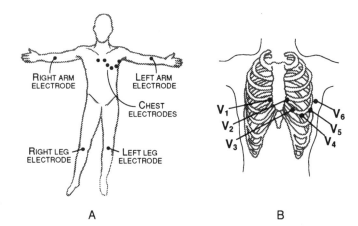

Figure 4.3. A. Standard positions of the EKG electrodes. **B.** Close-up view of chest electrode placement.

A   B

pole, and records an upward deflection when electrical activity is aimed in that direction.

In addition to these three unipolar limb leads, three **bipolar** leads are also part of the standard EKG recording (Fig. 4.4). Bipolar indicates that one limb electrode is the (+) pole and another *single* electrode provides the (−) reference. In this case, the EKG machine inscribes an upward deflection if elec-

Unipolar Limb Leads

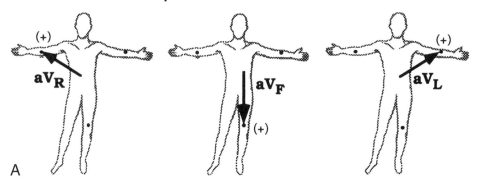

A

Bipolar Limb Leads

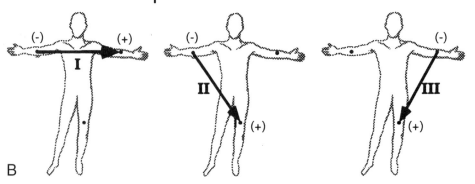

B

Figure 4.4. The six limb leads are formed from the electrodes placed on the arms and left leg. Each unipolar lead has a (+) designated electrode (for the unipolar leads, the (−) pole is an average of the other electrodes). Each bipolar lead has specific (−) and (+) designated electrodes.

trical forces are heading toward the (+) electrode, and records a downward deflection if the forces are heading toward the (−) electrode. A simple mnemonic to remember the placement of the bipolar leads is that the lead number indicates the number of L's in the placement sites. For example, lead III connects the *left* arm to the *left leg*, lead II connects the right arm to the *left leg*, and lead I connects the *left* arm to the right arm. Table 4.1 lists how the six limb leads are derived.

By overlaying the six limb leads together, a reference system is established (Fig. 4.5). In this figure, each lead is presented with its (+) pole designated by an arrowhead, and the (−) aspect by dashed lines. Note that each 30° sector of the circle falls along the (+) or (−) pole of one of the standard six electrocardiographic leads. Also note that the (+) pole of lead I points to 0° and that, by convention, measurement of the angles proceeds clockwise as +30°, +60°, etc. (This direction of measurement irks students of mathematics, but it is a tradition.) The complete EKG recording provides a simultaneous "snapshot" of the heart's electrical activity, taken from the perspective of each of these lead reference lines.

Figure 4.6 demonstrates how the magnitude and direction of electrical activity are represented by the EKG recording in each lead. Please study Figure 4.6 until the following four points are clear:

1. An electrical force directed toward the (+) pole of a lead results in an upward deflection on the EKG recording of that lead.

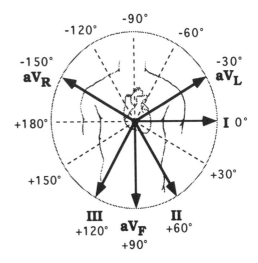

Figure 4.5. The axial reference system is created by combining together the leads shown in Figure 4.4. Each lead has a (+) region indicated by the arrowhead, and a (−) region indicated by the dashed line.

2. Forces that head away from the (+) electrode result in a downward deflection in that lead.
3. The magnitude of the deflection, either upward or downward, reflects how parallel the electrical force is to the axis of the lead being examined. The more parallel the electrical force is to the lead, the greater the magnitude of the deflection.
4. An electrical force directed perpendicular to an electrocardiographic lead does not register *any* activity by that lead (a "flat line" on the recording).

The six standard limb leads examine the electrical forces in the frontal plane of the body. However, since electrical activity travels in three dimensions, recordings from a perpendicular plane (Fig. 4.7A) are also essential. This is accomplished by the use of six electrodes placed on the anterior and left lateral aspect of the chest (Fig. 4.3B), creating the **chest** (or **precordial**) leads. The orientation of these leads around the heart is shown in Figure 4.7B. These are unipolar leads, and, as with the unipolar limb leads, electrical forces that are directed *toward* these individual (+) electrodes result in an upward deflection on the recording of that lead; forces heading *away* record a downward deflection.

TABLE 4.1. The Limb Leads

	(+) electrode	(−) electrode
Bipolar leads		
I	LA	RA
II	LL	RA
III	LL	LA
Unipolar leads		
aVR	RA	*
aVL	LA	*
aVF	LL	*

LA, left arm; LL, left leg; RA, right arm; *, (−) electrode constructed by combining all other electrodes together.

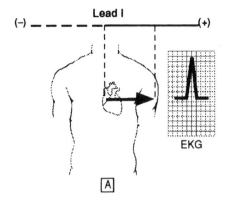

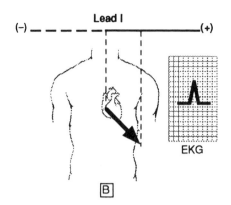

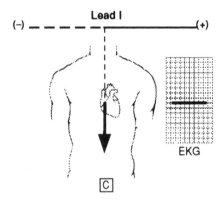

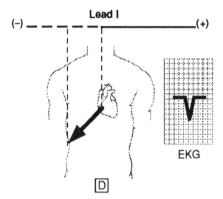

Figure 4.6. Relationship of the magnitude and direction of electrical activity to the EKG lead. A. The electrical vector is oriented parallel to lead I and aimed toward the (+) electrode; therefore, a tall, upward deflection is recorded by the lead. **B.** The vector is still oriented toward the (+) region of lead I, but not *parallel* to the lead so that only a component of the force is recorded. The recorded deflection is still upward, but less tall compared with **A. C.** The electrical vector is perpendicular to lead I so that no deflection is generated. **D.** The vector is directed toward the (−) region of lead I so that a downward deflection is recorded by the EKG.

The standard complete electrocardiogram prints samples from each of the six limb leads and each of the six chest leads, examples of which are presented later in this chapter.

SEQUENCE OF NORMAL CARDIAC ACTIVATION

Electrical conduction through the heart is an orderly process. The normal beat begins at the sinoatrial node at the junction of the right atrium and the superior vena cava (Fig. 4.8). The wave of depolarization rapidly spreads through the right and left atria and then reaches the AV node, where it encounters an expected delay. The impulse then travels rapidly through the bundle of His, and into the right and left bundle branches. These divide into the Purkinje fibers, which radiate toward the myocardial fibers, stimulating them to contract.

Each heart beat is represented on the EKG by three major deflections that record the sequence of electrical propagation (Fig. 4.8). The **P wave** represents depolarization of the atria. Following the P wave, the tracing returns to the flat baseline, due to the conduction delay at the AV node. The second deflection of the EKG, the **QRS complex,** represents depolarization of the ven-

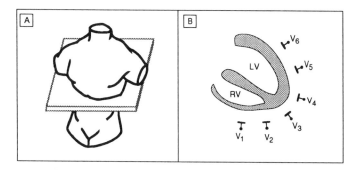

Figure 4.7. The chest (precordial) leads. A. The cross-sectional plane of the chest. **B.** Arrangement of the six chest electrodes shown in the cross-sectional plane.

tricular muscle cells. After the QRS complex, the tracing returns to baseline once again, and after a brief delay, repolarization of the ventricular cells is signaled by the **T wave.** Occasionally, an additional small deflection follows the T wave (the **U wave**), which is believed to represent late phases of ventricular repolarization.

The QRS complex may take one of several shapes, but can always be subdivided into individual components (Fig. 4.9). If the first deflection of a QRS complex is downward, it is known as a Q wave. However, if the initial deflection is upward, then that particular complex does *not* have a Q wave. The R wave is defined as the first upward deflection, whether or not a Q wave is present. Any downward deflection following the R wave is known as the S wave. Figure 4.9 demonstrates several variations of the QRS complex. In certain pathologic states, such as bundle branch blocks, additional deflections may be inscribed, as shown in the figure. Please study Figure 4.9 until you can confidently differentiate a Q from an S wave.

Let's now follow the course of normal

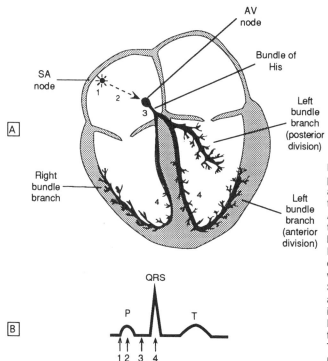

Figure 4.8. Cardiac conduction pathway. A. The electrical impulse begins at the sinoatrial (SA) node (1) then traverses the atria (2). After a delay at the AV node (3), conduction continues through the bundle of His and into the right and left bundle branches (4). The latter divide into Purkinje fibers, which stimulate contraction of the myocardial cells. **B.** Corresponding waveforms on the EKG recording: (1) The SA node discharges (too small to generate any deflection on EKG); (2) P wave inscribed by depolarization of the atria; (3) Delay at the AV node; (4) Depolarization of the ventricles generates the QRS complex. The T wave represents ventricular repolarization.

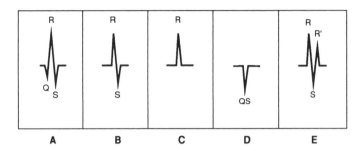

Figure 4.9. Examples of QRS complexes. A. The first deflection is downward (Q wave), followed by an upward deflection (R wave), and then another downward wave (S wave). **B.** Because the first deflection is upward, this complex does *not* have a Q wave; rather the downward deflection *after* the R is an S wave. **C.** A QRS complex without downward deflections lacks Q and S waves. **D.** QRS composed of only a downward deflection; this is a Q wave, but is often referred to as a QS complex. **E.** A second upward deflection (seen in bundle branch blocks) is labeled R'.

ventricular depolarization, and observe how it is recorded by two of the EKG leads, aV_F and aV_L (Fig. 4.10). In the resting state, the surface of the myocardial cells is positively charged compared with the inside, and the EKG leads record zero voltage, as electrical forces in any region are canceled by equal and opposite forces.

The initial portion of ventricular myocardium to depolarize is the mid portion of the interventricular septum, on the left side. Because depolarization reverses the cellular charge, the surface of that region becomes negative with respect to the inside, and an electrical current is generated (arrow). This initial force heads away from the left ventricle, toward the right ventricle. Because the force is heading *away* from the (+) pole region of lead aV_L, an initial *downward* deflection is recorded in that lead. At the same time, forces are heading *in* the direction of the (+) pole region of lead aV_F, so that an initial *upward* deflection is recorded there. As the wave of depolarization spreads through the myocardium, the sequence of net electrical charge is depicted by the series of arrows in Figure 4.10.

As the lateral walls of the ventricles are depolarized, the forces of the thicker left side start outweighing those of the right. Therefore, the arrow swings further and further toward the left ventricle (leftward and posteriorly). At the completion of depolarization, no further net electrical force is generated, and the EKG recording returns to baseline in both leads. Thus, in this ex-

ample of a normal heart, lead aV_L inscribes an initial small Q wave, followed by a tall R wave, whereas in lead aV_F, there is an initial upward deflection (R wave) followed by a downward S wave.

We can also record the sequence of depolarization in the cross-sectional plane of the body by studying the six chest leads (Fig. 4.11). Once again, recall that the first region to depolarize is the left ventricular aspect of the interventricular septum. The sequence of depolarization proceeds from the midventricular septum toward the anteriorly placed right ventricle, then toward the cardiac apex, and then around to the lateral walls of both ventricles. Because the initial forces are directed anteriorly—that is, toward the (+) pole of V_1—the initial deflection recorded by lead V_1 is upward. Since the same initial forces are heading *away* from V_6, an initial downward deflection is recorded there. As the wave of depolarization spreads, the forces of the left ventricle outweigh those of the right, and the vector swings posteriorly toward the bulk of the left ventricular muscle. As the forces swing *away* from lead V_1, the deflection there becomes *downward*, whereas it becomes more *upright* in lead V_6. Leads V_2 through V_5 record intermediate steps in this process, such that the R wave becomes progressively taller from lead V_1 through lead V_6 (Fig. 4.11E). Typically, the height of the R wave becomes greater than the depth of the S wave in lead V_3 or V_4; the lead in which this occurs is termed the "transition" lead.

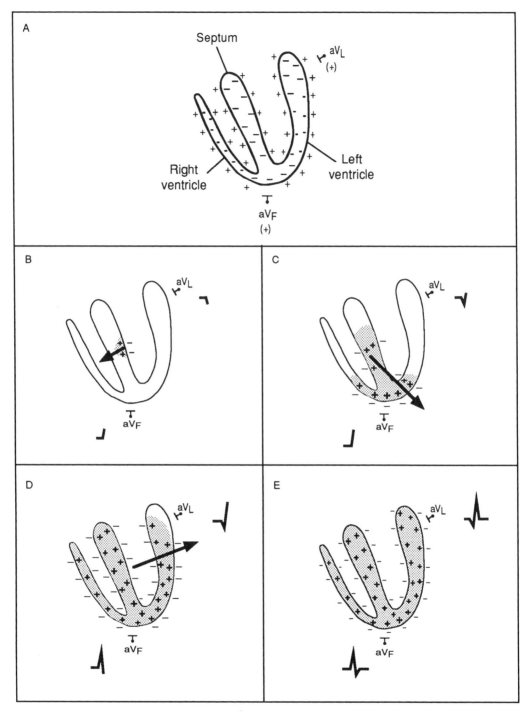

Figure 4.10. Normal ventricular depolarization as recorded by leads aV$_L$ and aV$_F$. A. In the resting state, the surface is homogeneously charged so that the leads do not record any electrical potential. **B.** The first area to depolarize is the left side of the ventricular septum. This results in forces heading away from aV$_L$ (downward deflection on aV$_L$ recording), but toward the (+) region of aV$_F$, such that an upward deflection is recorded by that lead. **C** and **D.** Depolarization continues; the forces from the thicker-walled left ventricle outweigh those of the right, such that the electrical vector swings leftward and posteriorly toward aV$_L$ (upward deflection) and away from aV$_F$. **E.** At the completion of depolarization, the surface is again homogeneously charged, and no further electrical voltage is recorded.

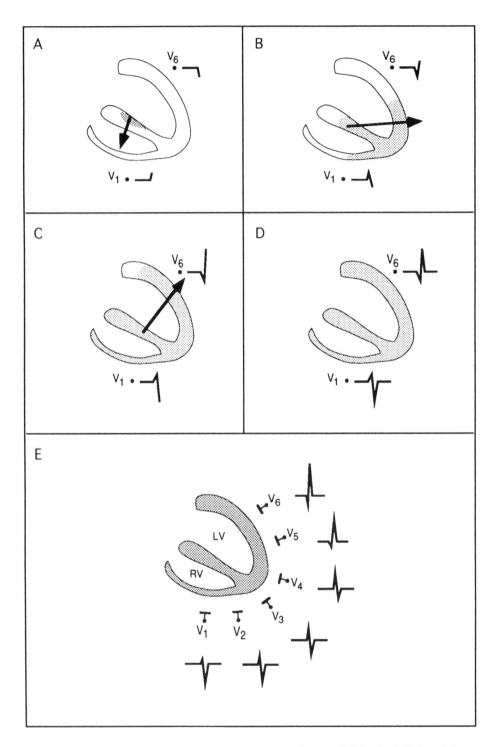

Figure 4.11. Sequence of depolarization recorded by the chest (precordial) leads. A–D. Depolarization begins at the left side of the septum, and the forces progress posteriorly toward the left ventricle. Thus, V_1, which is an anterior lead, records an initial upward deflection, followed by a downward wave, whereas V_6, a posterior lead, inscribes the opposite. **E.** Normal pattern of the QRS from V_1 to V_6: the R wave becomes progressively taller, and the S wave less deep.

A normal 12-lead EKG is shown at the end of the chapter (see Fig. 4.27).

Technical Considerations

EKG graph paper is divided into lines spaced 1 mm apart in both the horizontal and vertical directions. Each fifth line is made heavier to facilitate measurement. On the vertical axis, voltage is measured in millivolts (mV), and in the standard case, each 1 mm line separation represents 0.1 mV. The horizontal axis represents time. Because the standard paper speed is 25 mm per second, each 1 mm division represents 0.04 sec and each heavy line (5 mm) represents 0.2 sec (Fig. 4.12).

INTERPRETATION OF THE ELECTROCARDIOGRAM

Many cardiac disorders alter the morphology of the EKG recording in a diagnos-

tically useful way, and it is important to interpret each tracing in a standard fashion, so as to not miss subtle abnormalities. A commonly followed sequence of analysis is as follows:

1. Check voltage calibration
2. Heart rhythm
3. Heart rate
4. Intervals (PR, QRS, ST)
5. Mean QRS axis
6. Abnormalities of the P wave
7. Abnormalities of the QRS (hypertrophy, bundle branch block, infarction)
8. ST and T wave abnormalities

Calibration

EKG machines routinely inscribe a 1.0 mV vertical signal at the beginning or end of each 12-lead tracing, to document the voltage calibration of the machine. In the normal case, each 1 mm vertical box on the EKG paper represents 0.1 mV, so that the calibration sig-

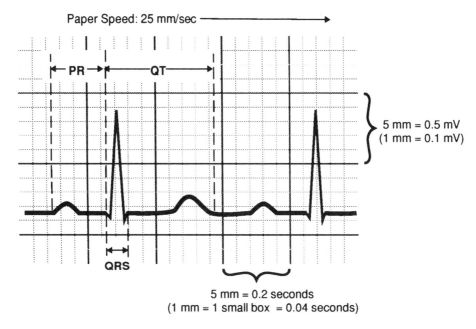

Figure 4.12.   Enlarged view of an EKG strip. The paper travels through the machine at 25 mm/sec, so that each 1 mm on the horizontal axis represents 0.04 sec. Each 1 mm on the vertical axis represents 0.1 millivolt. Interval measurements are: PR (from the beginning of the P wave to the beginning of the QRS) = 4 small boxes = 0.16 sec; QRS duration (from the beginning to the end of the QRS complex) = 1.75 small boxes = 0.07 sec; QT interval (from the beginning of the QRS to the end of the T waves) = 8 small boxes = 0.32 sec. The corrected QT $= \frac{QT}{\sqrt{R-R}}$. Since the R–R = 15 small boxes (0.6 sec), the corrected QT $= \frac{0.32}{\sqrt{0.6}} = 0.41$ sec.

nal records a 10 mm deflection (e.g., see Fig. 4.27). However, in patients with markedly increased voltage of the QRS complex (e.g., some patients with left ventricular hypertrophy or bundle branch blocks), the very large deflections would not fit on the EKG tracing. To facilitate interpretation in such a case, the recording is purposefully made at one-half of the standard voltage (i.e., each 1 mm box = 0.2 mV), and this is indicated on the EKG tracing by a change in the height of the 1.0 mV calibration signal (at one-half standard voltage, the signal would be 5 mm tall). It is important to check the height of the calibration signal on each EKG, so that the voltage criteria used to define specific abnormalities will be applicable.

Heart Rhythm

The normal cardiac rhythm is known as *sinus rhythm*, and is present if: 1) every P wave is followed by a QRS, 2) every QRS is preceded by a P wave, 3) the P wave is upright in leads I, II, and III, and 4) the PR interval is greater than 0.12 sec (three small boxes). In this situation, if the heart rate is between 60 and 100 beats/minute, then *normal* sinus rhythm is present. If less than 60 beats/minute, the rhythm is sinus *bradycardia*, and if greater than 100 beats/minute, sinus *tachycardia*. Other abnormal rhythms (termed "arrhythmias" or "dysrhythmias") are discussed in Chapters 11 and 12.

Heart Rate

The standard EKG paper speed is 25 mm/sec. Therefore,

Heart rate (beats/minute) =

$$\frac{25 \text{ mm/second} \times 60 \text{ seconds/minute}}{\text{mm/beat}}$$

or more simply:

$$\text{Heart rate} = \frac{1500}{\text{number of small boxes between two consecutive beats}}$$

It is rarely necessary, however, to determine the *exact* heart rate, and a more rapid

determination can be made, if you don't mind a bit of memorization. Simply "count off" the number of large boxes between two consecutive QRS complexes, using the sequence:

300—150—100—75—60—50,

which corresponds to the heart rate in beats/minute, and is illustrated in Figure 4.13.

When the rhythm is *irregular*, the heart rate may be approximated by taking advantage of the time markers, spaced 3 seconds apart, printed on the top of the EKG (Fig. 4.13, Method 3).

Intervals (PR, QRS, ST)

The PR interval, QRS duration, and QT interval are measured from the *limb* lead recordings (Fig. 4.12). For each of these intervals, first glance at all six of the limb lead recordings, and take the measurement in the lead where the interval is the *longest* in duration. The **PR interval** is measured from the onset of the P wave to the onset of the QRS. The **QRS interval** is measured from the beginning to the end of the QRS complex. The **QT interval** is measured from the beginning of the QRS to the end of the T wave. The normal ranges of the intervals are listed in Table 4.2, along with conditions associated with abnormal values.

Since the QT interval varies with heart rate (the faster the heart rate, the shorter the QT), a "corrected" QT is determined by dividing the measured QT by the square root of the R–R interval (see example in Fig. 4.12). When the heart rate is in the normal range (60 to 100 beats/min), a rapid rule can be applied: if the QT interval is visually less than half the interval between two consecutive QRS complexes, then the QT interval is within the normal range.

Mean QRS Axis

The mean QRS electrical axis represents the average of the instantaneous forces generated during the sequence of ventricular depolarization. The normal value is between −30° and +90° (Fig. 4.14). A mean axis that is more negative than $-30°$ implies **left axis deviation,** whereas an axis greater than $+90°$ represents **right axis deviation.** The axis can be accurately determined by plotting the QRS complexes of different leads on the axial reference diagram (Fig. 4.5), but this is tedious and rarely necessary. It is generally sufficient to note whether the axis is normal, deviated to the left, or deviated to the right. If a more precise measurement is needed, the simplified approach described below can be employed.

Please recall from Figure 4.5 that each EKG lead has a $(+)$ region and a $(-)$ region. Electrical activity directed toward the $(+)$ half results in an upward deflection, whereas activity toward the $(-)$ half results in a downward deflection on the EKG recording of that lead.

To determine whether the axis is normal or abnormal, examine the QRS complexes in limb leads I and II. If the QRS is primarily positive in both of these leads (upward deflection greater than downward deflection), then the mean vector falls within the normal range (Fig. 4.15). If the QRS in *either* lead I or II is not primarily upward, then the axis is *abnormal,* and the approximate axis should then be determined by the rapid method described here.

First, consider a special example (Fig. 4.16). A sequence of ventricular depolarization is represented in this figure by the arrows A through E. The initial deflection (representing left septal depolarization) points to the patient's right side. Because it is directed away from the $(+)$ pole of lead I, a strong downward deflection is recorded by the lead. As depolarization continues, the arrow swings downward and to the left, resulting in less-negative deflections in lead I. After arrow C, the electrical vector swings into the positive region of lead I so that upward deflections are recorded.

In this special example, in which electrical forces begin exactly opposite the $(+)$ electrode and terminate when pointed directly at that electrode, note that the mean electrical vector points straight downward (in the direction of arrow C), *perpendicular* to the lead I axis. Also note the configuration of the inscribed QRS complex. There is a

downward deflection, followed by an upward deflection of equal magnitude (when the upward and downward deflections of a QRS are of equal magnitude, it is termed an **isoelectric** complex). Thus, when an EKG lead inscribes an isoelectric QRS complex, it means that the average electrical axis of the ventricles is *perpendicular* to that lead.

Therefore, an easy way to determine the mean QRS axis is to glance at the six limb lead recordings, and observe which one has the most isoelectric-appearing complex: the mean axis is simply perpendicular to it. There is then one more step: When the mean axis is perpendicular to a lead, it could be perpendicular in either a clockwise *or* a counterclockwise direction. In our example, as the isoelectric complex appears in lead I, the mean vector could be at $+90°$, *or* it could be at $-90°$, since both are perpendicular. To determine which of these it is, the next step is to inspect the recording of the EKG lead that is perpendicular to the one inscribing the isoelectric complex (and is therefore parallel to the mean axis). If the QRS is predominantly upright in that perpendicular lead, then the mean vector points toward the $(+)$ pole of that lead. If it is predominantly negative, then it points away from the lead's $(+)$ pole. In our example, the isoelectric complex appears in lead I, and therefore, the next step is to inspect the perpendicular lead, which is aV_F (see Fig. 4.5 if this relationship is not clear). Because the QRS complex in aV_F is primarily upward, then the mean axis points toward its $(+)$ pole, which is in fact located at $+90°$.

To summarize, the mean QRS axis is calculated as follows:

1. Inspect limb leads I and II. If the QRS is primarily upward in both, then the axis is normal and you are done. If not, then proceed to the next step.
2. Inspect the six limb leads, and determine which one contains the QRS that is most isoelectric. The mean axis is perpendicular to that lead.
3. Inspect the lead that is perpendicular to the lead containing the isoelectric complex. If the QRS in that perpendicular lead is primarily upward, then the mean

---

Method 1

The standard paper speed = 25 mm/sec. So, count the number of mm between two QRS complexes (i.e., between 2 "beats"). Then:

Heart Rate (beats/min) $= \dfrac{(25 \text{ mm/sec } \times 60 \text{ sec/min})}{\text{number of mm between beats}} = \dfrac{1500}{\text{mm/beats}}$

On this strip for example, there are 23 mm between the first 2 beats:

23 mm between beats

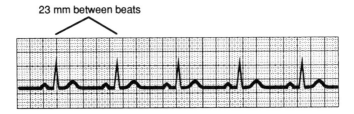

Therefore, the heart rate $= \dfrac{1500}{23} = 65$ beats/min

Method 1 is particularly helpful for measuring fast heart rates (>100 bpm).

Method 2

The "count-off" method requires memorizing the sequence:

300 - 150 - 100 - 75 - 60 - 50

In the example, count-off the number of large boxes between two consecutive beats:

start here   300 150 100 75 60

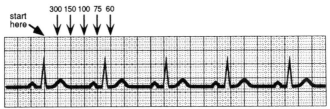

The second QRS falls between the "75" and "60" beats/min; therefore the heart rate is approximately mid-way between them, ≈ 67 beats/min. Knowing that the heart rate is *approximately* 60-70 beats/min is certainly close enough.

Figure 4.13. Methods to calculate the heart rate.

axis points to the (+) pole of that lead. If primarily negative, then the mean QRS points to the (−) pole of that lead.

Conditions that result in left or right axis deviation are listed in Figure 4.14. In addition, the vertical position of the heart in many normal children and adolescents may result in a rightward mean axis (> +90°).

Occasionally, isoelectric complexes are inscribed in *all* of the limb leads. That situation arises when the heart is tilted, so that the mean QRS is pointing straight forward

Method 3

EKG recording paper usually includes 3-second time markers at the top or bottom of the tracing:

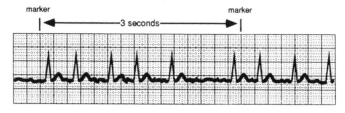

To calculate the heart rate, count the number of QRS complexes between the 3 second markers (= 6 beats in this example) and multiply by 20. Thus the heart rate here ≈ 120 beats/min.

It's even easier (and a bit more accurate) to count the number of complexes between the first and *third* markers on a strip (representing 6 seconds) and then multiply by 10 to determine the heart rate.

Method 3 is particularly helpful for measuring irregular heart rates.

Figure 4.13. (*continued*).

or back from the chest, as it may be in patients with chronic obstructive lung disease; in such a case, the mean axis is said to be "indeterminate."

Abnormalities of the P Wave

The P wave represents depolarization of the right atrium followed quickly by the left atrium; they are nearly superimposed on one another (Fig. 4.17). The P wave is usually best visualized in lead II, the lead that runs most parallel to the flow of electrical current through the atria from the sinoatrial to the AV node. When the *right* atrium is enlarged, the initial component of the P wave is larger than normal (taller than 2.5 mm in lead II).

Left atrial enlargement is best observed in

TABLE 4.2. **Electrocardiographic Intervals**

Interval	Normal	Decreased in	Increased in
PR	0.12–0.20 sec (3–5 small boxes)	• Pre-excitation syndrome • Junctional rhythm	• First-degree AV block
QRS	≤ 0.10 sec (≤ 2.5 small boxes)		• Bundle branch blocks • Ventricular ectopic beat • Toxic drug effect (e.g., quinidine) • Severe hyperkalemia
QT	Corrected QT[a] ≤ 0.44 sec	• Hypercalcemia • Tachycardia	• Hypocalcemia • Hypokalemia (↑ QU interval due to ↑ U wave) • Hypomagnesemia • Myocardial ischemia • Congenital prolongation of QT • Toxic drug-effect (e.g., quinidine)

[a]Corrected QT $= \dfrac{QT}{\sqrt{R-R}}$

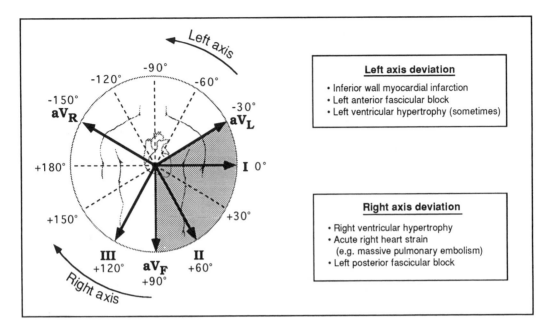

Figure 4.14. A normal mean QRS axis falls in the shaded area (between −30° and +90°). A mean axis more negative than −30° is termed "left axis deviation," whereas an axis > +90° is "right axis deviation." The table lists common conditions that result in axis deviation.

lead V_1. Normally, V_1 inscribes a P wave with an initial positive deflection reflecting right atrial depolarization (directed anteriorly), followed by a negative deflection, owing to the left atrial forces oriented posteriorly (see Fig. 1.2 for anatomic relationships). Left atrial enlargement is therefore manifest by a greater than normal negative deflection (at least 1 mm wide and 1 mm deep) in lead V_1 (Fig. 4.17).

Abnormalities of the QRS Complex

Ventricular Hypertrophy

Hypertrophy of the left or right ventricle results in greater than normal electrical forces generated by the hypertrophied chamber. Normally, the forces of the thicker-walled left ventricle are greater than those of the right. However, in **right ventricular hypertrophy** (RVH), the added right-sided forces may outweigh those of the left. Therefore, chest leads V_1 and V_2, which overlie the right ventricle, record greater than normal upward deflections: The R wave becomes

taller than the S wave in those leads, the reverse of the normal situation (Fig. 4.18). In addition, the increased right ventricular mass shifts the mean axis of the heart toward the right (greater than +90°).

In **left ventricular hypertrophy,** greater than normal forces are generated by the massive LV, which simply exaggerates the normal situation. Leads that overlie the left ventricle (chest leads V_5 and V_6, and limb leads I and aV_L) show taller R waves than normal. Leads on the other side of the heart (V_1 and V_2) demonstrate the opposite: deeper than normal S waves. Many criteria can be used for the diagnosis of left ventricular hypertrophy, and three of the most helpful are listed in Figure 4.18.

Bundle Branch Blocks

Interruption of conduction through the right or left bundle branches may develop from ischemic or degenerative damage to the fibers. As a result, the affected ventricle does not depolarize in the normal sequence. Rather than rapid uniform stimulation by

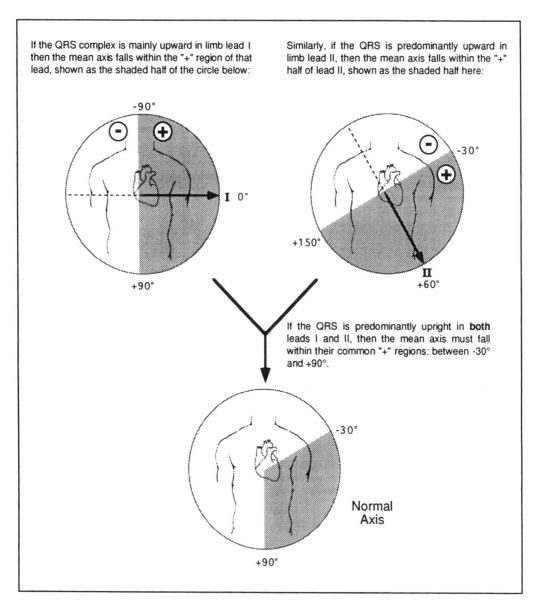

If the QRS complex is mainly upward in limb lead I then the mean axis falls within the "+" region of that lead, shown as the shaded half of the circle below:

Similarly, if the QRS is predominantly upward in limb lead II, then the mean axis falls within the "+" half of lead II, shown as the shaded half here:

If the QRS is predominantly upright in **both** leads I and II, then the mean axis must fall within their common "+" regions: between -30° and +90°.

Normal Axis

Figure 4.15. The mean axis is within the normal range if the QRS complex is predominantly upright in limb leads I and II.

the Purkinje fibers, the cells of that ventricle must rely on a more gradual myocyte-to-myocyte spread of electrical activity traveling from the unaffected ventricle. This is a slow process, which prolongs depolarization and widens the QRS complex (> 0.1 sec). When the QRS duration is between 0.10 and 0.12 sec (2.5 to 3 small boxes), *incomplete* bundle branch block is present. If greater than 0.12 sec (three small boxes), *complete* bundle branch block is identified.

In **right bundle branch block** (Fig. 4.19A; see also Fig. 4.28), initial depolarization of the ventricular septum (which is stimulated by a branch of the left bundle) is unaffected so that the normal small R wave in lead V_1 and small Q wave in lead V_6 are recorded. Furthermore, as the wave of depolarization spreads down the septum and into the left ventricular free wall, the sequence of depolarization is indistinguishable from normal, because LV forces *nor-*

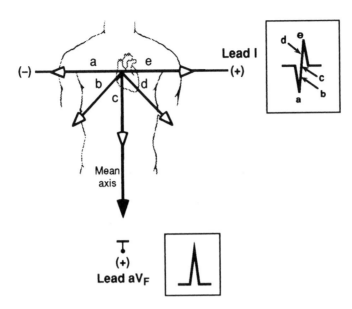

Figure 4.16. Sequence of ventricular depolarization when the mean axis is +90°. Because the mean axis is perpendicular to limb lead I, an isoelectric QRS complex (height of upward deflection = height of downward deflection) is recorded by that lead (see text for details).

mally outweigh those of the right. However, at the time when the LV has almost fully depolarized, the slow cell-to-cell spread finally reaches the right ventricle and depolarization of that chamber begins, unopposed by LV activity (since that chamber has nearly fully depolarized). Therefore, the QRS complex is widened by this prolonged depolarization process. Since the terminal portion of the QRS complex in this case represents right ventricular forces acting alone, there is a terminal *upward* deflection

(known as R′) over the RV (in lead V_1), and a downward deflection (S wave) in V_6 on the opposite side of the heart.

Left bundle branch block produces even greater QRS abnormalities. In that situation, normal initial depolarization of the left septum does *not* occur; rather, the right side of the ventricular septum is first to depolarize, through branches of the right bundle. Thus, the initial forces of depolarization are directed toward the left ventricle instead of the right (Fig. 4.19B; see also Fig. 4.29). There-

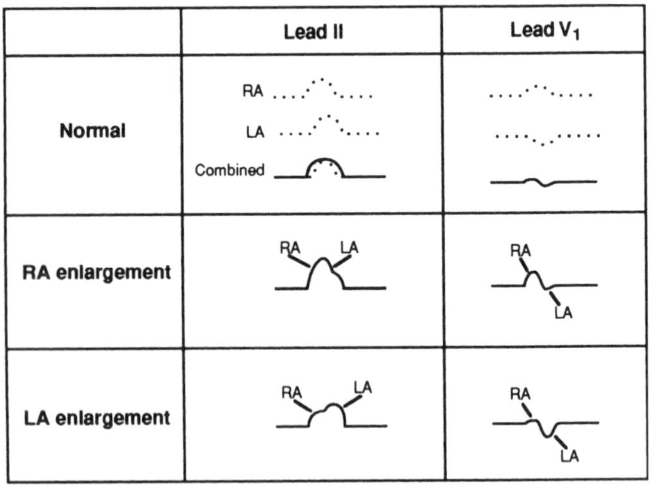

		Lead II	Lead V_1
Normal		RA ....⋯⋯.... LA ....⋯⋯..... Combined ⌒	....⋯...... ....⋅..... ‿
RA enlargement		RA LA ‿⌒‿	RA ‿⋀‿ LA
LA enlargement		RA LA ‿⌒⌒‿	RA ‿⋁‿ LA

Figure 4.17. The P wave represents superimposition of right atrial (RA) and left atrial (LA) depolarization. RA depolarization occurs slightly earlier than the LA. In RA enlargement, the initial component of the P is prominent (> 2.5 mm tall) in lead II. In LA enlargement, there is a large terminal downward deflection in lead V_1 (> 1 mm wide and > 1 mm deep).

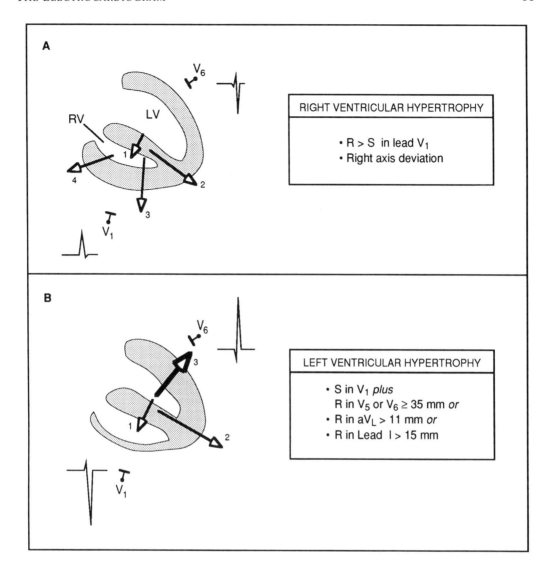

Figure 4.18.   Ventricular hypertrophy. The arrows indicate the sequence of average electrical forces during ventricular depolarization. **A.** Right ventricular (RV) hypertrophy. The RV forces outweigh those of the left, resulting in tall R waves in leads V_1 and V_2 and a deep S wave in lead V_6. **B.** Left ventricular (LV) hypertrophy exaggerates the normal pattern of depolarization, with stronger than usual forces directed toward the LV, resulting in tall R wave in V_6 and deep S in lead V_1.

fore, an initial *downward* deflection is recorded in V_1 and the normal small Q wave in V_6 is absent. Only after depolarization of the right ventricle does slow cell-to-cell spread reach the left ventricular cells. These slowly conducted forces inscribe a widened QRS complex with terminally upward deflections in the leads overlying the left ventricle (V_5 and V_6), as shown in Figure 4.19.

A more limited form of conduction block affects either the anterior or posterior fascicle (division) of the left bundle, resulting in left anterior or posterior fascicular block (also called "hemiblock"). Anatomically, the anterior fascicle of the left bundle runs anteriorly toward the anterior papillary muscle, whereas the posterior fascicle travels to the posterior papillary muscle. As a result, electrical activation of the LV normally spreads simultaneously from the base of the two papillary muscles. If conduction is impaired in one of these divisions, then initial LV depolarization arises exclusively from the unaffected zone. For

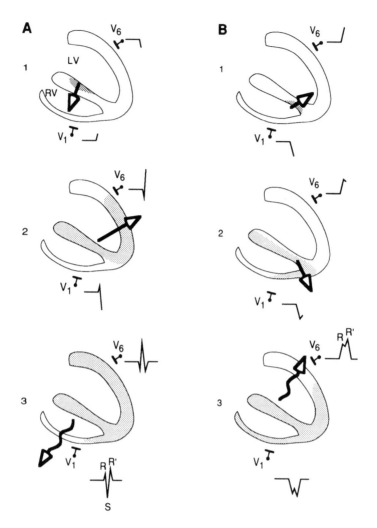

Figure 4.19. Bundle branch blocks. Interruption of conduction through the right (RBBB) or left (LBBB) bundles results in delayed, slowed activation of the respective ventricle and widening of the QRS complex. **A.** In RBBB there is normal initial activation of the septum (1) followed by depolarization of the left ventricle (2). Slow cell-to-cell spread activates the right ventricle (RV) *after* the left ventricle (LV) has nearly fully depolarized, so that the late forces generated by the RV are unopposed. Therefore, V_1 records an abnormal terminal upward deflection (R'), and V_6 records an abnormal, terminal deep S wave (3). **B.** In LBBB the initial septal depolarization is blocked, such that initial forces are oriented from right to left. Thus the normal initial R in V_1 and Q in V_6 are absent (1). After the RV depolarizes, late, slow activation of the LV results in a terminal upward deflection in V_6 and downward deflection in V_1 (3).

example, in the case of *left anterior fascicular block (LAFB)*, activation begins at the posterior papillary muscle, then spreads to the rest of the ventricle. Since the posterior papillary muscle is located below and medial to the anterior papillary muscle, the initial depolarization will be downward (i.e., toward the feet) and toward the patient's right side. This results in a positive deflection (initial R wave) in the inferior leads (II, III, aV_F) and a small Q wave in leads I and aV_L (Fig. 4.20).

As the electrical forces then spread upward and to the left, an R wave is inscribed in leads I and aV_L and an S wave in the inferior leads. The predominance of these leftward forces results in left axis deviation of the QRS mean axis.

In the much less common *left posterior fascicular block (LPFB)*, left ventricular activation starts at the base of the anterior papillary muscle, so the initial forces are directed upward and to the patient's left (creating an

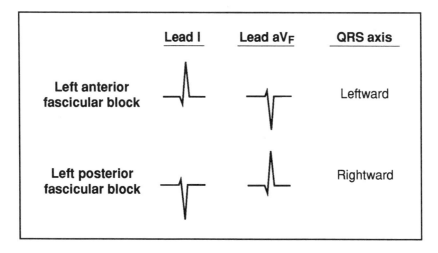

Figure 4.20. Electrocardiographic patterns in left anterior and left posterior fascicular blocks.

R in lead I and aV_L, and Q waves in the inferior leads). As the impulse spreads downward and to the right, an S wave is inscribed in I (and aV_L), while an R is recorded in II, III and aV_F. Since the bulk of these forces head rightward, right axis deviation of the QRS mean axis is expected.

LAFB and LPFB do not result in marked widening of the QRS (in distinction to right or left bundle branch blocks) because rapidly conducting Purkinje fibers bridge the territories served by the anterior and posterior fascicles. Therefore, although the sequence and pathway of conduction are altered, the total time required for depolarization is usually only slightly prolonged.

Myocardial Infarction

The hallmark of transmural myocardial infarction (MI) is the **pathologic Q wave.** Recall that an initial Q wave is normal in some leads. For example, initial septal depolarization routinely inscribes a small Q wave in leads V_6 and aV_L. *Normal* Q waves are of *short* duration (≤ 0.04 sec, or one small box) and of *low* magnitude (< 25% of the QRS total height). A pathologic Q wave is more prominent (Fig. 4.21), having a width ≥ one small box in duration, and a depth > 25% of the total height of the QRS. The EKG leads in which the pathologic Q

waves appear reflect the anatomic site of the infarction (Table 4.3; see also Fig. 4.23).

Pathologic Q waves develop in the leads overlying infarcted tissue because necrotic muscle does not generate electrical forces. Rather, the EKG electrode over that region records only the electrical currents from the healthy tissue on *opposite* regions of the ventricle, which are directed *away* from the infarct and the recording electrode, thus inscribing the downward deflection (Fig. 4.22). Q waves are permanent evidence of a transmural myocardial infarction; only rarely do they disappear over time.

Note in Table 4.3 that in the case of a pos-

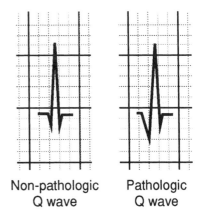

Non-pathologic Q wave   Pathologic Q wave

Figure 4.21. Compared with small Q waves generated during normal depolarization, pathologic Q waves are more prominent: their width is ≥ 1 mm (1 small box) and their depth > 25% of the height of the QRS complex.

TABLE 4.3. Localization of Myocardial Infarction

Anatomic Site	Leads with Abnormal EKG Complexes[a]	Coronary Artery Most Often Responsible
Inferior	II, III, aV_F	RCA
Antero septal	V_1–V_2	LAD
Antero apical	V_3–V_4	LAD (distal)
Antero lateral	V_5–V_6, I, aV_L	CFX
Posterior	V_1–V_2 [tall R, not Q]	RCA

[a]Pathologic Q waves in all of leads V_1–V_6 implies an "extensive anterior MI" usually associated with a proximal left coronary artery occlusion.

terior myocardial infarction (Fig. 4.23) it is not pathologic Q waves that are evident on the EKG. Because no standard electrodes are placed on the patient's back overlying the posterior wall, one must rely on other leads to indirectly indicate the presence of such an infarction. Since chest leads V_1 and V_2 are directly opposite the posterior wall, they record the *inverse* of what leads placed on the back *would* report. Therefore, *taller than normal R waves in leads V_1 and V_2* are the equivalent of a pathologic Q wave in the identification of a posterior wall MI. You may recall that right ventricular hypertrophy also produces tall R waves in leads V_1 and V_2, but unlike RVH, right axis deviation is not usually present in posterior wall MI.

It is important to note that if a pathologic Q wave appears only in a single EKG lead, it is not diagnostic for an infarction. True pathologic Qs should appear in the groupings listed in Table 4.3 and Figure 4.23. For example, if a pathologic Q wave is present in lead III, but not in II or aV_F, it likely does not indicate an infarction. Also, Q waves are *disregarded* in lead aV_R, as electrical forces are *normally* directed away from the right arm. Finally, in the presence of left bundle branch block, Q waves are usually not helpful in the diagnosis of myocardial infarction, because of the markedly abnormal pattern of depolarization in that condition.

The discussion thus far has considered infarctions in which Q waves develop, and these are therefore termed **Q-wave infarctions**. Pathologically, in such infarctions, the entire thickness of a myocardial segment is involved, so that this type of MI is

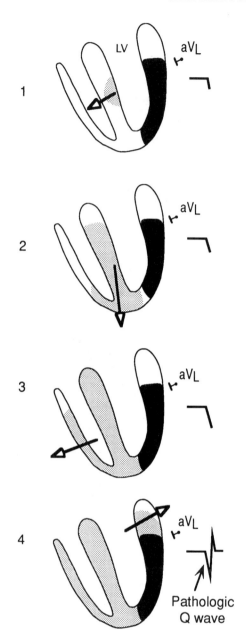

Figure 4.22. Sequence of depolarization recorded by lead aV_L, overlying a lateral wall infarction (black). A pathologic Q wave is recorded because the necrotic muscle does not generate electrical forces; rather, at the time when the lateral wall *should* be depolarizing (**panel 3**), the activation of the healthy muscle on the *opposite* side of the heart is unopposed, such that forces head away from aV_L. The terminal R wave recorded by aV_L reflects depolarization of the remaining viable myocardium beyond the infarct.

also termed a "transmural" infarct. As described in Chapter 7, infarctions are not always transmural, but may involve only the subendocardial layers of the myocardium.

A

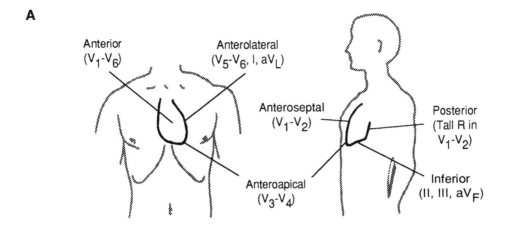

B

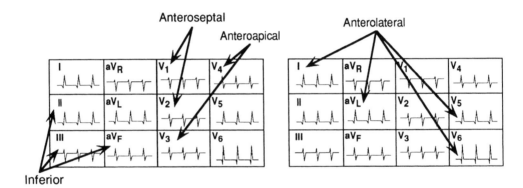

Figure 4.23. **A.** Cardiac anatomic regions. The leads listed in parentheses are those that reflect infarction within these regions. **B.** Miniaturized schematic drawings of a 12-lead EKG, showing the standard orientation of printed samples from each lead. The major anatomic groupings are indicated. Note that while the presence of pathologic Q waves in leads V_1 and V_2 are indicative of anteroseptal infarction, *tall initial R waves* in those leads are seen in posterior wall infarction.

In the latter case, pathologic Q waves do *not* develop, because the remaining viable cells are able to generate some electrical activity; such MIs are therefore called **non-Q-wave infarctions.** However, ST and T wave abnormalities evolve during both Q-wave and non-Q-wave infarctions, as discussed in the next section. The electrocardiographic differences between these types of MI are summarized here:

	Q waves	Acute ST deviation
Q-wave (transmural) MI	Yes	Upward
Non-Q-wave (nontransmural) MI	No	Downward

ST Segment and T Wave Abnormalities

Among the most common important abnormalities of the ST and T waves are those that represent myocardial ischemia and infarction. Because ventricular repolarization is very sensitive to myocardial perfusion, patients with coronary artery disease often demonstrate reversible deviations of the ST segments and T waves during transient myocardial ischemia.

Please recall from the last section that pathologic Q waves are indicative of a myocardial infarction, but do not differentiate

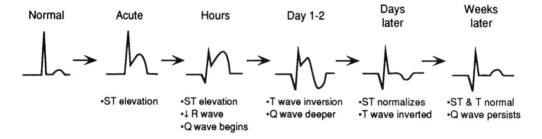

•ST elevation   •ST elevation   •T wave inversion   •ST normalizes   •ST & T normal
              •↓ R wave   •Q wave deeper   •T wave inverted   •Q wave persists
              •Q wave begins

Figure 4.24.   EKG evolution during acute Q-wave myocardial infarction.

between an acute event and an MI that had occurred weeks or years earlier. However, acute myocardial infarction does result in a sequence of ST and T wave abnormalities that permit this differentiation (Fig. 4.24).

The initial abnormality during an acute Q-wave MI is elevation of the ST segment, often with a peaked appearance of the T wave. At this early stage, myocardial cells are still viable and Q waves have not yet

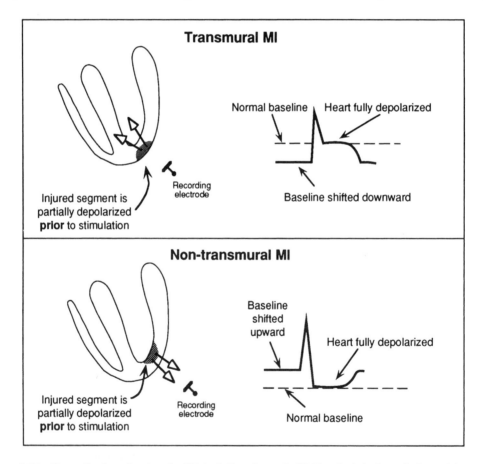

Figure 4.25.   Theoretical mechanism for ST deviations in acute MI. Top. Ionic leak results in partial depolarization of injured myocardium prior to electrical stimulation, which produces forces heading away from that site, and shifts the EKG baseline downward. This is not noticeable on the EKG because only relative, not absolute, voltages are recorded. Following stimulation, when the entire heart fully depolarizes, the voltage is "true" zero, but gives the appearance of ST elevation compared with the abnormally depressed baseline. **Bottom.** In nontransmural MI, the process is similar, but the ionic leak arises from the subendocardial tissue, so that the partial depolarization prior to stimulation is directed *toward* the exploring electrode; hence the baseline is shifted *upward*. When fully depolarized, the voltage is true zero, but the ST segment has the *appearance* that it is depressed, compared to the shifted baseline.

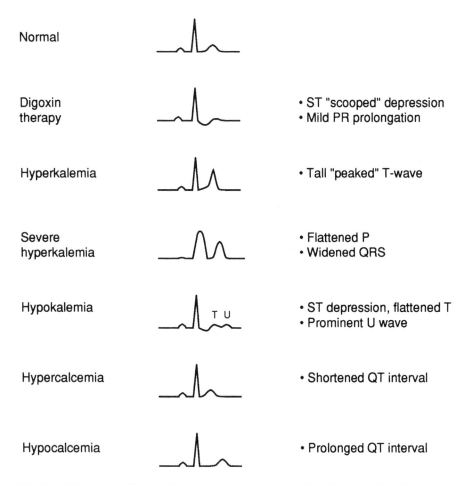

Normal

Digoxin
therapy
• ST "scooped" depression
• Mild PR prolongation

Hyperkalemia
• Tall "peaked" T-wave

Severe
hyperkalemia
• Flattened P
• Widened QRS

Hypokalemia
T U
• ST depression, flattened T
• Prominent U wave

Hypercalcemia
• Shortened QT interval

Hypocalcemia
• Prolonged QT interval

Figure 4.26. Conditions that alter repolarization of myocytes, and therefore result in ST segment and T wave abnormalities.

developed. Within several hours, however, myocyte death leads to loss of the amplitude of the R wave, and pathologic Q waves begin to be inscribed by the EKG leads positioned over the infarct territory. During the first 1 to 2 days following infarction, the ST segments remain elevated, the T wave inverts, and the Q wave deepens. Several days later, the ST segment elevation returns to baseline, but the T waves remain inverted. Weeks or months following the infarct, the ST segment and T waves have often returned to normal, but the pathologic Q waves persist, a permanent marker of the MI. If the ST segment *remains* elevated several weeks later, it is likely that a bulging fibrotic scar (ventricular aneurysm) has developed at the site of infarction.

These evolutionary changes of the QRS, ST, and T waves are recorded by the leads overlying the zone of infarction (Table 4.3). Typically, "reciprocal" changes are seen in leads opposite to that site. For example, in acute anteroseptal MI, ST segment elevation is expected in chest leads V_1 and V_2; simultaneously, however, reciprocal changes (ST *depression*) may be inscribed by the leads overlying the opposite (inferior) region, namely in leads II, III, and aV_F.

The mechanism by which ST segment elevation develops during acute MI has not been established with certainty. It is believed, however, that the abnormality results from injured myocardial cells immediately adjacent to the infarct zone producing abnormal systolic or diastolic currents. One explanation contends that these

TABLE 4.4. Summary: Sequence of EKG Interpretation

1. **Calibration**
   - Check 1.0 mV vertical box inscription (normal standard = 10 mm)
2. **Rhythm**
   - Sinus rhythm is present, if:
     - each P wave is followed by QRS
     - each QRS is preceeded by a P wave
     - the P wave is upright in leads I, II, & III
     - the PR interval is > 0.12 sec (3 small boxes)
   - If these criteria are not met, determine type of arrythmia (Chapter 12)
3. **Heart rate**
   - Use one of three methods:
     - 1500/(number of mm between beats)
     - Count off method: 300—150—100—75—60—50
     - Number of beats in 6 seconds × 10
   - Normal rate = 60–100 beats/min (bradycardia < 60, tachycardia > 100)
4. **Intervals**
   - Normal PR = 0.12–0.20 sec (3–5 small boxes)
   - Normal QRS ≤ 0.10 sec (≤ 2.5 small boxes)
   - Normal QT ≤ one-half if the R–R interval, if heart rate normal
5. **Mean QRS axis**
   - Normal if QRS is primarily upright in leads I and II (+90° to −30°)
   - Otherwise, determine axis by isoelectric/perpendicular method
6. **P wave abnormalities**
   - Inspect P in leads II and V_1 for left and right atrial enlargement
7. **QRS wave abnormalities**
   - Inspect for left and right ventricular hypertrophy
   - Inspect for bundle branch blocks (BBB)
   - Inspect for pathologic Q waves: What anatomic distribution?
8. **ST segment/T wave abnormalities**
   - Inspect for ST elevations:
     - transmural infarct pattern
     - pericarditis (described in Chapter 14)
   - Inspect for ST depressions/T wave inversions:
     - subendocardial ischemia or infarct
     - commonly accompany ventricular hypertrophy or BBBs
     - metabolic/chemical abnormalities (Fig. 4.26)
9. **Compare** with patient's previous EKGs

cells are capable of depolarization, but are abnormally "leaky" so that they never fully repolarize (Fig. 4.25). As a result, in the resting state, partial depolarization of these cells results in forces heading away from the injured segment, causing the baseline of the overlying EKG lead to shift in a *downward* direction. Since the EKG machine records only *relative* position, rather than absolute voltages, the deviation of the

baseline is not noticed. Following ventricular depolarization (the QRS complex), after *all* of the myocardial cells have fully depolarized, including those of the injured zone, the net electrical potential surrounding the heart is *true* zero. However, compared with the abnormally displaced (downward) baseline, there is the *appearance* of ST segment elevation. As the cells repolarize, the injured cells return to the abnormal state of diastolic leak, and the EKG again inscribes the abnormally depressed baseline owing to the abnormal forces heading away from the electrode. Thus, the appearance of ST elevation in acute MI may in part reflect an abnormal shift of the recording baseline.

In non-Q-wave myocardial infarctions, it is ST segment *depression*, rather than elevation, that develops in the leads overlying the infarct. In this situation, the diastolic leak of injured cells adjacent to the infarct generates electrical forces heading from the inner endocardium to the outer epicardium and therefore toward the EKG electrode. Thus, the baseline of the EKG is shifted *upward* (Fig. 4.25). Following full cardiac depolarization, the electrical potential of the heart returns to true zero, but relative to the abnormal baseline, gives the appearance of ST segment depression.

Other common causes of ST segment and T wave abnormalities due to alterations in myocyte repolarization are illustrated in Figure 4.26.

SUMMARY

The electrocardiogram provides a wealth of important information regarding the structure and integrity of the heart and remains one of the simplest but most important diagnostic tools in cardiology. With the knowledge of this chapter in hand, you should be well suited to practice reading electrocardiograms in any of the excellent texts listed below. Table 4.4 summarizes the suggested sequence of EKG interpretation. Some sample EKGs follow, with their interpretations, in Figures 4.27 through 4.34.

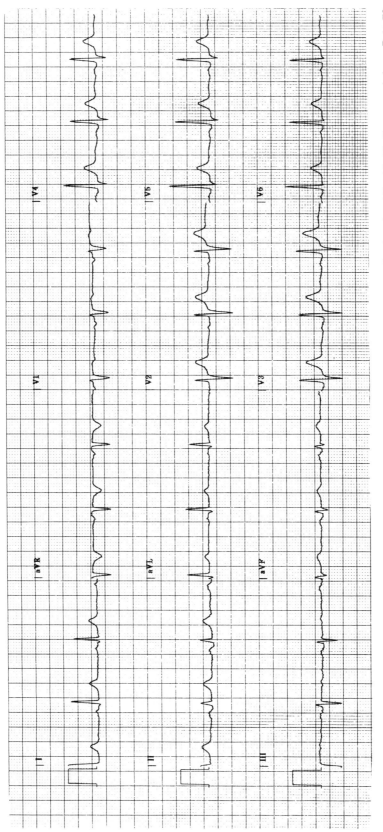

Figure 4.27. 12-lead EKG (normal). The rectangular upward deflection at the beginning of each line is the voltage calibration signal (1 mV). *Rhythm:* normal sinus. *Rate:* 70 bpm. *Intervals:* PR 0.17, QRS 0.06, QT 0.40 msec. *Axis:* 0° (QRS is isoelectric in lead aV$_F$). The P wave, QRS complex, ST segment, and T waves are normal. Note the gradual increase in R wave height between leads V$_1$ through V$_6$.

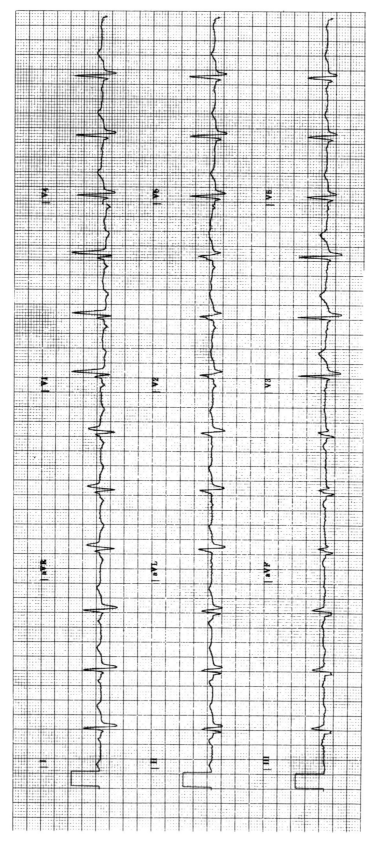

Figure 4.28. 12-lead EKG (abnormal). *Rhythm:* normal sinus. *Rate:* 75 bpm. *Intervals:* PR 0.16, QRS 0.15, QT 0.42 msec. *Axis:* indeterminate (isoelectric in all limb leads). *P wave:* left atrial enlargement (1 mm wide and 1 mm deep in lead V_1). *QRS:* widened with RSR' in lead V_1, consistent with right bundle branch block (RBBB). Also, pathologic Q waves in leads II, III, and aV_F, consistent with inferior wall myocardial infarction (an old one, because the ST segments do not demonstrate an acute injury pattern).

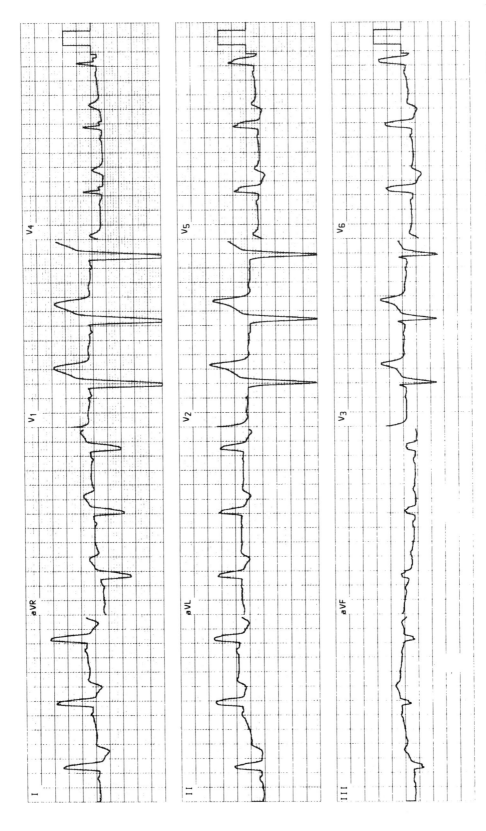

Figure 4.29. 12-lead EKG (abnormal). *Rhythm:* normal sinus. *Rate:* 68 bpm. *Intervals:* PR 0.16, QRS 0.16, QT 0.40 msec. *Axis:* +15°. *P wave:* normal. *QRS:* widened with RR' in lead V_4–V_6 consistent with left bundle branch block (LBBB). The *ST segment and T wave abnormalities are secondary to LBBB.

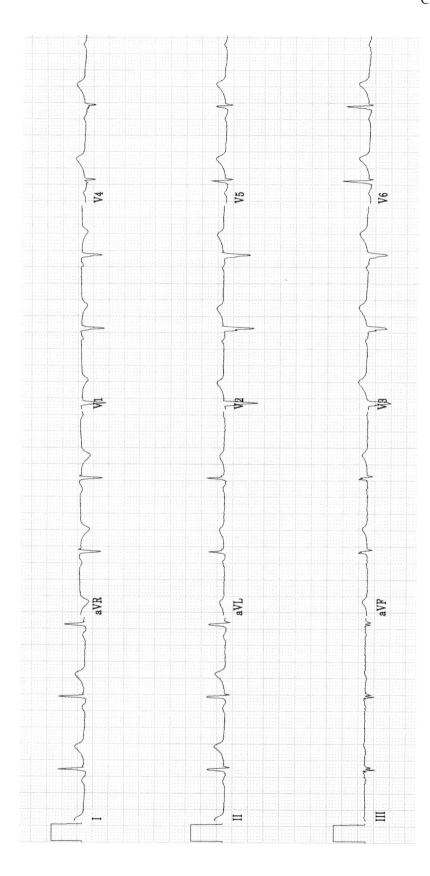

Figure 4.30. 12-lead EKG (abnormal). *Rhythm:* normal sinus. *Rate:* 66 bpm. *Intervals:* PR 0.16, QRS 0.08, QT 0.40 msec. *Axis:* +10°. *P wave:* normal. *QRS:* pathologic Q waves in leads V_1–V_4, consistent with anteroseptal and anteroapical myocardial infarction (MI). The *ST segment and T waves* do not demonstrate an acute injury pattern, so that the MI is old.

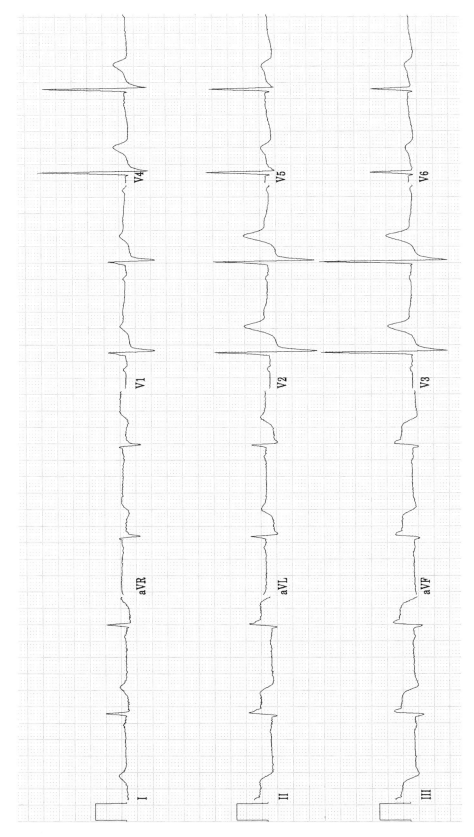

Figure 4.31. 12-lead EKG (abnormal). *Rhythm:* sinus bradycardia. *Rate:* 55 bpm. *Intervals:* PR 0.20 (in aV$_F$), QRS 0.10, QT 0.44 msec. *Axis:* normal (QRS is predominantly upright in leads I and II). *P wave:* normal. *QRS:* prominent voltage in chest leads, but does not meet criteria for ventricular hypertrophy; pathologic Q waves are present in II, III. aV$_F$, indicative of inferior wall MI, and the tall R waves in V$_1$ and V$_2$ are consistent with posterior MI involvement as well. There is marked *ST segment elevation* in II, III, aVF, indicating that this is an *acute* MI.

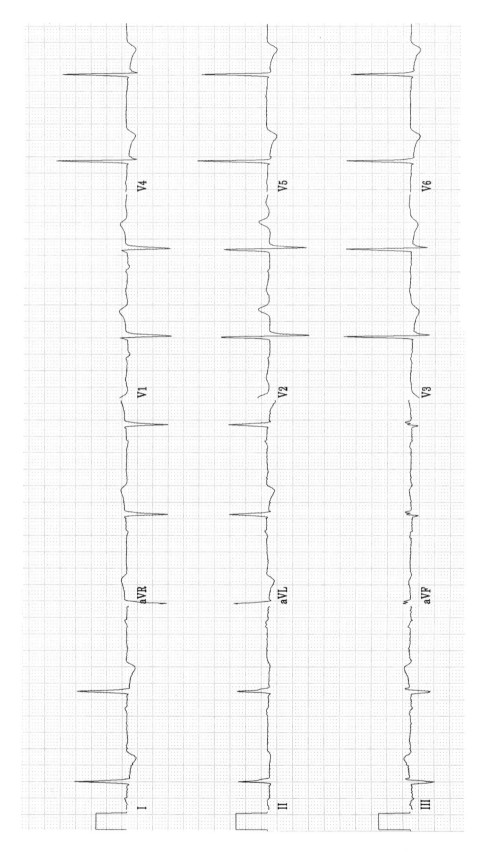

Figure 4.32. **12-lead EKG (abnormal).** *Rhythm:* sinus bradycardia. *Rate:* 55 bpm. *Intervals:* PR 0.24 (first-degree AV block—see Chapter 12), QRS 0.09, QT 0.44 msec. *Axis:* 0°. *P wave:* normal. *QRS:* left ventricular hypertrophy (LVH): S in V_1 (14 mm) + R in V_5 (22 mm) > 35 mm. There are pathologic Q waves in leads III and aV_F raising the possibility of an old inferior MI. The *ST segment depression* and *T wave inversion* are secondary to abnormal repolarization seen in LVH.

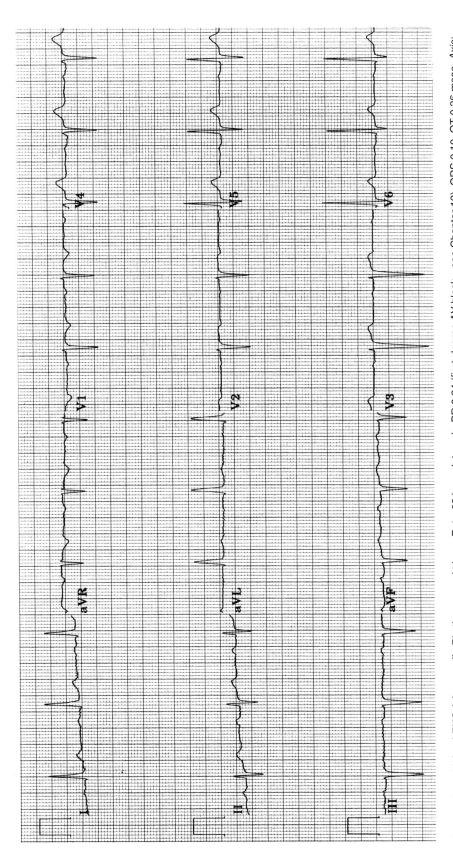

Figure 4.33. 12-lead EKG (abnormal). *Rhythm:* normal sinus. *Rate:* 68 bpm. *Intervals:* PR 0.24 (first-degree AV block—see Chapter 12), QRS 0.10, QT 0.36 msec. *Axis:* −45° (left axis deviation). *P wave:* left atrial enlargement (terminal deflection of P wave in V_1 is 1 mm wide and 1 mm deep—just barely). *QRS:* pattern of left anterior fascicular block (LAFB; see Fig. 4.20). The abnormally small R waves in leads V_2–V_4 are associated with LAFB, due to the reduction of initial anterior forces. The *ST segment and T waves* are unremarkable.

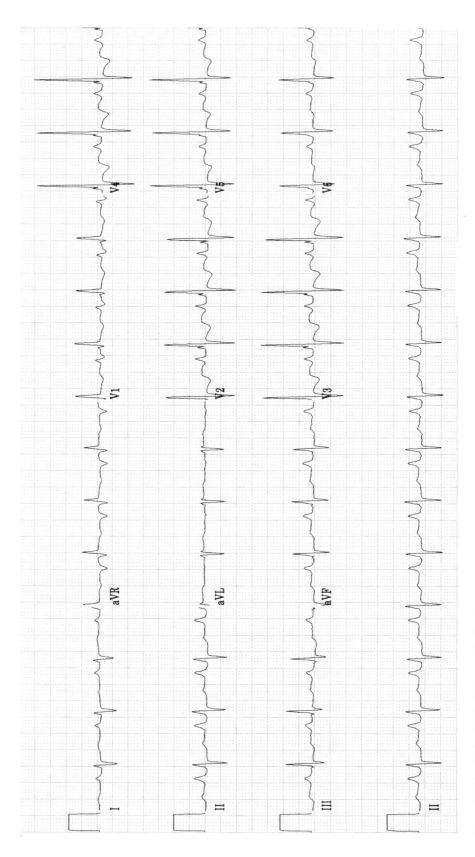

Figure 4.34.   12-lead EKG (abnormal). *Rhythm:* normal sinus. *Rate:* 95 bpm. *Intervals:* PR 0.20, QRS 0.10, QT 0.34 msec. *Axis:* +160° (right axis deviation (RAD)). *P wave:* right atrial enlargement (P in II is > 2.5 mm tall). *QRS:* right ventricular hypertrophy (RVH): R > S in V$_1$ with RAD. The *T waves* are inverted in the anterior leads, at least in part reflecting abnormal repolarization due to RVH.

Disturbances of the cardiac rhythm (arrhythmias) are discussed in Chapters 11 and 12.

ADDITIONAL READING

Dubin D. Rapid Interpretation of EKGs. 4th ed. Tampa, FL: Cover Publishing Co., 1989.

Goldberger AL, Goldberger E. Clinical electrocardiography: A Simplified Approach. 5th ed. St. Louis: Mosby Year Book, 1994.

Huang PL. Introduction to Electrocardiography. Philadelphia: WB Saunders Co., 1993.

Mudge GH. Manual of Electrocardiography. 2nd ed. Boston: Little, Brown & Co., 1991.

Shamroth L. The 12-lead Electrocardiogram. London: Blackwell Scientific Publications, 1989.

Stein E. Rapid Analysis of Electrocardiograms: A Self-Study Course. 2nd ed. Baltimore: Williams & Wilkins, 1992.

Wagner GS. Marriott's Practical Electrocardiography. 9th ed. Baltimore: Williams & Wilkins, 1994.

Atherosclerosis

Gopa Bhattacharyya and Peter Libby

Atherosclerosis is a disease of muscular arteries, in which the inner layer becomes thickened by fatty deposits and fibrous tissue. Often referred to as "hardening of the arteries," this condition frequently involves the coronary and cerebral vessels, leading to myocardial infarctions and strokes. As a result, atherosclerosis is responsible for the majority of deaths in industrialized societies, including more than half of the yearly mortality in the United States. Although it is so prevalent, and its pathologic hallmarks have been recognized for more than a century, the mechanisms by which atherosclerosis develops remain incompletely understood.

This chapter describes the pathologic lesions of atherosclerosis, reviews the epidemiologic risk factors associated with this condition and focuses on the cellular and biochemical processes that may contribute to its development.

THE ARTERIAL WALL

The wall of normal muscular arteries consists of three layers (Fig. 5.1): the intima (closest to the arterial lumen and therefore most "intimate" with the blood), the media (the middle layer), and the outer adventitia.

The **intima** is composed of a single layer of endothelial cells that rests on a bed of connective tissue. The endothelium forms a barrier that contains circulating blood within the lumen of the vessel, and in the normal artery, serves many additional metabolic and signaling functions that help maintain the integrity of the vessel wall. When atherosclerotic lesions develop, they form within the intimal layer.

The **media** is the thickest layer of the normal arterial wall, and is separated from the intima and adventitia by the internal and external elastic laminae, respectively. These laminae contain openings between elastic fibers through which cells can pass. The media is composed mainly of smooth muscle cells in a matrix of collagen, elastin, and proteoglycans. In large elastic arteries (such as the aorta and its primary branches), the media stretches during systole from the high pressure generated by the heart, then recoils during diastole such that blood is propelled forward throughout the cardiac cycle. In the smaller muscular arteries, the degree of contraction of the smooth muscle cells within the media determines the resistance of the vessel, and therefore regulates blood flow through the lumen.

The outermost layer of the arterial wall, the **adventitia,** contains fibroblasts and collagen, as well as blood vessels (vasa vasorum), nerves, and lymphatics that service

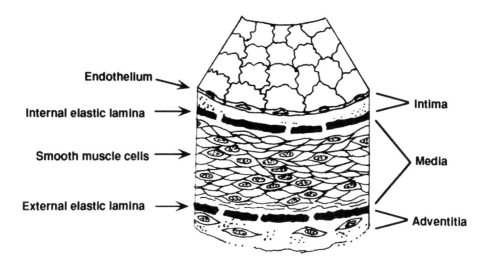

Figure 5.1.   Schematic diagram of the arterial wall. The intima is the innermost layer and is separated from the muscular media by the internal elastic membrane. The external elastic lamina separates the media from the outer adventitia. (Modified from Ross R, Glomset J. The pathogenesis of atherosclerosis. N Engl J Med 1976;295:369.)

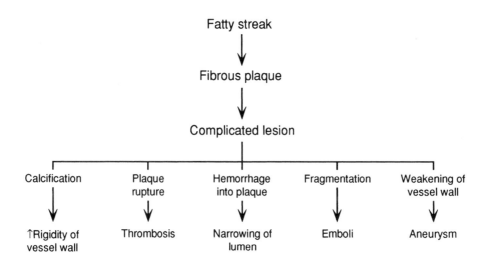

Figure 5.2.   Sequence of lesion development in atherosclerosis. Complications of the fibrous plaque lead to clinical manifestations of the disease.

the artery. The adventitia is not thought to be directly involved in the development of atherosclerotic lesions.

PATHOLOGIC LESIONS OF ATHEROSCLEROSIS

The pathological hallmarks of atherosclerosis are the **fatty streak** and the **fibrous plaque.** Figure 5.2 summarizes the developmental sequence by which these abnormalities ultimately lead to clinically apparent disease.

Fatty Streak

Fatty streaks represent the earliest visible lesions of atherosclerosis. At the gross level, they are areas of yellow discoloration on the inner surface of the artery. They often appear as spots less than 1 mm in diameter or streaks 1 to 2 mm wide and up to 1 cm long (Fig. 5.3). They do not protrude

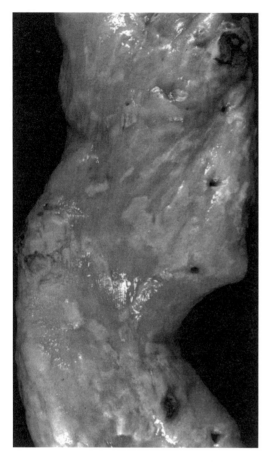

Figure 5.3. Gross specimen of an aorta with extensive fatty streak formation. (Courtesy of Dr. Frederick Schoen, Brigham & Women's Hospital, Boston, MA.)

into the arterial lumen, and do not disturb blood flow.

When examined microscopically, fatty streaks are characterized by the subendothelial accumulation of large "**foam cells**" filled with intracellular lipid (Fig. 5.4). Using monoclonal antibody techniques, it has been demonstrated that the majority of foam cells in fatty streaks are derived from macrophages, with a lesser contribution by smooth muscle cells.

Fatty streaks develop early in life and can be found in the aorta and coronary arteries of most individuals by age 20. They do not cause symptoms, and in some locations in the vasculature, they may regress over time. However, in other locations such as the coronary arteries, fatty streaks appear to be precursors of the more ominous fibrous plaques.

Fibrous Plaque

Fibrous plaques are more advanced lesions of atherosclerosis and are the source of the clinical manifestations of the disease. Fibrous plaques appear to develop from fatty streaks, and are located in coronary arteries and other vessels at the same sites where fatty streaks typically appear. Grossly, the fibrous plaque (Fig. 5.5) is a firm, pale gray, elevated lesion. It may project into the arterial lumen and, if sufficiently large, constitute a clinically significant stenosis that reduces blood flow through the vessel.

Histologically, most of the arterial

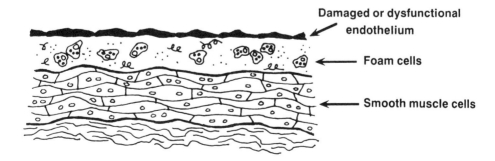

Figure 5.4. Schematic representation of the fatty streak. There is the subendothelial accumulation of large lipid-laden cells, known as foam cells, primarily of macrophage origin.

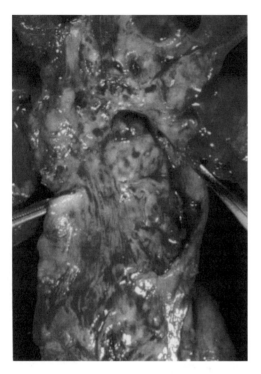

Figure 5.5.   Gross specimen of an abdominal aorta with extensive fibrous plaque formation. (Courtesy of Dr. Frederick Schoen, Brigham & Women's Hospital, Boston, MA.)

changes of the fibrous plaque occur in the intimal layer, where there is an accumulation of monocytes, lymphocytes, foam cells, and connective tissue. Unlike the fatty streak, most of the foam cells appear to be of smooth muscle origin. Fibrous plaques often contain a necrotic core of cell debris, degenerating foam cells, and cholesterol crystals, and are separated from the arterial lumen by a **fibrous cap,** largely composed of extracellular connective tissue matrix with embedded smooth muscle cells (Fig. 5.6).

Fibrous plaques are not distributed homogeneously throughout the vasculature in affected individuals. They are most common within the abdominal aorta, followed in frequency by the coronary arteries, popliteal arteries, descending thoracic aorta, internal carotid arteries, and the vessels that compose the circle of Willis of the brain. The regions perfused by these vessels are the ones most likely to suffer the consequences of atherosclerosis.

The clinical impact of fibrous plaques is that complications may ensue that restrict blood flow through the artery or alter the integrity of the vessel wall (Fig. 5.2). These complications can result from:

1. Calification of fibrous plaque, imparting a pipelike rigidity to the vessel wall, increasing its fragility.
2. Rupture or ulceration of the fibrous plaque, which exposes thrombogenic material to circulating blood, causing a thrombus to form at that site. Such thrombosis can occlude the vessel, resulting in, for example, myocardial infarction or stroke. Alternatively, the thrombus material can also be incorporated into the plaque, enlarging its size.
3. Hemorrhage into the fibrous plaque from rupture of the fibrous cap or of the tiny capillaries that vascularize the plaque. The resulting hematoma may further narrow the vessel lumen.
4. Embolization of fragments of disrupted atheroma to distal sites
5. Weakening of the vessel wall, as the fibrous plaque subjects the neighboring medial layer to increased pressure, which may provoke atrophy and loss of elastic tissue, with subsequent dilatation of the artery (i.e., formation of an aneurysm).

The clinical significance of these complications are described later, in Chapters 6, 7, and 15.

EPIDEMIOLOGIC RISK FACTORS

By examining whom atherosclerosis strikes, we can learn something about its pathogenesis. It has long been known that the prevalence of clinically significant atherosclerosis is highest in societies with a large meat consumption, and much less so among populations where less fatty diets are the staple. For example, the death rate due to coronary artery disease has historically been much lower in Japan than in the United States. This fact is possibly related to dietary differences, because studies of Japanese individuals who have moved to the United States and follow an American diet and lifestyle show a significant increase

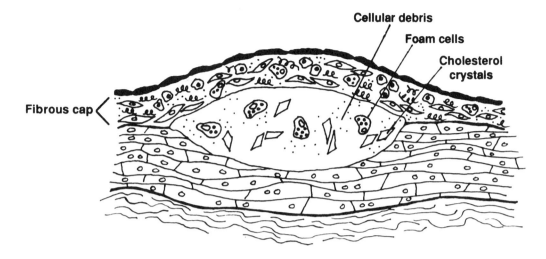

Figure 5.6.   Schematic representation of the fibrous plaque. A necrotic core of cell debris, foam cells, and cholesterol crystals is present under a fibrous cap of connective tissue and smooth muscle cells within the intima.

in total cholesterol levels and the frequency of coronary-related death.

Several large epidemiological studies in the United States and in Europe have provided much information about the habits or traits that correlate with the development of atherosclerosis and ischemic heart disease. One of these is the Framingham Heart Study, in which residents of a Massachusetts town have been observed for several decades to identify the relationship between certain risk factors and the development of coronary disease. Another is the Multiple Risk Factor Intervention Trial (MRFIT), in which more than 325,000 men were evaluated for the relationship between risk factors and subsequent cardiovascular disease and mortality. Through such studies it has been possible to identify four major, potentially modifiable risk factors associated with atherosclerosis: 1) aberrant levels of circulating lipids (termed "dyslipidemia"), 2) hypertension, 3) cigarette smoking, and 4) diabetes mellitus.

Several major nonmodifiable risk factors have also been identified, including advanced age, male sex, and a history of the development of coronary disease among family members at a young age (i.e., male family members before age 55 or female family members before age 65). Additional "minor" risk factors that are potentially

modifiable include obesity, a sedentary lifestyle, and stressful emotional behavior. An elevated circulating level of the amino acid homocysteine has also recently been identified as an independent risk factor, as described below.

Dyslipidemia

A large body of evidence indicates that abnormal circulating lipid levels are a major risk factor for the development of atherosclerosis. Observational studies have shown that societies with relatively high total cholesterol levels have the highest mortality rates due to coronary artery disease. For example, in countries with low saturated fat intake and low serum cholesterol levels (e.g., Japan and certain Mediterranean states) the mortality due to coronary artery disease is low, compared with the United States and other societies where fat consumption and cholesterol levels are higher. Similarly, data from the Framingham Study and many other trials have shown that the risk of ischemic heart disease increases with higher cholesterol levels: The coronary risk is approximately twice as high for an individual with a total cholesterol of 240 mg/dl than for one with a cholesterol of 200 mg/dl. However, not *all* cholesterol is "bad," as revealed by reviewing the various forms of circulating lipids and their functions.

Pathways of Cholesterol Transport

Lipoproteins are the carriers for lipids in the bloodstream. They consist of a lipid core surrounded by soluble phospholipid and free cholesterol, and apoproteins, which serve a role in directing the lipoproteins to specific organ and tissue receptors. There are five major classes of lipoproteins, which are differentiated by their densities, lipid constituents, and associated apoproteins (Table 5.1).

Figure 5.7 summarizes the major lipoprotein pathways in the circulation. Fats ingested in the diet enter a cycle known as the **exogenous pathway.** When cholesterol and triglycerides are consumed, they are absorbed in the intestine, incorporated into chylomicrons in intestinal epithelial cells, and transported through the lymphatics and then into the venous circulation. These large, triglyceride-rich particles are hydrolyzed by the enzyme lipoprotein lipase, which releases fatty acids into peripheral tissues, such as adipose tissue and muscle cells. The metabolic remnants of the chylomicrons that remain in the circulation are composed largely of cholesterol. These remnants are absorbed by the liver, which releases the lipid as either free cholesterol or bile acids back into the intestine.

In the **endogenous pathway,** very low density lipoprotein (VLDL) is released by the liver into the circulation. Although the major lipid constituent of VLDL is triglyc-

eride with a much smaller proportion of cholesterol, this is the main route by which cholesterol enters into the bloodstream from the liver. Lipoprotein lipase acts on VLDL at muscle cells and adipose tissue to release free fatty acids into the cells, and the lipoprotein residue in the circulation is termed an intermediate density lipoprotein (IDL) remnant, which contains mostly esterified cholesterol. Further processing of IDL in the circulation results in the formation of cholesterol-rich low density lipoprotein (LDL) particles. Approximately 75% of the circulating LDL is eventually taken up by the liver and extrahepatic cells through LDL receptor-mediated mechanisms. The remainder is degraded independently of classical LDL receptor mechanisms, largely by monocyte scavengers.

Cholesterol released back into the circulation by peripheral tissue cellular turnover is thought to be transported by high density lipoprotein (HDL) particles, which ultimately return cholesterol to the liver via IDL and LDL (by a process termed *reverse cholesterol transport*) for recycling into lipoproteins or excretion into the bile. In this way, HDL appears to serve a protective role against the potential accumulation of lipids in atherosclerotic lesions. In large epidemiologic studies, the circulating HDL level correlates *inversely* with the development of atherosclerosis. Thus HDL is often referred to as "good" cholesterol in contrast to the "bad" LDL.

Seventy percent of the cholesterol in the plasma is transported as LDL, and elevated LDL levels correlate closely with atherosclerosis development. In the late 1970s, Drs. Brown and Goldstein demonstrated

---

TABLE 5.1. Plasma Lipoproteins (In Order of Increasing Density)

Type	Source	Major Lipid Component	Associated Apoproteins
Chylomicrons	GI tract	Triglcerides	A-I, A-II, A-IV, B-48, C-1, C-II, C-III, E
VLDL	Liver	Triglycerides	B-100, C-I, C-II, C-III, E
IDL	Remnant of VLDL	Cholesterol	B100, E
LDL	Metabolism of IDL	Cholesterol	B100
HDL	Liver, GI tract	Cholesterol	A-I, A-II, C-I, C-II, C-III, E

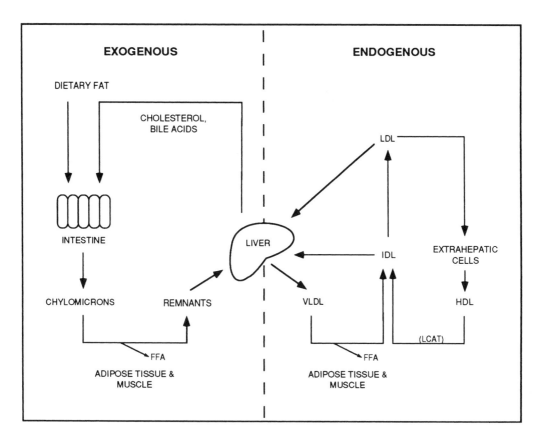

Figure 5.7. Overview of the lipoprotein transport system. In the exogenous pathway, dietary fats are incorporated into chylomicrons in the GI tract, and enter the circulation through the lymphatic system. Free fatty acids (FFAs) are removed at peripheral cells (e.g., adipose tissue and muscle), and the lipoprotein remnant returns to the liver, where the cholesterol content can be re-exported to the GI tract, or used for other hepatic processes. In the endogenous pathway, triglyceride-rich very low density lipoproteins (VLDLs) are released from the liver, and their FFAs are removed and deposited in peripheral adipose cells and muscle. The resultant intermediate density lipoprotein (IDL) is converted to low density lipoprotein (LDL), the major transport lipoprotein for cholesterol in the circulation. The majority of LDL is taken up by the liver and other peripheral cells via receptor-mediated endocytosis. Cholesterol released into the circulation by cellular turnover is transported by high density lipoproteins (HDLs), and is delivered to IDL by the action of circulating lecithin:cholesterol acyltransferase (LCAT), for ultimate return to the liver. (Modified from Brown MS, Goldstein JL. The hyperlipo-proteinemias and other disorders of lipid metabolism. In: Wilson JE, et al., eds. Harrison's principles of internal medicine. 12th ed. New York: McGraw Hill, 1991:1816.)

the central role of the LDL receptor for the delivery of cholesterol to tissues and clearance of cholesterol from the bloodstream. Expression of the LDL receptor is regulated by negative feedback inhibition: Normal or high intracellular cholesterol levels suppress expression of the LDL receptor at the transcriptional level, whereas reduced intracellular cholesterol increases expression of the receptor with subsequent enhanced cellular uptake of LDL. Patients with genetic defects in the LDL receptor (usually heterozygotes with one normal and one de-

fective gene for the receptor) cannot remove LDL from the circulation efficiently, have high plasma LDL levels, and are prone to develop premature atherosclerosis. This condition is called *familial hypercholesterolemia*. Homozygotes for the *total* absence of LDL receptors are only rarely encountered, but such individuals may sustain a myocardial infarction as early as the first decade of life.

Recently, subclasses of LDL have been identified, based on the buoyant densities of the particles. Individuals with smaller, denser LDL particles (a characteristic that is determined by genetic and environmental factors) have a greater risk of myocardial infarction than those with the less dense varieties. It is not yet clear why denser LDL particles confer more risk, but this attribute may relate to the greater susceptibility of dense particles to oxidation, a key aspect of atherogenesis, as described below.

There is increasing evidence that serum triglycerides, carried largely as VLDL and IDL, may also be important in the development of atherosclerotic lesions. It is not yet clear whether this is a direct effect, or because the triglyceride level generally varies inversely with the circulating HDL level. Adult-onset diabetes mellitus is one common clinical condition associated with hypertriglyceridemia and low HDL levels, often accompanied by obesity and hypertension. This clustering of risk factors, which may relate to a state of insulin-resistance (discussed in Chapter 13) is particularly atherogenic.

Benefits of Treatment of Dyslipidemia

Many recent studies of patients with coronary disease have shown that dietary or pharmacological reduction of serum cholesterol can prevent progression of coronary atherosclerotic lesions. Some data has actually shown modest *regression* of the narrowings within coronary arteries in patients treated with certain anticholesterol drugs. More important, pharmacologic reduction of LDL cholesterol has been shown to result in a significant fall in the incidence of myocardial infarction and mortality in treated patients, *out of proportion* to the benefit expected by the improvement in arterial narrowings. The most pronounced benefit has been demonstrated with drugs that competitively inhibit hydroxymethyl glutaryl CoA reductase (HMG CoA reductase), the rate-limiting enzymatic step in cholesterol synthesis. These potent reducers of circulating LDL are thought to improve outcome by reducing the lipid content of atherosclerotic plaques, thus reducing the vulnerability of such lesions to rupture. The remarkable beneficial clinical outcome of lipid-lowering is consistent with the proposed pathogenetic role of LDL cholesterol in the development of atherosclerosis.

Current national guidelines recommend that cholesterol screening be performed in all adults. For the general population, the desired total serum cholesterol level is less than 200 mg/dL, the LDL cholesterol level ≤ 130 mg/dL and an HDL level ≥ 35 mg/dL. Dietary and often pharmacologic therapy is recommended for individuals who do not meet these goals, particularly if major risk factors for atherosclerosis development are known to be present. Even lower target values of LDL cholesterol (≤ 100 mg/dL) are recommended for those with known coronary disease or previous myocardial infarction.

Elevated Lipoprotein (A) as a Risk Factor for Atherosclerosis

Another independent lipoprotein-associated cardiovascular risk factor has been identified, known as lipoprotein (a). Lipoprotein (a), the level of which is primarily genetically determined, is similar to the LDL particle, but it is linked to a specific apoprotein known as apo(a) by a disulfide bridge. Apo(a) structurally resembles plasminogen, a plasma protein that is important for the endogenous lysis of fibrin clots (see Chapter 7). It has been postulated that the detrimental effect of increased lipoprotein (a) levels may relate to inhibition of the normal thrombolytic activity of plasminogen.

Effect of Estrogen

Before menopause, women have a lower incidence of coronary events than men. After menopause, however, the coronary risk is equal between the sexes, and cardiovascular events are the major cause of mortality in women, significantly outweighing the number of deaths from other conditions, including breast cancer. A normal serum estrogen level lowers LDL and lipoprotein (a) and raises HDL cholesterol levels, which may partly explain its protective role against coronary lesions. Estrogen also demonstrates potentially beneficial antioxident and antiplatelet actions.

Since estrogen levels fall after menopause, treatment of postmenopausal women with hormone replacement therapy is often undertaken, particularly if hypercholesterolemia and other cardiac risk factors are present. However, estrogen replacement therapy may increase the risk of endometrial cancer. The addition of a progestin-containing hormone supplement reduces that cancer risk, and does not appear to attenuate the beneficial cardiovascular effect of estrogen alone.

Tobacco Smoking

Tobacco smoking is perhaps the most preventable of all cardiac risk factors. Numerous studies have shown an increased risk of atherosclerosis, ischemic heart disease, and sudden death among smokers. The relative risk of dying from coronary disease has ranged between 1.35 and 2.40 in studies of all smokers, and between 1.43 and 3.50 in heavy smokers. Tobacco smoking is a cardiac risk factor in its own right, and can also potentiate the cardiovascular complications associated with other known risk factors.

The amount of nicotine and other chemicals absorbed by a smoker are highly variable, so that it is difficult to directly relate the number of cigarettes smoked with the risk of atherosclerosis. It is clear, however, that even minimal tobacco smoking increases cardiac risk, and that the danger is greatest among the heaviest smokers. Studies also indicate that low-tar and low-nicotine cigarettes do not significantly decrease the risk of myocardial infarction compared with regular cigarettes.

It is not precisely known why cigarette smoking leads to atherosclerotic events and coronary heart disease. Potential mechanisms include: decreases in circulating HDL levels, inappropriate stimulation of the sympathetic nervous system by nicotine, displacement of oxygen by carbon monoxide from hemoglobin, increased platelet ad-

hesiveness, and endothelial dysfunction due to cigarette smoke constituents.

Fortunately, some of this adverse potential is reversible. Epidemiologic studies have shown that people who stop smoking reduce their incidence of coronary heart disease compared with those who continue to smoke. In one study, after three years of cessation, the risk for the development of coronary artery disease became similar to subjects who never smoked.

Hypertension

Elevated blood pressure (either systolic or diastolic) is a risk factor for the development of atherosclerosis, coronary heart disease, and stroke (see Chapter 13). There is not a specific threshold above which an elevated pressure is associated with cardiovascular disease; rather there is a continuum of risk associated with progressively higher pressures. The mechanism by which hypertension contributes to atherosclerosis is not known. However, animal studies have shown that elevated blood pressure injures vascular endothelium, and may increase the permeability of the vessel wall to lipoproteins.

Dietary or pharmacological reduction of hypertension reduces the risk of stroke, and to a lesser degree coronary vascular complications. It is widely believed that recognition and treatment of hypertension have significantly contributed to the 57% decline in mortality from stroke and 50% decline in mortality from coronary heart disease in the United States over the past two decades.

Diabetes Mellitus

Diabetes is also a risk factor for atherosclerosis, but measuring that risk is difficult, because diabetics frequently also suffer from other atherogenic conditions such as hypertension and dyslipidemia. It has been postulated that the increased risk relates to glycosylation of lipoproteins in diabetics (which may enhance uptake of cholesterol by scavenger macrophages, as discussed below) or to the increased platelet adhesiveness present in this condition. It has not yet been established whether tight control of serum glucose levels in diabetics reduces the risk of atherosclerotic lesions, as has been shown for the microvascular complications (e.g., retinopathy) of this disease.

Homocysteinemia

In addition to the traditional risk factors indicated above, recent studies have shown a significant relationship between circulating levels of the amino acid homocysteine and the incidence of coronary, cerebral, and peripheral artery disease. The risk of a myocardial infarction is approximately threefold higher in individuals with the highest levels of homocysteine compared with patients with the lowest values. The mechanism by which homocysteine increases atherosclerotic risk is not known, but current evidence suggests that abnormally high amounts of this amino acid may injure endothelial cells in the arterial wall. Supplementation of the diet with folic acid and other B vitamins can reduce the level of homocysteine, but it is not yet known whether such treatment reduces the coronary risk.

CELLULAR ELEMENTS OF THE VESSEL WALL

The participation of key cells within the arterial wall is necessary for the development of atherosclerotic lesions. Among the most important are endothelial cells of the arterial intima, and the vascular smooth muscle cells.

Endothelial Cells

Endothelial cells line the intima of blood vessels and serve critically important structural, metabolic, and paracrine functions in the normal state (Table 5.2). First, they form a barrier that contains circulating blood within the lumen of the vessel. The endothelial cells are joined firmly together, limiting the passage of large molecules from the circulation into the subendothelial space.

Second, the endothelium resists clot formation because of the expression of antithrombotic surface molecules (e.g., heparan sulfate, thrombomodulin, and plasminogen activators, as described in Chapter 7), and through the release of platelet inhibitors, including prostacyclin and endothelium-derived relaxing factor. The latter substance has been identified as nitric oxide, or a closely related derivative, and will be referred to as EDRF-NO in the remainder of this text. The actions of these important mediators are described in Chapter 6.

Third, endothelial cells secrete vasoactive substances that directly modulate contraction of the smooth muscle cells in the underlying medial layer. In the normal artery, the effect of certain vasodilator substances predominate (e.g., prostacyclin and EDRF-NO), contributing to relaxation of the smooth muscle, which increases the diameter of the vessel.

Finally, through secretion of specific products (such as heparan sulfate and EDRF-NO), endothelial cells inhibit smooth muscle cell migration and proliferation, which may also serve an important antiatherosclerotic role, as we will examine. Thus, in its normal state, the endothelial layer of the intima provides a protective nonthrombogenic surface, is metabolically active, and produces vasoactive substances.

In distinction, when endothelial cells become injured or dysfunctional, their activity is modified in ways that may contribute to atherosclerosis (Table 5.2). First, the permeability of the injured endothelial layer may increase, such that the cells no longer serve as a barrier to the passage of cells and large molecules from the circulation into the subendothelial space. Second, injured endothelial cells may lose their antithrombotic properties because of reduced production of prostacyclin and EDRF-NO. Third, the reduced secretion of vasodilators (e.g.,

TABLE 5.2. Endothelial Cell Functions

Activity	Normal endothelium	"Injured" endothelium
Barrier function	Forms tight barrier that restricts passage of large molecules and cells into subendothelial space	Demonstrates increased permeability
Antithrombotic activity	Resists thrombosis through actions of heparan sulfate, thrombo-modulin, plasminogen activators and secretion of platelet inhibitors (prostacyclin, EDRF-NO)	Reduced antithrombotic properties (e.g., decreased secretion of prostacyclin and EDRF-NO)
Effect on vascular tone	Promotes vasodilation through secretion of prostacyclin and EDRF-NO	Promotes vasoconstriction because of impaired secretion of prostacyclin and EDRF-NO
Effect on arterial smooth muscle cells	Inhibits smooth muscle cell migration and proliferation (via heparan sulfate and EDRF-NO)	Promotes smooth muscle cell migration and proliferation (decreased secretion of EDRF-NO, increased secretion of PDGF)

EDRF-NO, endothelium-derived relaxing factor–nitric oxide; PDGF, platelet-derived growth factor.

prostacyclin and EDRF-NO) impairs smooth muscle cell relaxation in the arterial media, resulting in relative vasoconstriction. Fourth, injured endothelial cells secrete increased amounts of mitogenic substances, such as platelet-derived growth factor (PDGF) that recruit smooth muscle cells into the intima and stimulate their replication. Finally, the injured endothelium secretes chemotactic factors that attract other key cells toward the intima, including circulating monocytes, which are involved in the development of atherosclerotic lesions, as discussed below.

Vascular Smooth Muscle Cells

Current evidence suggests that a key event in atherogenesis involves proliferation of smooth muscle cells within the arterial intima, and that the muscle cells are derived primarily from the medial layer. Stimuli for movement and proliferation of these cells will be described below.

Smooth muscle cells within the vessel wall exhibit phenotypic heterogeneity, both in physiologic and in disease states (Fig. 5.8). In the normal artery, smooth muscle cells of the "*contractile*" phenotype contain large numbers of contractile proteins, to serve the role of myofibril shortening and cellular contraction. Smooth muscle cells in

this state express receptors for many vasoactive substances such as angiotensin II, catecholamines, and endothelin. When a vasoactive ligand binds to its specific receptor, myocyte contraction or relaxation follows, thus altering the diameter of the vessel's lumen and blood flow through it.

In contrast, smooth muscle cells of the "*synthetic*" phenotype are characterized by less abundant myofibrils in the cytoplasm. Rather, there is prominent rough endoplasmic reticulum and Golgi apparatus, reflecting active protein synthesis. Smooth muscle cells of this phenotype produce the collagen, elastin, and proteoglycans that form the matrix of the blood vessel media. They also express receptors for chemotactic and mitogenic factors such as PDGF, in response to which smooth muscle cells migrate from the media into the intima and proliferate. "Synthetic" smooth muscle cells can also produce their own mitogenic factors (including PDGF), possibly leading to autostimulation and proliferation.

There is evidence that smooth muscle cells within atherosclerotic lesions have changed from the contractile to the synthetic phenotype. This alteration in cellular function may be crucial to the responsiveness to key agonists, extracellular matrix formation, and smooth muscle cell proliferation that characterize developing atherosclerotic plaques.

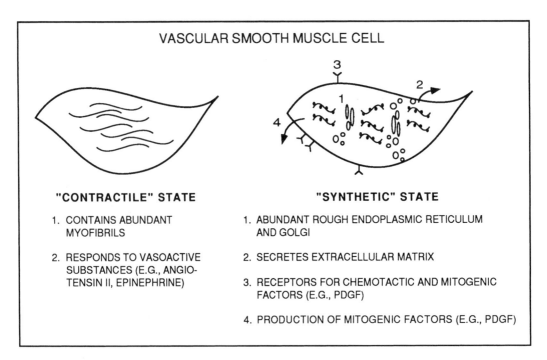

Figure 5.8.   Phenotypic modulation of the vascular smooth muscle cell. The features of the "synthetic" state likely contribute to the atherosclerotic process. PDGF, platelet-derived growth factor.

PATHOGENESIS OF ATHEROSCLEROSIS

Although the events that lead to atherosclerotic lesions remain incompletely understood, several key steps have been identified (Fig. 5.9). Atherogenesis requires the participation of cells within the vessel wall (endothelial cells and smooth muscle cells), circulating blood elements (monocytes, platelets), lipoproteins, and certain chemical mediators (termed cytokines).

Endothelial Dysfunction

Many researchers believe that *the primary event in atherogenesis is "injury" to the arterial endothelium.* There are several lines of evidence to support this conclusion. For example, it has been observed that advanced atherosclerotic lesions do not occur randomly within blood vessels, but are most common at arterial branch points. These are the areas of turbulence where the greatest possibility for endothelial trauma exists. The second

line of evidence is derived from the known risk factors of atherosclerosis discussed above. A common mechanism is that each of the risk factors can cause abnormal function of endothelial cells. Cigarette smoking, for example, causes increased circulating carbon monoxide levels and tissue hypoxia, which can injure the endothelium. High LDL or low HDL concentrations can lead to excess cholesterol available to be taken up by, and damage, the intimal layer. Hypertension directly increases the hemodynamic stress on endothelial cells. A third line of evidence that implicates endothelial injury as an initial event in atherogenesis is that in animal models, atheromatous lesions have been shown to develop in response to endothelial injury.

Until recently, it was thought that the type of endothelial injury that triggers atherogenesis requires physical trauma to, and loss of, endothelial cells. It is now known that structural disruption of endothelial cells is actually *not* necessary. In fact, several of the early changes in the developing atherosclerotic lesion, including

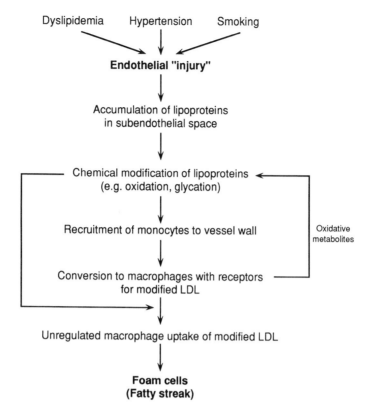

Figure 5.9.   The modified response-to-injury hypothesis of atherosclerosis. Endothelial "injury" is triggered by a large number of conditions, including dyslipidemia (high LDL or low HDL), hypertension, and cigarette smoking. Endothelial dysfunction permits accumulation of lipoproteins in the subendothelial space, where chemical modification of LDL can occur. Modified LDL recruits monocytes into the vessel wall, where these cells are converted to macrophages that engulf the modified lipoproteins. The unregulated uptake of modified LDL results in large foam cells, a prominent characteristic of the fatty streak.

the accumulation of lipids within the arterial wall, and entry of monocytes, occur through an *intact* surface of endothelial cells. As we will examine, these early features rely on specific biochemical modifications and cellular signaling pathways, rather than structural disruption of the endothelial cell layer.

Many of the risk factors associated with atherosclerosis (high LDL cholesterol, smoking, hypertension, diabetes) predispose to endothelial dysfunction. Even before atherosclerotic lesions are physically apparent, such dysfunction may be manifest by: 1) impairment of the endothelium's role as a permeability barrier, 2) interference with normal antithrombotic properties, and 3) altered release of vasoactive substances (e.g., prostacyclin and EDRF-NO), affecting the tone of the underlying smooth

muscle. These undesired effects of endothelial dysfunction lay the groundwork for subsequent events in atherosclerosis development.

Recently, certain infectious agents (e.g., herpesvirus group, chlamydia) have been observed in some atherosclerotic lesions, raising the question of their potential role in atherogenesis. Although this relationship has not been proved, some researchers believe that infectious agents are an additional source of endothelial injury that could initiate atherogenesis.

The process by which endothelial injury and dysfunction are presumed to be the initiating event in atherogenesis is known as the modified **response-to-injury hypothesis.** The sequence of events that follow endothelial injury remains the subject of ongoing research, and this discussion (and the schematic presented in Figure 5.9) should be considered a general framework, the specific details of which will likely undergo refinement as further knowledge evolves.

Lipoprotein Entry and Modification

When the endothelium becomes dysfunctional, it no longer serves as an effective barrier to the passage of circulating substances into the arterial wall. For example, increased endothelial permeability allows the transport of low-density lipoprotein into the intima, a process facilitated by an elevated circulating LDL concentration. Once within the intima, LDL accumulates in the subendothelial space by binding to components of the extracellular matrix. This "trapping" increases the residence time of LDL within the vessel wall, where the lipoprotein may undergo chemical modifications that appear critical to the development of atherosclerotic lesions.

A major modification of LDL that occurs in the subendothelial space is *oxidation* of the lipoprotein by local oxygen free radicals and enzymes. The source of the oxidizing substances is likely the overlying endothelial cells, and later macrophages that penetrate the vessel wall. In diabetics with sustained hyperglycemia, glycation of LDL is another way in which the lipoprotein can be biochemically modified.

The biochemical modification of LDL has two major consequences: 1) modified LDL (mLDL) acts as a chemoattractant that recruits circulating monocytes to the vessel wall, and 2) unlike normal LDL particles, mLDL can be ingested by macrophages and other cells in large quantities. Recall that normal organ uptake of circulating LDL is regulated by LDL-receptors that are subject to negative feedback inhibition. For example, when the internal cholesterol content of a liver cell increases, the number of LDL receptors on the surface of the cell decreases, with a subsequent reduction of further uptake of the lipoprotein. Conversely, LDL that has been biochemically modified (by oxidation or glycation) is not recognized by the LDL receptor and cannot be internal-

ized by that mechanism. Rather, mLDL is recognized by, and taken up by means of "scavenger" receptors on macrophages and other cells, and this internalization pathway is *not* regulated by negative feedback inhibition. Therefore, very large amounts of modified LDL can be ingested by such cells in an unregulated fashion, contributing to the development of the large "foam cells" of the fatty streak.

Recruitment of Leukocytes

Following the entry and biochemical modification of LDL, a subsequent key step in atherogenesis is the attraction of leukocytes, primarily monocytes and T lymphocytes, toward the vessel wall. Factors that contribute to this process are: 1) the chemoattractant nature of mLDL, 2) the expression of specific cytokines (e.g., tumor necrosis factor (TNF) and monocyte chemoattractant protein (MCP) secreted by the injured endothelial cells), and 3) the expression of adhesion molecules on the luminal surface of the injured endothelial cells. Examples of adhesion molecules include vascular cell adhesion molecule (VCAM-1) and intercellular adhesion molecule (ICAM-1), members of the immunoglobulin gene superfamily, and P-selectin, a distinct leukocyte receptor molecule. Constituents of oxidatively modified LDL have been shown to contribute to the expression of the VCAM gene, mechanistically linking the accumulation of lipid in the arterial intima with leukocyte recruitment. The likely importance of adhesion molecules in monocyte recruitment has been confirmed in animal experiments. For example, consumption of an atherogenic diet by rabbits results in the expression of VCAM preceding monocyte adhesion to the vessel wall.

After monocytes have adhered to the luminal surface of the intima, they may penetrate into the subendothelial space by slipping between the junctions of the endothelial monolayer. Once localized beneath the endothelium, monocytes differentiate into macrophages, the phagocytic cells that are able to ingest modified LDL in large quantities by the scavenger pathway described above. In doing so, macrophages become lipid-laden foam cells, the primary constituent of the fatty streak.

T lymphocytes, the principal mediators of the cellular immune system, also appear to play an important role in early atherosclerosis. T cells constitute a relatively small fraction of the cells within an atheromatous plaque, outnumbered by macrophages and smooth muscle cells. However, T cells become activated during atherogenesis, and produce cytokines that may modulate lesion formation.

Recruitment of Smooth Muscle Cells

The transition from fatty streak to fibrous plaque involves the migration of smooth muscle cells from the arterial media into the injured intima, proliferation of the smooth muscle cells within the intima, and secretion of large amounts of connective tissue by the smooth muscle cells. Substances re-

sponsible for smooth muscle cell migration and proliferation are produced chiefly by the foam cells, activated platelets, and endothelial cells (Fig. 5.10).

Foam cells elaborate several factors that contribute to smooth muscle cell recruitment. For example, they release platelet-derived growth factor (PDGF), which stimulates the migration of smooth muscle cells into the intimal subendothelial space, and their subsequent replication there. Foam cells also release cytokines and growth factors (e.g., tumor necrosis factor-α, interleukin-1, fibroblast growth factor, and transforming growth factor-β) that additionally stimulate smooth muscle cell proliferation and the production of extracellular matrix proteins. The increase in the smooth muscle cell mass growing from the medial layer into the diseased intima and the development of the surrounding fibrous cap of extracellular matrix tissue characterize the fibrous plaque of advanced atherosclerotic disease.

Foam cells also produce large amounts of tissue factor, a thrombogenic substance that can activate the coagulation pathway when

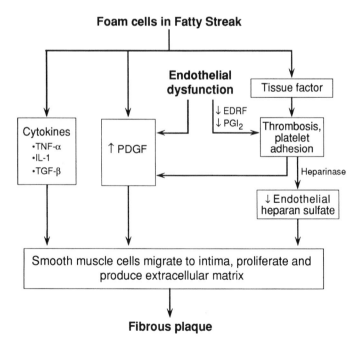

Figure 5.10.   The transition from fatty streak to fibrous plaque involves the migration and proliferation of smooth muscle cells and production of extracellular matrix. Substances released from foam cells, dysfunctional endothelial cells and platelets contribute to this process. TNF-α, tumor necrosis factor-α; IL-1, interleukin-1; TGF-β, transforming growth factor-β.

contact is made with circulating blood. Since the atheromatous plaque is covered by a fibrous cap and endothelium, the thrombogenic core containing tissue factor is usually "hidden" from the circulating blood. However, small breaches in the integrity of advanced atherosclerotic lesions may expose tissue factor, and microthrombi rich in platelets can then adhere to areas of the interrupted endothelium. The activated platelets within such microthrombi release potent factors that also contribute to smooth muscle cell migration and proliferation. These factors include PDGF (the actions of which are described above), and heparinase. The latter degrades heparan sulfate, a polysaccharide in the extracellular matrix that normally *inhibits* smooth muscle cell migration and proliferation.

For its part, the injured endothelial cell also plays a role in smooth muscle cell activities in the developing atheroma. The damaged endothelial cells may secrete increased amounts of PDGF and elaborate less EDRF-NO and prostacyclin, actions that further contribute to smooth muscle cell recruitment and proliferation.

Fibrous plaques often contain a central core of necrotic tissue. Cellular death may result from the toxic effects of highly oxidized LDL and the accumulation of oxygen-free radicals. The core lesion often contains degenerating foam cells, and the latter release cholesterol crystals, which may be-come engulfed by smooth muscles cells growing into the lesion.

Thus, atherosclerosis is currently considered to be a chronic inflammatory process of the arterial wall that develops in response to triggers that result in endothelial dysfunction, accumulation of lipids within the intima, recruitment of leucocytes and smooth muscle cells to the vessel wall, and deposition of extracellular matrix.

It should be noted that, in addition to this modified response-to-injury hypothesis, other theories of atherogenesis have been put forward, including those in which endothelial injury is not the primary event, but a secondary result. For example, the "monoclonal hypothesis" suggests that the initial event in atherogenesis is smooth muscle cell migration and proliferation into the intima, induced by genetic, chemical, or viral stimuli. The finding that the cells within some human atherosclerotic plaques appear to descend from a single smooth muscle cell support this view.

COMPLICATIONS OF ATHEROSCLEROSIS

Atherosclerotic plaques usually grow gradually and come to attention only when a lesion sufficiently restricts blood flow to an organ or alters the integrity of an artery such that clinical symptoms develop. The

TABLE 5.3. Complications of Atherosclerosis

Complication	Mechanism	Examples
Narrowing and calcification of vessel	Progressive development of fibrous plaque Organization of microthrombi within lesion Hemorrhage into plaque	Myocardial ischemia (see Ch. 6) Limb claudication (see Ch. 15)
Thrombus formation with occlusion of lumen	Plaque ulceration or rupture Plaque hemorrhage with rupture	Myocardial infarction or unstable angina Thrombotic stroke (cerebral infarction)
Peripheral emboli	Fragmentation and passage of atheromatous material from large proximal vessel to smaller peripheral vessels	Embolic stroke Atheroembolic renal failure
Weakening of vessel wall	Pressure on neighboring medial layer promotes atrophy of muscle cells and loss of elastic tissue	Aortic aneurysms (see Ch. 15)

major manifestations of atherosclerosis arise from complications of the fibrous plaque as demonstrated in Figure 5.2 and Table 5.3. For example, as described in the next chapter, atherosclerotic lesions within the coronary arteries may impair perfusion to the myocardium and produce intermittent chest discomfort (angina pectoris), the classic symptom of coronary artery disease. In other instances, a fibrous plaque may become complicated by a superimposed thrombus that fully obstructs a coronary artery, resulting in a sudden acute myocardial infarction (as described in Chapter 7).

Recent studies have shown that the degree of coronary artery narrowing (e.g., observed by coronary angiography) does not correlate well with the subsequent occurrence of myocardial infarction at sites of the highest grade stenosis. This supports the hypothesis that plaque rupture with superimposed thrombosis is the primary mechanism for acute coronary events, rather than vessel occlusion from gradual, progressive enlargement of fibrous plaque. The "culprit lesions" that lead to acute thrombosis (and a clinical event) are often unimpressive angiographically.

Factors that make such a plaque more susceptible to rupture include a relatively thin fibrous cap separating the foam cells (which contain tissue factor, the powerful procoagulant) from the circulating blood elements (Fig. 5.11). These "vulnerable"

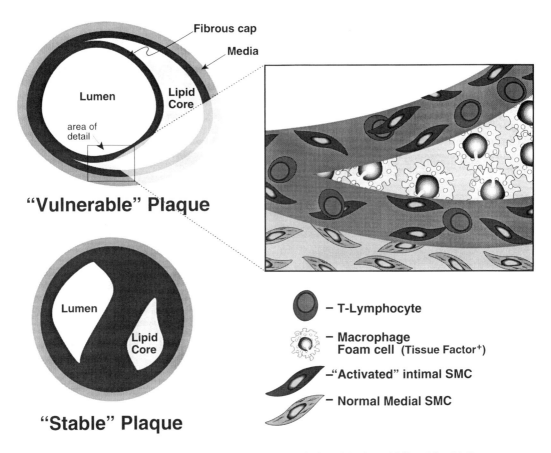

Figure 5.11. Schematic diagram demonstrating characteristics of "vulnerable" and "stable" atherosclerotic plaques. The vulnerable plaque usually has a substantial lipid core and a thin fibrous cap separating the thrombogenic macrophages (bearing tissue factor) from the blood. At sites of lesion disruption, smooth muscle cells (SMCs) are often activated. In contrast, the stable plaque has a thick fibrous cap protecting the lipid core from contact with the blood. Clinical data suggest that stable plaques more often show luminal narrowing detectable by angiography than do vulnerable plaques. (Reproduced with permission from Libby P. Molecular bases of the acute coronary syndromes. Circulation. 1995;91:2844–2850, copyright 1995, American Heart Association.)

plaques often grossly appear quite minor and do not impede luminal blood flow as much as chronic, stable plaques with thick fibrous caps that are less susceptible to rupture. The vulnerable sites are distinguished by a very rich lipid core and a high concentration of inflammatory cells (macrophages and T lymphocytes). The macrophages in such lesions are often localized at the borders of the plaque where it abuts normal tissue (the "shoulder regions") and release mediators of inflammation, as well as enzymes that can degrade and weaken the fibrous cap, making it more susceptible to rupture. In addition, gamma interferon, a T cell-derived mediator elaborated in response to chronic inflammation within plaque, can inhibit collagen synthesis by smooth muscle cells, and impede the ability of these cells to maintain and repair the fibrous cap that protects the plaque from rupture. Lesions that are able to synthesize and maintain a thick fibrous cap are less prone to rupture.

As indicated above, recent clinical trials of antilipid drug therapy have shown a dramatic reduction in coronary events, out of proportion to achieved reductions in coronary artery narrowing. It is postulated that the marked clinical benefit relates to reduction of the lipid burden within atherosclerotic plaque and therefore "stabilization" of the lesion, rendering it less likely to rupture.

SUMMARY

Atherosclerosis causes more deaths than any other disease in industrialized society. During atherogenesis, fatty deposits and fibrous tissue accumulate in the intima of muscular arteries. The earliest pathologic sign of atherosclerosis is the fatty streak, which may evolve into a fibrous plaque. The development of atherosclerotic lesions appears to involve the complex interplay between cells of the vessel wall (endothelial cells, smooth muscle cells), circulating cells (leukocytes, platelets), lipoproteins, and many cytokines and growth factors. Clini-

cal manifestations of atherosclerosis result from narrowing of the lumen and calification of vessel wall, plaque fissure or rupture leading to superimposed thrombus formation, intraplaque hemorrhage, and weakening of the arterial wall.

Major risk factors for the development of atherosclerosis include dyslipidemia (high LDL or low HDL), hypertension, smoking, a family history of premature coronary disease, and diabetes. Aggressive recognition of and correction of the modifiable risk factors are key to the practice of contemporary preventive cardiology, and will likely contribute to a continued decline in cardiovascular morbidity and mortality.

The next two chapters consider two of the most important complications of atherosclerosis: chronic ischemic heart disease and acute myocardial infarction.

ADDITIONAL READING

Berliner JA, et al. Atherosclerosis: basic mechanisms: oxidation, inflammation, and genetics. Circulation 1995;91:2488–2496.

Fuster V, Badimon L, Badimon JJ, et al. The pathogenesis of coronary artery disease and the acute coronary syndromes. N Engl J Med 1992;326:242–250 (Part I),326:310–318 (Part II).

Goldstein JL, Brown MS. A receptor-mediated pathway for cholesterol homeostasis. Science 1986;232: 34–47.

Grundy SM. Role of low-density lipoproteins in atherogenesis and development of coronary heart disease. Clin Chem 1995;41:139–146.

Hajjar DP, Nicholson AC. Atherosclerosis. Am Scientist 1995;83:460–467.

Levine GN, Keaney JF, Vita JA. Cholesterol reduction in cardiovascular disease. N Engl J Med 1995;332: 512–521.

Libby P. Molecular bases of acute coronary syndromes. Circulation 1995;91:2844–2850.

O'Keefe JH Jr, Conn RD, Lavie CJ Jr., et al. The new paradigm for coronary artery disease: altering risk factors, atherosclerotic plaques, and clinical prognosis. Mayo Clin Proc. 1996;71:957–965.

Ross R. The pathogenesis of atherosclerosis: a perspective for the 1990s. In: Braunwald E, ed. Heart Disease: A Textbook of Cardiovascular Medicine. Philadelphia: WB Saunders, 1997:1105–1125.

Summary of the Second Report of the National Cholesterol Education Project Expert Panel on Detection, Evaluation, and Treatment of High Blood Cholesterol in Adults. JAMA 1993;269:3015–3023.

Acknowledgments The previous edition of this chapter was written by Rushika Fernandopulle, MD, and Joseph Loscalzo, MD, PhD.

Ischemic Heart Disease

Marc S. Sabatine, Patrick T. O'Gara, and Leonard S. Lilly

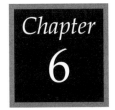
In 1772, the British physician William Heberden reported a disorder in which patients developed an uncomfortable sensation in the chest upon walking. Labeling it "angina pectoris," Heberden noted that this discomfort would disappear soon after the patient stood still, but would worsen again with exertion. Although he didn't know the cause of this sensation, it is likely that his report was the first to describe the symptoms of ischemic heart disease, a condition of insufficient myocardial perfusion, that now afflicts millions of Americans and accounts for more than 600,000 deaths annually.

The clinical presentation of ischemic heart disease is highly variable. It may be accompanied by the exertional symptoms originally described by Heberden, still known as angina pectoris. In other cases, ischemia may occur without any symptoms, a condition termed "silent" ischemia. This chapter describes the spectrum of syndromes associated with ischemic heart disease (Table 6.1), and the mechanisms by which they occur.

ETIOLOGY AND PATHOGENESIS OF ANGINA PECTORIS

The most common manifestation of ischemic heart disease, angina pectoris, literally means "strangling in the chest." Although many intrathoracic diseases may lead to similar chest discomfort, "angina" refers to that condition which arises from an imbalance between myocardial oxygen supply and demand. By far, the leading cause of that imbalance is coronary artery disease, in which a reduction in oxygen supply is due to atherosclerotic narrowings in one or more of the coronary arteries.

In the normal heart, there is a continuous match between the oxygen requirements of the myocardium and coronary arterial supply. Even during vigorous exercise, when the heart's metabolic needs increase, so does the delivery of oxygen to the myocardial cells, so that the balance is maintained. The following sections review the key determinants of myocardial oxygen supply and demand in normal individuals (Fig.

TABLE 6.1. Clinical Definitions

Syndrome	Description
Ischemic heart failure	Condition in which imbalance between myocardial oxygen supply and demand results in myocardial hypoxia and accumulation of waste metabolics; most often due to atherosclerotic disease of the coronary arteries ("coronary artery disease")
Angina pectoris	Uncomfortable sensation in the chest and neighboring anatomic structures produced by myocardial ischemia
Stable angina	Chronic pattern of transient angina pectoris, precipitated by physical activity or emotional upset, relieved by rest within a few minutes; episodes often associated with temporary depression of the ST segment, but permanent myocardial damage does not result
Variant angina	Typical anginal discomfort, usually *at rest*, which develops because of coronary artery spasm, rather than an increase of myocardial oxygen demand; episodes often associated with transient shifts of the ST segment (usually ST elevation)
Unstable angina	Pattern of increased frequency and duration of angina episodes, produced by less exertion, or at rest; high frequency of progression to myocardial infarction if untreated
Silent ischemia	Asymptomatic episodes of myocardial ischemia; can be detected by EKG and other laboratory techniques
Myocardial infarction (see Chapter 7)	Region of myocardial necrosis usually due to prolonged cessation of blood supply; most often results from acute thrombus at site of coronary atherosclerotic stenosis; may be first clinical manifestation of ischemic heart disease, or there may be a history of angina pectoris

6.1) and how they are altered by the presence of coronary artery disease.

Myocardial Oxygen Supply

The supply of oxygen to the myocardium depends on the **oxygen-carrying capacity** of the blood, and the rate of **coronary blood flow.** The oxygen-carrying capacity is determined by the hemoglobin content of the blood and systemic oxygenation. In the absence of anemia or lung disease, oxygen-carrying capacity remains fairly constant. However, coronary blood flow is much more dynamic, and regulation of that flow is responsible for matching the oxygen supply with metabolic requirements.

As in all blood vessels, coronary artery flow (Q) is directly proportional to the vessel's perfusion pressure (P) and is inversely proportional to coronary vascular resistance (R). This is expressed as $Q \propto P/R$.

However, unlike other arterial systems in which the greatest blood flow occurs during systole, *the coronary vessels demonstrate maximal flow during diastole.* This is so because systolic flow is compromised by compression of the coronaries by the contracting myocardium, as well as by the dynamics of left ventricular ejection into the aorta: During systole, rapid blood flow across the aortic valve produces a Venturi effect, in which there is a localized drop in pressure along the sides of the proximal aorta. This causes the systolic pressure within the aortic sinuses and coronary ostia to be lower than that of the aorta itself, and therefore reduces the perfusion pressure into the coronary arteries.

Coronary flow is unimpaired in diastole, because the pressure-lowering Venturi effect does not occur when the aortic valve is closed and rapid flow has ceased, and because the relaxed myocardium exerts little external compression on the coronary vessels. Thus in the case of the coronaries, the **perfusion pressure** is approximated by the aortic diastolic pressure. Conditions that decrease aortic diastolic pressure (e.g., hypotension or aortic regurgitation) decrease coronary artery perfusion pressure, and may impair myocardial oxygen supply.

Coronary vascular resistance is the other major determinant of coronary blood flow. In the normal artery, this resistance is dynamically modulated by: 1) forces that externally compress the coronary arteries,

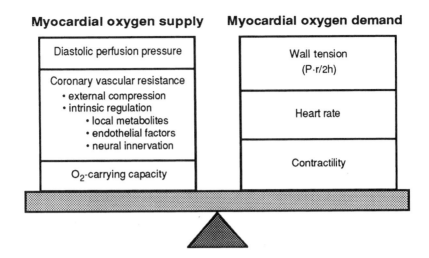

Myocardial oxygen supply

| Diastolic perfusion pressure |
| Coronary vascular resistance
• external compression
• intrinsic regulation
    • local metabolites
    • endothelial factors
    • neural innervation |
| O$_2$-carrying capacity |

Myocardial oxygen demand

| Wall tension
(P·r/2h) |
| Heart rate |
| Contractility |

Figure 6.1. Major determinants of myocardial oxygen supply and demand. P, ventricular systolic pressure; r, ventricular radius; h, ventricular wall thickness.

and 2) factors that affect intrinsic coronary tone.

External Compression

External compression is exerted on the coronary vessels during the cardiac cycle by contraction of the surrounding myocardium. The degree of compression is directly related to intramyocardial pressure, and is therefore greatest during systole, as indicated in the previous section. Moreover, when the myocardium contracts, the subendocardium, adjacent to the high intraventricular pressure, is subjected to greater force than the outer muscle layers. This is one reason why the subendocardium is the region most vulnerable to ischemic damage.

Intrinsic Control of Coronary Tone

Unlike most tissues, the heart cannot increase oxygen extraction on demand because in its basal state it removes nearly as much oxygen as it can from its blood supply. Thus, *any additional oxygen requirement must be met by an increase in blood flow,* and autoregulation of coronary vascular resistance is the most important mediator of this process. Factors that participate in the regulation of coronary vascular resistance include the accumulation of local metabolites, endothelium-derived substances, and neural innervation.

Metabolic Factors

The accumulation of local metabolites markedly affects coronary vascular tone, and acts to modulate myocardial oxygen supply to meet changing metabolic demands. Two of the key regulators are 1) *oxygen*, which acts as a vasoconstrictor, and 2) *adenosine*, which serves as a vasodilator. Molecular oxygen is thought to cause precapillary sphincters to contract. Thus, as perfusion decreases, so too does oxygen tension, leading to dilatation of precapillary sphincters and an increase in blood flow and oxygen supply.

During states of hypoxemia, aerobic metabolism and oxidative phosphorylation in the mitochondria are inhibited. High-energy phosphates, including ATP, cannot be regenerated. Consequently, adenosine diphosphate (ADP) and monophosphate (AMP) accumulate and are subsequently degraded to adenosine. Adenosine is a potent vasodilator and is thought to be the prime metabolic mediator of vascular tone. By binding to receptors on vascular smooth muscle, adenosine decreases calcium entry into cells, which leads to relaxation, vasodilatation, and increased coronary blood flow. Other metabolites that act locally as vasodilators include lactate, acetate, hydrogen ions, and carbon dioxide.

Endothelial Factors

Endothelial cells of the arterial wall produce a number of vasoactive substances that contribute to the regulation of vascular tone. *Vasodilators* produced by the endothelium include endothelium-derived relaxing factor and prostacyclin. Endothelin-1 is an example of a natural endothelium-derived *vasoconstrictor.*

The identification and important actions of **endothelium-derived relaxing factor** are described in Box 6.1. This factor has been identified as **nitric oxide** or a closely related substance, and is therefore referred to as EDRF-NO in this text. EDRF-NO regulates vascular tone by relaxing neighboring arterial smooth muscle by a cyclic GMP-dependent mechanism. The production of EDRF-NO by normal endothelium occurs in the basal state and is additionally stimulated by many substances and conditions. For example, it is released in an increased quantity when the endothelium is exposed to acetylcholine (ACh), thrombin, products of aggregating platelets (e.g., serotonin and ADP), or the shear stress of blood flow. Although the *direct* effect of many of these substances on vascular smooth muscle is *vasoconstriction,* the induced release of EDRF-NO from the normal endothelium results in *vasodilatation* instead (Fig. 6.2).

Prostacyclin, an arachidonic acid metabolite, has vasodilator properties that are similar to EDRF-NO (Fig. 6.2). It is released from endothelial cells in response to many stimuli, including hypoxia, shear stress, acetylcholine, and platelet products (e.g., serotonin). It causes relaxation of vascular smooth muscle by a cyclic AMP dependent mechanism.

Endothelin-1 is a potent vasoconstrictor produced by endothelial cells, and it partially counteracts the vasodilating properties of EDRF-NO and prostacyclin. Its expression is stimulated by several factors, including thrombin, angiotensin II, epinephrine, and the shear stress of blood flow.

Under normal circumstances, the healthy endothelium promotes vascular smooth muscle *relaxation* (vasodilatation) through elaboration of EDRF-NO and prostacyclin, the influences of which predominate over the endothelial vasoconstrictors (Fig. 6.2). As we shall see, however, dysfunctional endothelium (e.g., as is apparent in atherosclerosis) secretes reduced amounts of vasodilators, such that the balance shifts toward vasoconstriction instead.

Neural Factors

The neural control of vascular resistance has both sympathetic and parasympathetic components. Under normal circumstances, the contribution of the parasympathetic nervous system appears minor, but *sympathetic receptors* play an important role. Coronary vessels contain both α-adrenergic and β₂-adrenergic receptors. Stimulation of α-adrenergic receptors results in vasoconstriction. Conversely, β₂-receptor stimulation promotes vasodilatation.

It is the interplay between the metabolic, endothelial, and neural regulating factors that determines the net impact on coronary vascular tone. For example, catecholamine stimulation of the heart may initially cause coronary *vasoconstriction* via the α-adrenergic receptor neural effect. However, catecholamine stimulation also increases myocardial oxygen consumption through increased heart rate and contractility (β₁-adrenergic effect) and the resulting increased production of local metabolites induces net coronary *dilatation* instead.

Myocardial Oxygen Demand

There are three major determinants of myocardial oxygen demand: 1) ventricular wall stress, 2) heart rate, and 3) contractility (the inotropic state). Additionally, very small amounts of oxygen are consumed to provide energy for basal cardiac metabolism and electrical depolarization.

Ventricular **wall stress (σ)** is the tangential force acting on the myocardial fibers, tending to pull them apart, and energy is expended in opposing that force. Wall

Box 6.1: Endothelium-derived Relaxing Factor and Nitric Oxide

Normal arterial endothelial cells synthesize potent vasodilator substances that contribute to the modulation of vascular tone. These include prostacyclin (an arachidonic acid metabolite) and endothelium-derived relaxing factor (EDRF).

EDRF was first described in the 1970s. In experimental preparations, it was shown that acetylcholine (ACh) has two opposite actions on blood vessels: Its direct effect on vascular smooth muscle cells is to cause vasoconstriction, but when an intact endothelial lining overlies the smooth muscle cells, vasodilation occurs instead. Subsequent eloquent experiments showed that ACh causes the endothelial cells to release a chemical mediator (that was termed EDRF) that quickly diffuses to the adjacent smooth muscle cells and results in their relaxation with subsequent vasodilation of the vessel.

More recent studies have shown that the mysterious EDRF is actually *nitric oxide* (NO) or a closely related substance. When ACh (or other endothelial-dependent vasodilators such as serotonin or histamine) binds to endothelial cells, intracellular free calcium increases, which activates the enzyme nitric oxide synthase (NOS). NOS catalyzes the formation of NO from the amino acid L-arginine (see figure). NO diffuses from the endothelium to the adjacent smooth muscle, where it activates guanylyl cyclase (G-cyclase). G-cyclase in turn forms cyclic guanosine monophosphate (cGMP) from guanosine triphosphate (GTP). The increase in intracellular cGMP results in smooth muscle cell relaxation through mechanisms that involve a reduction in cytosolic Ca^{++}. The increase in cGMP is also associated with antimigratory effects of the smooth muscle cells.

In distinction to the endothelial-dependent vasodilators, a few agents cause smooth muscle relaxation *independent* of the presence of endothelial cells. For example, the drugs sodium nitroprusside and nitroglycerin result in vasodilation by providing an exogenous source of NO to vascular smooth muscle cells, thereby activating G-cyclase and forming cGMP without endothelial cell participation.

In the cardiac catheterization laboratory, the intracoronary administration of ACh into a normal individual causes vasodilation of the vessel, presumably through the release of EDRF-NO. However, in conditions of endothelial dysfunction, such as atherosclerosis, intracoronary ACh administration results in paradoxical vasoconstriction instead. This likely reflects reduced production of EDRF-NO by the dysfunctional endothelial cells, such that there is unopposed direct vasoconstriction of the smooth muscle by ACh. Of particular interest is that the loss of vasodilatory response to infused ACh is evident in individuals with certain cardiac risk factors (e.g., elevated LDL cholesterol, hypertension, cigarette smoking) even before the physical appearance of atheromatous plaque. Thus the impaired release of EDRF-NO may be an early and sensitive predictor for the later development of atherosclerotic lesions.

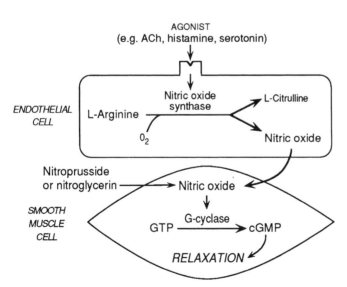

(Modified from Furchgott, RF. The discovery of endothelium-derived relaxing factor and its importance in the identification of nitric oxide. JAMA 1996; 276:1186–1188.)

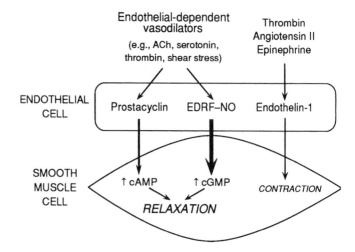

Figure 6.2. Endothelium-derived vasoactive substances and their regulators. Endothelium-derived vasodilators are shown on the left and include endothelium-derived relaxing factor/nitric oxide (EDRF-NO) and prostacyclin. Endothelin is an endothelium-derived vasoconstrictor. In the normal state, the vasodilator influence predominates over that of vasoconstriction. Ach, acetylcholine.

stress is related to intraventricular pressure (P), the radius of the ventricle (r) and ventricular wall thickness (h). Approximated by LaPlace's relationship,

$$\sigma = \frac{P \cdot r}{2h}$$

Thus, wall stress is directly proportional to the radius of the left ventricle. Conditions that augment left ventricular filling (e.g., mitral or aortic regurgitation) increase the ventricular radius, and raise wall stress and oxygen consumption. Conversely, any physiologic or pharmacologic maneuver that decreases left ventricular filling and size (e.g., nitrate therapy) decreases wall stress and myocardial oxygen consumption.

Wall stress is also proportional to systolic ventricular pressure. Circumstances that increase pressure development in the left ventricle, such as aortic stenosis or hypertension, increase the wall stress and myocardial oxygen consumption. Conditions that decrease ventricular pressure, such as antihypertensive therapy, reduce myocardial oxygen consumption.

Finally, wall stress is *inversely* proportional to ventricular wall thickness, since the force is spread out among a greater muscle mass. A hypertrophied heart has lower wall stress and oxygen consumption per gram of tissue than a thinned-wall heart. Thus when hypertrophy develops in conditions of chronic pressure overload,

such as aortic stenosis, it serves a compensatory role in reducing oxygen consumption.

The second major determinant of myocardial oxygen demand is **heart rate.** If the heart rate accelerates, the number of contractions and the amount of ATP consumed per minute increases, and oxygen requirements rise. Conversely, slowing the heart rate (e.g., using a β-blocking drug) decreases ATP utilization and oxygen consumption.

The third major determinant of myocardial oxygen demand is myocardial **contractility,** a measure of the force of contraction (described in Chapter 9). Circulating catecholamines or the administration of positive inotropic drugs directly increases the force of contraction, and increases oxygen utilization. Conversely, negative inotropic effectors, such as β-adrenergic blocking drugs, decrease myocardial oxygen consumption.

In summary, in the normal state, autoregulatory mechanisms adjust coronary tone so as to match myocardial oxygen supply with oxygen requirements. In the absence of obstructive coronary disease, the autoregulatory mechanisms maintain a fairly constant rate of coronary flow, as long as the aortic perfusion pressure is approximately 60 mm Hg or greater. In the setting of advanced coronary atherosclerosis, however, the fall in perfusion pressure distal to the arterial stenosis, and dysfunction of the endothelium of the involved segment, set the stage for a mismatch between the available blood supply and myocardial metabolic demands.

PATHOPHYSIOLOGY OF ISCHEMIA

The traditional view has been that myocardial ischemia in coronary artery disease results from fixed atherosclerotic plaques that narrow the vessel's lumen and limit myocardial blood supply. However, recent research has demonstrated that the reduction of blood flow results from the *combination* of fixed vessel narrowing *and* abnormal vascular tone, contributed to by atherosclerosis-induced endothelial cell dysfunction.

Fixed Vessel Narrowing

The hemodynamic significance of atherosclerotic coronary artery stenoses relates to both the fluid mechanics and the anatomy of the vascular supply.

Fluid Mechanics

Poiseuille's law states that for flow through a vessel,

$$Q = \frac{\Delta P \pi r^4}{8 \eta L}$$

in which Q is flow, ΔP is the pressure difference between the points being measured, r is the vessel radius, h is the fluid viscosity, and L is the vessel length. By analogy to Ohm's law, flow is also equal to the pressure difference divided by the resistance (R) to flow:

$$Q = \frac{\Delta P}{R}$$

By combining these two formulas, resistance to blood flow in a vessel can be expressed as:

$$R = \frac{8 \eta L}{\pi r^4}$$

Thus, vascular resistance is governed, in part, by the geometric component L/r^4.

Therefore, the hemodynamic significance of a stenotic lesion depends on its length and, far more important, on the degree of vessel narrowing (i.e., the reduction of r) that it causes.

Anatomy

The coronary arteries consist of large, proximal epicardial segments and smaller, distal resistance vessels. The proximal vessels are subject to overt atherosclerosis that results in stenotic plaques. The distal vessels are usually free of flow-limiting plaques and can adjust their vasomotor tone in response to metabolic needs. These resistance vessels serve as a reserve, increasing their diameter with exertion to meet increasing oxygen demand and dilating even at rest if a proximal stenosis is sufficiently severe.

The hemodynamic significance, and hence the pathophysiological consequences, of varying degrees of coronary artery narrowing depends on both the degree of stenosis of the epicardial portion of the vessel and the amount of *compensatory vasodilatation* of the distal resistance vessels (Fig. 6.3). If a stenosis narrows the lumen diameter by less than 60%, the maximal potential blood flow through the artery is not significantly altered, and, in response to exertion, the resistance vessels can dilate to provide adequate blood flow. When a stenosis narrows the diameter by more than approximately 70%, the impediment to flow is such that the resistance vessels need to fully dilate, even at rest, in order to achieve adequate perfusion. In this situation, when oxygen demand increases (e.g., from the elevated heart rate and force of contraction during physical exertion), there is little coronary flow reserve available, and maximal vessel flow is reduced. Thus oxygen demand exceeds supply and myocardial ischemia results. If the stenosis compromises the vessel lumen by more than approximately 90%, blood flow may be inadequate to meet basal requirements even with maximal dilatation of the resistance vessels, and ischemia can develop *at rest*.

Although collateral channels (see Chap-

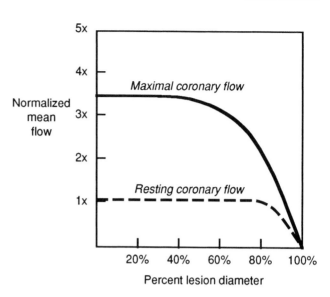

Figure 6.3. Resting and maximal coronary blood flow are affected by the magnitude of proximal arterial stenosis (percent lesion diameter). The dotted line indicates resting blood flow, whereas the solid line represents maximal blood flow (i.e., when there is full dilatation of the distal resistance vessels). Compromise of maximal blood flow is evident when then proximal stenosis reduces the coronary lumen diameter by more than ~70%. Resting flow may be compromised if the stenosis exceeds ~90%. (Modified from Gould KL, Lipscomb K. Effects of coronary stenoses on coronary flow reserve and resistance. Am J Cardiol 1974;34:50.)

ter 1) may become apparent between non-obstructed coronaries and sites distal to atherosclerotic stenoses, and such flow can buffer the fall in myocardial oxygen supply, it is usually not sufficient to prevent ischemia during exertion in critically narrowed vessels.

Endothelial Cell Dysfunction

In addition to fixed vessel narrowing, the other major contributor to reduced myocardial oxygen supply in chronic coronary artery disease is endothelial dysfunction. Abnormal endothelial cell function can contribute to the pathophysiology of ischemia in two ways: 1) by inappropriate vasoconstriction of coronary arteries, and 2) through loss of normal antithrombotic properties.

Inappropriate Vasoconstriction

In normal individuals, physical activity or mental stress results in measurable coronary artery *vasodilatation.* This effect is thought to be regulated by activation of the sympathetic nervous system, with increased blood flow and shear stress stimulating the release of endothelial-derived vasodilators, such as EDRF-NO. It is postu-

lated that in normal individuals, the relaxation effect of EDRF-NO outweighs the direct α-adrenergic constrictor effect of catecholamines on arterial smooth muscle, such that vasodilatation results. However, in patients with dysfunctional endothelium (e.g., atherosclerosis), an *impaired release of endothelial vasodilators* leaves the direct catecholamine effect unopposed, such that relative *vasoconstriction* occurs instead. The resultant decrease in coronary blood flow and myocardial oxygen supply contributes to ischemia. Of note, in patients with risk factors for coronary artery disease such as hypercholesterolemia, diabetes mellitus, hypertension, and cigarette smoking, impaired endothelial-dependent vasodilation is noted even in *anatomically normal* coronary arteries, suggesting that endothelial dysfunction occurs very early in the atherosclerotic process. In patients with impaired endothelial function, even the vasodilatory effect of local metabolites (such as adenosine and hypoxia) is attenuated, thus uncoupling the regulation of vascular tone from metabolic demands.

In acute coronary syndromes (e.g., unstable angina), inappropriate vasoconstriction also appears to be important. The cause of unstable angina is commonly attributed to disruption of atherosclerotic plaque, with superimposed platelet aggregation and thrombus formation. In normal individuals, the products of platelet aggregation in a developing clot (e.g., serotonin, ADP) result in vasodilatation, because they stimulate the endothelial release of EDRF-NO. However, with dysfunctional endothelium, the direct *vasoconstricting* actions of platelet products predominate, and constriction occurs instead (Fig. 6.4), leading to reduced flow through the arterial lumen.

Platelet Aggregation

Factors released from endothelial cells, including EDRF-NO and prostacyclin serve antithrombotic roles, as they interfere with platelet aggregation (Fig. 6.4). However, in states of endothelial cell dysfunction, there is reduced release of these substances, and

therefore, the antithrombotic effect is attenuated. Thus, in syndromes characterized by thrombosis (e.g., unstable angina, acute myocardial infarction), the loss of EDRF and prostacyclin allows platelets to aggregate and to secrete procoagulants and potential vasoconstrictors, promoting further interference with blood flow.

Other Causes of Myocardial Ischemia

In addition to coronary artery disease (CAD), other conditions may result in an imbalance between myocardial oxygen supply and demand and result in ischemia. Causes of decreased myocardial oxygen supply include: 1) decreased aortic perfu-

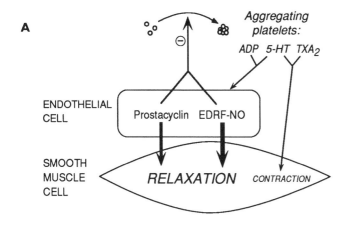

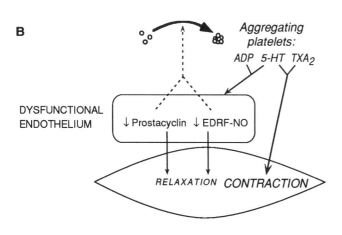

Figure 6.4. **The interaction between platelets and endothelial cells. A.** Normal endothelium. Aggregating platelets release thromboxane (TXA$_2$) and serotonin (5-HT), the direct vascular effects of which cause contraction of vascular smooth muscle and vasoconstriction. However, platelet products (e.g., ADP, 5-HT) also stimulate the endothelial release of the potent vasodilators EDRF-NO and prostacyclin, such that the net effect is smooth muscle relaxation. Endothelial production of EDRF-NO and prostacyclin also serve antithrombotic roles, which limit further platelet aggregation. **B.** Dysfunctional endothelium demonstrates impaired release of the vasodilator substances, such that net smooth muscle contraction and vasoconstriction supervene. The reduced endothelial release of EDRF-NO and prostacyclin diminishes their antiplatelet effect, such that thrombosis proceeds unchecked.

sion pressure (e.g., due to hypotension or aortic regurgitation), and 2) a severe decrease in blood oxygen-carrying capacity (e.g., anemia or hypoxemia). For example, a patient with massive bleeding from the gastrointestinal tract may develop myocardial ischemia and angina pectoris, even in the absence of atherosclerotic coronary disease, because of a reduction in tissue oxygen delivery owing to the loss of hemoglobin.

On the other side of the balance, a profound increase in myocardial oxygen demand can cause ischemia, in the absence of coronary atherosclerosis or otherwise impaired myocardial oxygen supply. This can occur, for example, with severe aortic stenosis, in which there is markedly increased wall stress due to the greatly elevated left ventricular systolic pressure.

ISCHEMIC SYNDROMES

Myocardial ischemia occurs when there is a mismatch between myocardial oxygen supply and demand. Yet depending on the contributions of various pathophysiologic processes, different clinical syndromes may be manifest (Fig. 6.5).

Stable Angina (Fig. 6.5B)

When atherosclerotic stenoses narrow a coronary artery lumen diameter by more

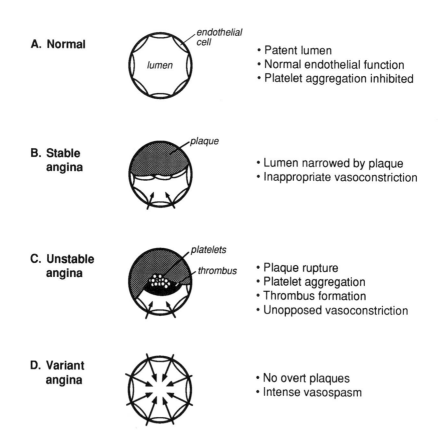

Figure 6.5. Pathophysiologic findings in anginal syndromes. A. Normal coronary arteries are widely patent, and the endothelium functions normally. **B.** In stable angina, atherosclerotic plaque and inappropriate vasoconstriction (due to dysfunctional endothelium) reduce the vessel lumen's size and coronary blood flow. **C.** In unstable angina, disruption of the plaque (e.g., rupture) triggers platelet aggregation, thrombus formation, and vasoconstriction, all of which contribute to reduced coronary blood supply. **D.** In variant angina, atherosclerotic plaques are absent; rather ischemia is due to intense vasospasm that reduces myocardial oxygen supply.

than approximately 70%, the reduced flow capacity may be sufficient to serve the low cardiac oxygen needs at rest, but is insufficient to compensate for any significant increase in oxygen demand (Fig. 6.3). During physical exertion, for example, activation of the sympathetic nervous system results in increased heart rate, blood pressure and contractility, all of which contribute to augmented myocardial oxygen consumption. During the period that oxygen demand exceeds available supply, myocardial ischemia results, often accompanied by the chest discomfort of angina pectoris. The ischemia and symptoms persist until the increased demand is alleviated and oxygen balance is restored. A pattern of chronic, predictable transient angina during exertion or emotional stress is termed "stable angina."

Potentially contributing to the inadequate oxygen supply in stable angina is inappropriate coronary vasoconstriction due, at least in part, to atherosclerosis-associated endothelial dysfunction. In a normal individual, the increased myocardial oxygen demand during exertion is balanced by an increased supply of blood as the accumulation of local metabolites induces vasodilatation. With endothelial cell dysfunction, however, vasodilatation is impaired and the vessels may paradoxically vasoconstrict in response to exercise-induced catecholamine stimulation of α-adrenergic receptors on the coronary arteries.

As a result, the extent of coronary artery narrowing in patients with atherosclerosis is not necessarily constant. Rather, it can vary from moment to moment because of changes in the superimposed coronary vascular tone. For some patients with stable angina, alterations in tone play a minimal role in the decreased myocardial oxygen supply, and the level of physical activity required to precipitate angina is fairly constant. These patients have "fixed-threshold" angina. In other cases, however, the degree of dynamic obstruction caused by vasoconstriction or vasospasm plays a more prominent role, and such patients may have "variable-threshold" angina. For example, on a given day, such a patient can exert her-self or himself without chest discomfort, but on another day, the same degree of myocardial oxygen demand *does* produce symptoms—the difference reflects alterations in vascular tone over the sites of fixed stenosis.

Unstable Angina

A patient with chronic, stable angina may experience a sudden increase in the tempo and duration of ischemic episodes, occurring with lesser degrees of exertion and even at rest. This acceleration of symptoms is known as unstable angina, and is often a precursor to acute myocardial infarction. Although the majority of patients with unstable angina have severe atherosclerotic disease, it occasionally develops in those with only minor coronary obstructions. Therefore, the pathogenesis of unstable angina is likely multifactorial. Most commonly, the key event is probably *fissuring and disruption of an atherosclerotic plaque* (Fig. 6.5C). The resultant platelet activation and thrombus formation at the site of the plaque fissure may lead to further obstruction of the lumen, thereby worsening the already reduced coronary blood supply.

Compounding the reduced blood supply in unstable angina is the vasoconstricting effect of the aggregating platelets and thrombus. In normal vessels, vasoactive substances released from platelets, such as thrombin and serotonin, usually elicit an endothelium-mediated vasodilatory response (Fig. 6.4). With dysfunction of the endothelium (and impaired elaboration of EDRF-NO and prostacyclin), these platelet factors, as well as thrombin within the clot, promote vasoconstriction instead. Furthermore, in the setting of dysfunctional endothelium, inhibition of platelet aggregation by endothelial antagonists (EDRF-NO and prostacyclin) no longer occurs, and a key defense against thrombosis in unstable angina is lost.

Variant Angina

A small minority of patients manifest episodes of focal *coronary artery spasm* in the absence of overt atherosclerotic lesions, and this syndrome is known as "variant" or "Prinzmetal's" angina. In this case, intense vasospasm alone reduces coronary oxygen supply and results in angina (Fig. 6.5D). The mechanism by which such profound spasm develops is not definitively known. It is thought that many of these patients may have early atherosclerosis manifested only by a dysfunctional endothelium, as the response to many endothelium-dependent vasodilators (e.g., ACh and serotonin) is abnormal in patients with this condition.

Variant angina often occurs *at rest* because ischemia in this case is due to transient marked reduction in the coronary oxygen supply, rather than an increase in myocardial oxygen demand.

Silent Ischemia

Episodes of cardiac ischemia sometimes occur *in the absence* of perceptible discomfort or pain, and such instances are referred to as "silent ischemia." These asymptomatic episodes can occur in patients who on other occasions experience typical *symptomatic* angina, but in some individuals, silent ischemia may be the *only* manifestation of CAD. As you can imagine, it may be difficult to diagnose silent ischemia, but its presence can be detected by laboratory techniques such as continuous ambulatory electrocardiography or elicited by exercise stress testing (described below). One study estimated that silent ischemic episodes occur in 40% of patients with stable symptomatic angina and in 2.5% to 10% of asymptomatic middle-aged men. When considering the importance of anginal discomfort as a physiologic warning signal, the asymptomatic nature of silent ischemia becomes all the more alarming.

The reason why some episodes of ischemia are "silent" whereas others are symptomatic has not been elucidated. The degree of ischemia cannot fully explain the disparity, as even myocardial infarction may present without symptoms in some patients. It is, however, particularly common among diabetics, possibly related to impaired pain sensation due to peripheral neuropathy.

Syndrome X

This term refers to patients with typical symptoms of angina pectoris who have no evidence of significant atherosclerotic coronary stenoses on coronary angiograms. Some of these patients may show definite laboratory signs of ischemia during exercise testing. The pathogenesis of ischemia in this situation may be related to inadequate vasodilator reserve of the coronary resistance vessels. It is thought that the resistance vessels (which are too small to be visualized during coronary angiography) in such patients may not dilate appropriately during periods of increased myocardial oxygen demand. These patients have a better prognosis than patients with overt atherosclerotic disease.

CONSEQUENCES OF ISCHEMIA

The consequences of intermittent ischemia reflect the inadequate myocardial oxygenation and local accumulation of metabolic waste products. During ischemia, the myocytes convert from aerobic to anaerobic metabolic pathways. The reduced generation of ATP impairs the interaction of the contractile proteins and results in a transient reduction of both ventricular systolic contraction and diastolic relaxation. In addition, the products of anaerobic metabolism (e.g., lactate, serotonin, adenosine) accumulate locally. It is suspected that one or more of these compounds activate peripheral pain receptors in the C7 through T4 distribution, and may be the mechanism by which angina is produced.

During the pain of an acute ischemic attack, generalized sympathetic and parasympathetic stimulation may result in tachycardia, diaphoresis, and nausea. Because ischemia results in a sudden decrease in myocardial diastolic relaxation, the left ventricle transiently stiffens, and its diastolic pressure rises. The elevated pressure is transmitted to the pulmonary vasculature and may precipitate dyspnea and pulmonary congestion. Additionally, transient abnormalities of myocyte ion transport and accumulation of local metabolites may precipitate dangerous ventricular arrhythmias.

Once the acute ischemic episode has resolved (i.e., once the balance between oxygen supply and demand has been restored), the symptoms of angina fully abate, and, if the ischemic insult was brief, no permanent damage is sustained by the myocardium.

CLINICAL FEATURES

The most important part of the clinical evaluation of ischemic heart disease is the history described by the patient. Because chest pain is such a common complaint, it is important to focus on those characteristics that help distinguish myocardial ischemia from other causes of discomfort. From a diagnostic standpoint, it would be ideal to interview and examine a patient *during* an actual episode of angina, but most individuals are asymptomatic during the routine office or clinic examination. Therefore, a careful history probing several features of the discomfort should be elicited.

Quality

Most often angina is described as a "pressure," "tightness," "heaviness," or "constriction" in the chest. It is rare that the sensation is actually described as a pain, and often a patient will correct the physician who refers to the anginal symptom as such. Anginal discomfort is neither sharp nor stabbing, and it does not vary significantly with inspiration or movement of the chest wall. It is a steady discomfort that lasts a few minutes, yet rarely more than 5 to 10. It *always* lasts more than a second or two, and this helps to differentiate it from sharper musculoskeletal pains. Occasionally, a patient likens the sensation to "an elephant sitting on my chest."

While describing angina, the patient may place a clenched fist over his or her sternum, referred to as **Levine's sign,** as if defining the constricting discomfort by that tight grip. As noted above, frequently associated symptoms that accompany angina include dyspnea, diaphoresis, and nausea.

Location

Anginal discomfort is usually *diffuse* rather than localized to a single point. It is most often located retrosternally or in the left precordium, but may occur anywhere in the chest, back, arms, neck, lower face, or upper abdomen. It often radiates to the shoulders and inner aspect of the arms, especially on the left side.

Precipitants

Angina, when not due to pure vasospasm, is precipitated by those factors that increase myocardial oxygen demand (e.g., increased heart rate, contractility, or wall stress). These include physical exertion, anger, and other emotional excitement. Other factors that increase myocardial oxygen demand and precipitate anginal discomfort in patients with coronary artery disease include a large meal or cold weather. The latter induces peripheral vasoconstriction, which in turn augments myocardial wall stress as the left ventricle contracts against the increased resistance.

Angina is generally relieved within minutes after the cessation of the activity that precipitated it, and even more quickly (within 3 to 5 minutes) by sublingual nitroglycerin. This response can help differentiate myocardial ischemia from many of the other conditions that produce chest discomfort.

Patients who experience angina primarily due to increased coronary artery tone or vasospasm often develop symptoms at rest, independent of those activities that increase myocardial oxygen demand. Sometimes patients awake during the night with angina precipitated by this mechanism or because of the emotional stress (and increased oxygen demand) of a bad dream.

Frequency

Although the level of exertion necessary to precipitate angina may remain fairly constant, the frequency of episodes varies considerably, because patients quickly learn which activities cause their discomfort and avoid them. It is thus important to inquire about reductions in activities of daily living when taking the history.

Risk Factors

In addition to the description of the chest discomfort, a careful history should uncover risk factors that predispose to atherosclerosis and CAD, including cigarette smoking, hypercholesterolemia, hyperten-

sion, diabetes, and a family history of premature coronary disease (see Chapter 5).

DIAGNOSIS

Several conditions can mimic angina pectoris, including gastroesophageal reflux, esophageal spasm, biliary pain, pericarditis, and musculoskeletal conditions such as chest wall pain, spinal osteoarthritis, and cervical radiculitis. The history remains of paramount importance in distinguishing myocardial ischemia from these disorders. In contrast to angina pectoris, gastrointestinal causes of recurrent chest pain are often precipitated by certain foods and are unrelated to exertion. Musculoskeletal causes of chest pain tend to be more superficial or can be localized to a discrete spot (i.e., the patient can point to the pain with one finger), and often vary with changes in position. Useful differentiating features are listed in Table 6.2.

TABLE 6.2. Causes of Recurrent Chest Pain

Condition	Differentiating Features
Cardiac	
Myocardial ischemia	• Retrosternal tightness or pressure; typically radiates to neck, jaw, or left shoulder and arm
	• Lasts a few minutes (usually < 10 min)
	• Brought on by exertion, relieved by rest
	• Relieved by nitroglycerin
	• EKG: transient ST depressions or elevations
Pericarditis	• Sharp, pleuritic pain that varies with position; friction rub on auscultation
	• Can last for hours to days
	• EKG: diffuse ST elevations and PR depression
Gastrointestinal	
Gastroesophageal reflux	• Retrosternal burning
	• Precipitated by certain foods, worsened by supine position, unaffected by exertion
	• Relieved by antacids, not by nitroglycerin
Peptic ulcer disease	• Epigastric ache or burning
	• Occurs after meals, unaffected by exertion
	• Relieved by antacids, not by nitroglycerin
Esophageal spasm	• Retrosternal pain accompanied by dysphagia
	• Precipitated by meals, unaffected by exertion
	• May be relieved by nitroglycerin
Biliary colic	• Constant, deep right upper quadrant pain
	• Brought on by fatty foods, unaffected by exertion
	• Not relieved by antacids or nitroglycerin
Musculoskeletal	
Costochondral syndrome	• Sternal pain worsened by chest movement
	• Costochondral junctions tender to palpation
	• Relieved by anti-inflammatory drugs, not by nitroglycerin
Cervical radiculitis	• Constant ache or shooting pains, may be in a dermatomal distribution
	• Worsened by neck motion

Physical Examination

If it is possible to examine a patient *during* an anginal attack, several transient physical signs may be detected (Fig. 6.6). Increases in heart rate and blood pressure are common because of the increased sympathetic response. Myocardial ischemia may lead to papillary muscle dysfunction and therefore mitral regurgitation, as well as regional ventricular contractile abnormalities, which can sometimes be detected as an abnormal bulging impulse on palpation of the left chest. Ischemia may decrease ventricular compliance, producing a stiffened ventricle and therefore an S_4 gallop during atrial contraction (see Chapter 2). However, if the patient is free of chest discomfort during the examination, there may be *no* abnormal physical findings.

Diagnostic Studies

Once angina is suspected, several diagnostic tests may be helpful in confirming myocardial ischemia as the etiology. Many of these tests are costly so that it is important to choose the appropriate studies for each patient.

Electrocardiogram

One of the most useful tools is an EKG obtained *during* an anginal episode. Although this is easy to arrange when symptoms occur in hospitalized patients, it may not be possible to "catch" episodes in individuals seen on an outpatient basis. During myocardial ischemia, ST segment and T wave changes can be seen (Fig. 6.7). Acute ischemia usually results in transient horizontal or downsloping ST segment depressions and T wave flattening or inversions. Occasionally, ST segment *elevations* are seen; this is suggestive of more severe transmural myocardial ischemia and can also be seen with the intense vasospasm of "variant" angina. In distinction to an acute MI, the ST deviations quickly normalize with resolution of the patient's symptoms. If the EKG is obtained during a period free of ischemia, it may be normal, or "nondiagnostic" ST and T wave abnormalities may be present. Evidence of a previous myocardial infarction (e.g., pathologic Q waves) on the EKG also points to the presence of underlying coronary disease.

Exercise Stress Test

An EKG obtained during or between episodes of chest discomfort may be normal

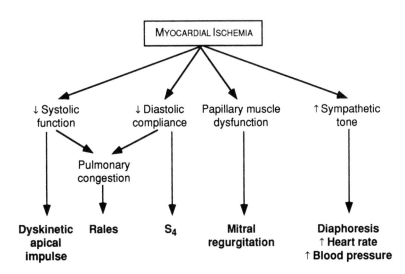

Figure 6.6. Pathophysiology of physical signs during acute myocardial ischemia.

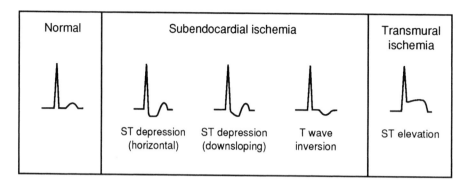

Figure 6.7. Common transient EKG abnormalities during ischemia. Subendocardial ischemia results in ST segment depressions and/or T wave flattening or inversions. Severe transient transmural ischemia can result in ST segment elevations, similar to the early changes in acute myocardial infarction. When transient ischemia resolves, so do the electrocardiographic changes.

and does not rule out the diagnosis of is-chemic heart disease. For this reason, the **exercise stress test** (also termed exercise tolerance test) is a valuable diagnostic aid. During this test, the patient exercises on a treadmill or a stationary bicycle to progressively higher workloads. He or she is observed for chest discomfort or inordinate dyspnea. Heart rate and EKG tracings are continuously recorded, and blood pressure is checked at regular intervals. The test is continued until angina develops, signs of myocardial ischemia appear on the EKG, a target heart rate is achieved, or the patient becomes too fatigued to continue.

The test is considered *positive* for ischemic heart disease if the patient's typical chest discomfort is reproduced or if EKG abnormalities consistent with ischemia develop (i.e., ≥ 1 mm horizontal or downsloping ST segment depressions). By these criteria, the test has approximately 65%–80% sensitivity and 65%–75% specificity in detecting patients with anatomically significant coronary disease. The stress test is considered *markedly positive* if one or more of the following signs of *severe* ischemic heart disease occur: 1) the ischemic EKG changes develop in the first 3 minutes of exercise or persist 5 minutes after exercise has stopped; 2) the magnitude of the ST segment depressions ≥ 2 mm; 3) the systolic blood pressure *decreases* during exercise (i.e., due to ischemia-induced impairment of contractile function); 4) high-grade ventricular ar-

rhythmias develop; or 5) the patient cannot exercise for at least 2 minutes because of cardiopulmonary limitations. Patients with markedly positive tests are more likely to have severe, multivessel coronary disease.

The utility of a stress test may be affected by the patient's medications. For example, β-blockers or certain calcium channel blockers may blunt the ability to achieve the target heart rate. In these situations, one must consider the purpose of the stress test. If it is to determine whether ischemic heart disease is present, then those medications are withheld for 24–48 hours before the test. On the other hand, if the patient has known ischemic heart disease and the purpose of the test is to assess the efficacy of the current medical regimen, then testing is performed while the patient takes his or her usual antianginal medications.

Nuclear Exercise Studies

As the standard exercise stress test relies on ischemia-related changes on the EKG, the test is less useful in patients with baseline abnormalities of the ST segments (e.g., as seen in left bundle branch block or left ventricular hypertrophy). In addition, the standard exercise stress test sometimes yields equivocal results in patients for whom the clinical suspicion of ischemic heart disease is high. In these situations, radionuclide imaging can be combined with exercise stress testing to overcome these limitations and to increase the sensitivity and specificity of the test.

During myocardial perfusion scintigraphy (described further in Chapter 3), a radionuclide (usually either thallium-201 or technetium-99m-sestamibi) is injected intravenously at peak exercise and immediate imaging is performed. The radionuclide accumulates in proportion to the degree of perfusion of viable myocardial cells. Therefore, areas of poor perfusion (i.e., areas of ischemia) during exercise do not accumulate radionuclide and will appear as "cold spots" on the image. However, irreversibly infarcted areas also do not take up the radionuclide, and they too will appear as cold spots. To differentiate between transient ischemia and infarcted tissue, repeat imaging is performed several hours later. If the cold spot fills in, a region of *transient ischemia* has been identified. If the cold spot remains unchanged, then a region of irreversible *infarction* is likely. These radionuclide techniques are approximately 90% sensitive and 80%–90% specific for the presence of clinically significant CAD. Because these techniques are expensive, myocardial perfusion scintigraphy should be restricted to patients whose abnormal baseline EKG precludes interpretation of a standard exercise test, or to improve testing sensitivity in a patient for whom the clinical suspicion and standard stress test results are discordant.

Exercise Echocardiography

At some centers, exercise testing with *echo*cardiographic imaging is an alternative technique used to demonstrate exercise-induced abnormalities of myocardial contraction as a manifestation of transient ischemia.

Pharmacologic Stress Tests

For patients unable to exercise (e.g., patients with severe arthritis), *pharmacologic* stress testing can be performed using various agents including the inotrope *dobutamine* (which increases myocardial oxygen demand by stimulating the heart rate and

force of contraction), or *dipyridamole*. Dipyridamole blocks the uptake and degradation of adenosine from the circulation. The resultant increased concentration of adenosine induces coronary vasodilatation, which increases flow to the myocardium perfused by healthy coronary arteries. As ischemic regions are already maximally dilated (because of the accumulation of local metabolites), this action tends to "steal" blood away from the diseased segments and therefore renders them as cold spots on scintigraphy. Pharmacologic stress testing can also be performed in conjunction with echocardiography in place of nuclear imaging.

Coronary Angiography

The most direct means to identify coronary artery stenoses is by coronary angiography, in which atherosclerotic plaques are visualized radiographically, following the injection of radiopaque contrast material into the artery (Fig. 6.8; also see Chapter 3). The risk of this procedure is low, but signif-

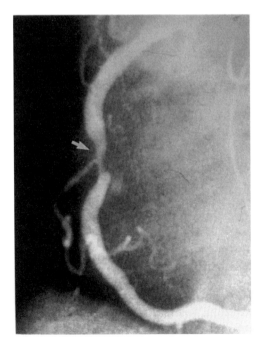

Figure 6.8.   Example of coronary angiography.
Injection of the right coronary artery demonstrates a stenosis in the midportion of the vessel, indicated by the arrow. (Courtesy of Dr. William Daley.)

icantly greater than that of the noninvasive studies described above.

The diagnosis of CAD can be made in most affected patients by history supplemented by noninvasive studies. If, however, the diagnosis is unclear, symptoms do not respond to medical therapy, the patient has an unstable presentation, or the results of noninvasive tests are so abnormal that severe CAD warranting revascularization is likely, then cardiac catheterization and angiography are undertaken.

Although coronary angiography is considered the "gold standard" in the diagnosis of CAD, it should be noted that it provides only anatomic information. The clinical significance of lesions detected by angiography depends not only on the degree of narrowing, but also on the physiologic consequences. Therefore, treatment decisions are made not only on the finding of such stenoses, but even more so on their functional effects, manifest by the patient's symptoms, the viability of the myocardium segment served by stenotic vessels, and the degree of ventricular contractile dysfunction (see below). Furthermore, standard arteriography does not reveal the composition of the atherosclerotic plaque or its vulnerability to rupture.

NATURAL HISTORY

The patient with chronic angina may show no change in the stable pattern of ischemia for many years. In some individuals, however, the course may be punctuated at any time by the occurrence of unstable angina, myocardial infarction, or sudden ischemic death. These complications are often related to acute thrombosis at the site of disrupted atherosclerotic plaque (as described in Chapter 7). Why some individuals, but not others, sustain these complications remains a subject of intense clinical and basic science investigation, and may relate to the vulnerability of plaque to rupture.

Prior to the current era of sophisticated pharmacotherapy, coronary angioplasty, and surgical procedures, studies showed

that the annual mortality rate of patients with CAD corresponded to the number of vessels containing significant stenoses (Table 6.3). For example, patients with advanced stenoses within a single coronary vessel could expect an annual mortality rate of < 4%. Those with two involved vessels had an annual mortality rate of 7% to 10%, and those with advanced, three-vessel disease showed a 10% to 12% mortality rate. If the left main artery was significantly stenosed, the mortality rate was markedly increased (15% to 25%). These outcomes were worse in corresponding patients with decreased systolic contractile function.

More recent studies have continued to show that the location and extent of coronary stenoses are important, but that other critical predictors of mortality are: 1) the degree of impaired left ventricular contractile function, 2) poor exercise capacity, and 3) the magnitude of clinical anginal symptoms. These predictors are taken into account when contemplating treatment decisions.

Of note, the mortality associated with CAD has declined significantly over the past three decades; the age-adjusted death rate has fallen by more than 50%. This is likely related to: 1) atherosclerotic risk reduction through improved lifestyle changes (less tobacco use, less dietary fat consumption, and more exercise, for example), 2) improved therapeutic strategies and longevity following acute MI (see Chapter 7), and 3) advances in the medical and surgical therapies of chronic CAD.

TABLE 6.3. Natural History of Angina Pectoris (Prior to current aggressive medical/surgical era)

Number of Stenosed Vessels	Annual Mortality (%)*
1	<4
2	7–10
3	10–12
Left main stenosis	15–25

*Prognosis is worse in patients with impaired left ventricular function.
Reprinted with permission from Humphries JO. Expected course of patients with coronary artery disease. In: Rahimtoola SH, ed. Coronary Bypass Surgery. Philadelphia: FA Davis, 1977.

TREATMENT

The goal of therapy in chronic ischemic heart disease is to improve the patient's quality of life by decreasing the frequency of anginal attacks, to prevent acute myocardial infarction, and to prolong survival. A long-term crucial step is to address those risk factors that have contributed to the development of atherosclerotic coronary disease. Accordingly, measures must be aimed at managing hypertension, controlling diabetes mellitus, lowering cholesterol and fat intake, eliminating tobacco use, reducing stress, and controlling body weight. Recent studies have shown a marked reduction in coronary events and mortality in patients who significantly lower their serum LDL-cholesterol levels through dietary and pharmacologic means (see Chapter 5).

The strategy underlying current therapy of ischemic symptoms is to restore the balance between myocardial oxygen supply and demand and to prevent complications of fibrous plaque.

Treatment of an Acute Episode of Angina

Upon experiencing angina, the patient should cease physical activity. Sublingual nitroglycerin, an organic nitrate, is the drug of choice. Placed under the tongue, this medication produces a slight burning sensation as the nitroglycerin is absorbed through the mucosa. The drug takes effect in 1 to 2 minutes and relieves ischemia primarily through vascular smooth muscle relaxation, particularly venodilatation. Venodilatation reduces venous return to the heart, such that there is a subsequent decline in left ventricular volume (a determinant of wall stress), which causes myocardial oxygen consumption to fall.

A second action of nitrates is to dilate the coronary vasculature with subsequent augmentation of coronary blood flow. This effect may be of minimal value in the common individual with angina in whom the accumulation of local metabolites has already resulted in maximal dilatation. However, when coronary vasospasm plays a role in the development of ischemia, nitrate-induced coronary vasodilatation may be beneficial.

Prevention of Recurrent Ischemic Episodes

In the prevention of anginal attacks, pharmacologic agents are also usually the first line of defense. The goal of these agents is to decrease the cardiac workload, and thus reduce myocardial oxygen demand, and to increase myocardial perfusion. The three classes of medications typically employed are the organic nitrates, β-adrenergic blockers, and calcium channel blockers (Table 6.4).

Organic nitrates (e.g., nitroglycerin, isosorbide dinitrate, isosorbide mononitrate), as discussed above, relieve ischemia primarily through venodilatation (i.e., lower wall stress results from a smaller ventricular radius), and possibly through coronary vasodilatation. The organic nitrates are the oldest of antianginal drugs and come in several preparations. Sublingual nitroglycerin tablets or spray are the forms employed in the treatment of acute attacks because of their rapid onset of action. In addition, by taking a dose immediately before engaging in those activities known to provoke anginal symptoms, these rapidly acting nitrates are useful as *prophylaxis* against anginal attacks.

Longer-acting anginal prevention can be achieved through a variety of nitrate preparations including oral tablets of isosorbide dinitrate (or mononitrate) or a transdermal nitroglycerin patch, which is applied once a day. A limitation to chronic nitrate therapy is the development of drug tolerance (i.e., a decrease in the effectiveness of the drug during continued administration), which occurs to some degree in most patients. This undesired effect can be overcome by providing a nitrate-free interval for several hours each day, usually while the patient sleeps.

There is no evidence that nitrates im-

TABLE 6.4. **Pharmacologic Agents in the Treatment of Angina**

Drug Class	Mechanism of Action	Adverse Effects
Organic Nitrates	↓ *Myocardial O_2 demand* 　↓ Preload ↑ O_2 *supply* 　↑ Coronary perfusion 　↓ Coronary vasospasm	• Headache • Hypotension • Reflex tachycardia
β-blockers	↓ *Myocardial O_2 demand* 　↓ Contractility 　↓ Heart rate	• Excessive bradycardia • (↓) LV contactile function • Bronchoconstriction • May worsen diabetic control • Fatigue
Calcium channel blockers 　(agent specific — see key)	↓ *Myocardial O_2 demand* 　↓ Preload 　↓ Wall stress (↓BP) 　↓ Contractility (V, D) 　↓ Heart rate (V, D) ↑ O_2 *supply* 　↑ Coronary perfusion 　↓ Coronary vasospasm	• Headache, flushing • (↓) LV contraction (V, D) • Marked bradycardia (V, D) • Edema (esp. N, D) • Constipation (esp. V)
Aspirin	↓ *Platelet aggression*	• GI irritation or bleeding

V, verapamil; D, diltiazem; N, nifedipine and other dihydropyridine Ca^{++} channel antagonists

prove survival or prevent infarctions in patients with chronic CAD, and they are used purely for symptomatic relief. Common side effects include headache, lightheadedness, and palpitations induced by reflex sinus tachycardia. The latter can be prevented by combining a β-blocker with the nitrate regimen.

β-**blockers** (described further in Chapter 17) exert their antianginal effect by reducing myocardial oxygen demand. They are directed against β-receptors, of which there are two classes. $β_2$ adrenergic receptors are located throughout peripheral blood vessels and the bronchial tree, and $β_1$ adrenergic receptors are restricted to the myocardium. The stimulation of $β_1$ adrenergic receptors by catecholamines and sympathomimetic drugs increases heart rate and contractility. Thus, β-adrenergic antagonists decrease the force of ventricular contraction and heart rate, thereby reducing myocardial oxygen demand and relieving ischemia.

In addition to the beneficial effects of β-blockers in the suppression of chronic angina, several recent studies have shown that this group of drugs decreases the rates of recurrent infarction and mortality following an acute MI (see Chapter 7). Moreover, β-blockers have been shown to reduce the likelihood of a first myocardial infarction in patients with hypertension. Thus, β-blockers are considered first-line therapy in the treatment of coronary artery disease.

Beta-blockers are generally well-tolerated, but have several potential side effects. For example, they may precipitate bronchospasm in patients with underlying asthma by antagonizing $β_2$ receptors in the bronchial tree. Although β-1-*selective* blockers are theoretically less likely to exacerbate bronchospasm in such patients, drug selectivity for the β-1 receptor is not complete, and in general, all beta-blockers should be avoided in patients with obstructive airways disease.

Beta-blockers are also generally not used in patients with moderate or severely reduced ventricular contractile function, because a further decrease in contractility could precipitate congestive heart failure. Similarly, they are relatively contraindicated in patients with bradycardia or heart blocks, to avoid additional impairment of electrical conduction. Beta-blockers sometimes cause fatigue and sexual dysfunction, and can worsen control of serum glucose levels in diabetic patients. They could theoretically decrease myocardial perfusion by blocking the vasodilating β_2 adrenergic receptors on the coronary arteries. However, this effect is usually attenuated by autoregulation and *vasodilation* of the coronary vessel owing to the accumulation of local metabolites.

Calcium channel blockers (see Chapter 17) antagonize voltage-gated L-type calcium channels, but the actions of the individual drugs of this group vary. The dihydropyridines (e.g., nifedipine) are potent vasodilators. They relieve myocardial ischemia by: 1) decreasing oxygen demand (*venodilatation* reduces ventricular filling and size; *arterial dilatation* reduces the resistance against which the left ventricle contracts—both actions reduce wall stress) and by 2) increasing myocardial oxygen supply via coronary dilatation. By the latter mechanism, they are also potent agents for the relief of coronary artery vasospasm.

The calcium channel blockers verapamil and diltiazem are also vasodilators, but are not as potent in this regard as the dihydropyridine group of drugs. However, these agents have additional beneficial antianginal effects: They reduce the force of ventricular contraction (inotropy) and slow the heart rate. Accordingly, verapamil and diltiazem also decrease myocardial oxygen demand by these mechanisms.

Recent reports have raised questions about the safety of *short-acting* dihydropyridine calcium channel blocking drugs in the treatment of ischemic heart disease. In meta-analyses of randomized trials, these drugs have been associated with an *increased* incidence of myocardial infarction and mortality. If such findings are confirmed, the adverse effect may relate to the rapid hemodynamic effects and blood pressure swings induced by the short-acting agents. Therefore, only *long-acting* calcium-channel blocking drugs are recommended in the treatment of chronic angina today, generally as second-line drugs, if symptoms are not controlled by β-blockers and nitrates.

The three groups of antianginal drugs can be used alone or in combination. However, care should be taken in combining a β-blocker with a nondihydropyridine calcium channel blocker (i.e., verapamil or diltiazem) because the combined negative chronotropic effect can cause excessive bradycardia and the combined negative inotropic effect can precipitate congestive heart failure.

Although useful in controlling symptoms of angina, none of the antianginal drug groups has been shown to slow or reverse the atherosclerotic process responsible for the arterial lesions of chronic CAD. There is recent evidence, however, that reduction of serum LDL-cholesterol by antilipid pharmacologic therapy may achieve this goal (see Chapter 5).

Antiplatelet therapy with aspirin is a standard addition to the regimen of drugs used to treat CAD. Platelet aggregation and thrombosis have been implicated in acute myocardial infarction (see Chapter 7) and unstable angina. Aspirin inhibits platelet aggregation (and therefore reduces the subsequent release of platelet-derived procoagulants and vasoconstrictors) and has been shown to reduce the risk of myocardial infarction in patients with chronic angina. Unless contraindications are present (e.g., allergy, gastric irritation), aspirin is continued indefinitely in patients with known coronary artery disease, especially following an MI. Given the critical role of platelet aggregation and thrombosis in coronary syndromes, newer and more potent antiplatelet agents are in development.

Patients with angina that becomes asymptomatic after initiation of medical therapy are usually followed clinically with continued attention to their cardiac risk factors. However, more aggressive **mechanical revascularization** is considered if: 1) the angina is refractory to drug therapy, 2) unacceptable side effects of medications has occurred, or 3) the patient is known to have a specific pattern of severe disease for which surgical revacularization is known to improve survival (see below). The two most common techniques used to accomplish mechanical revascularization are percutaneous transluminal coronary angioplasty and coronary artery bypass graft surgery.

Percutaneous transluminal coronary angioplasty (PTCA) is a procedure performed under fluoroscopy in which a balloon-tipped catheter is inserted through a peripheral artery (usually a femoral or brachial artery) and maneuvered into the stenotic segment of a coronary vessel. The balloon at the end of the catheter is then inflated under high pressure to dilate the stenosis and thereby increase coronary perfusion, after which the catheter is removed from the body. The improvement in the size of the coronary lumen develops through compression of the plaque, and often by creating a fracture within the plaque and stretching the underlying media. Only certain types of stenoses are amenable to balloon dilation, but successful angioplasty is achieved in approximately 90% of such cases. The risk of MI during the procedure is less than 5%, and mortality is approximately 1% or less. Unfortunately, about a third of dilated vessels restenose within 6 months and require a second angioplasty procedure.

In addition to balloon angioplasty, several other percutaneous coronary revascularization procedures are in use. *Directional coronary atherectomy* involves positioning a windowed cylindrical housing against a stenosis as an attached balloon is inflated against the opposite wall. A rotating metal blade is then advanced within the housing and used to shave plaque from the vessel wall and extract the fragments through the catheter tip. *Rotational atherectomy* uses a rapidly spinning burr to penetrate calcified or fibrotic plaque. Percutaneous *excimer laser* catheter techniques are used to "vaporize" atherosclerotic plaques. Unfortunately, none of these advanced techniques have proved superior to standard balloon angioplasty at maintaining vessel patency over the long term.

The most recent advance in percutaneous catheter technique involves the implantation of *coronary stents*—slender, cagelike, stainless-steel support devices that in their collapsed configuration can be threaded into the region of stenosis by a catheter. Once in position, the stent is expanded into its open position by inflating a high-pressure balloon in its interior. The balloon is then removed, but the stent is left permanently in place to serve as a scaffold to maintain arterial patency. Recent data indicate that stenting results in larger luminal diameters, significantly decreases restenosis rates, and reduces the need for repeat angioplasty. Current strategies are testing potent new antithrombotic agents in conjunction with stent deployment to further reduce the thrombosis and restenosis rates.

Coronary artery bypass graft (CABG) surgery entails grafting portions of native blood vessels to bypass obstructed coronary arteries. Two types of surgical grafts are used (Fig. 6.9). The first employs a section of the saphenous vein—a "superfluous" vessel removed from the leg—which is sutured from the base of the aorta to a coronary segment downstream from the stenosis. In the second method, an internal mammary artery (a branch of the subclavian artery) can be directly anastomosed distal to the stenotic site. Because the internal mammary artery (yet another "superfluous" vessel) has been found to remain patent over time in a greater percentage of patients, compared with vein grafts, it is desirable to use this vessel in reperfusing sites of critical flow, such as the left anterior descending artery. The patency rate of the internal mammary graft is 90% at 10 years. Conversely, vein grafts have a patency rate of up to 80% at 12 months, but by 10 years following surgery more than 50% have occluded. There is recent evidence however, that aggressive lipid-lowering drug therapy after CABG can improve the long-term patency rates of venous bypass grafts.

Following CABG, angina is relieved in the vast majority of patients, and exercise performance is generally improved. Large clinical trials have shown a survival advantage of CABG over medical therapy of CAD only in certain subsets of individuals, most notably: 1) patients with significant stenosis of the left main coronary artery, and 2) patients with major blockages in all three main

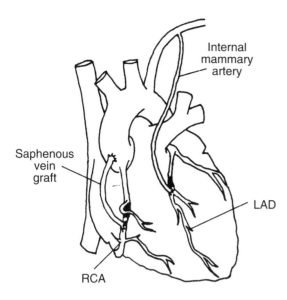

Figure 6.9. Coronary artery bypass surgery.
A. The left internal mammary artery originates from the left subclavian artery, and in this schematic, is anastomosed to the left anterior descending coronary artery distal to a tight stenosis. **B.** One end of a saphenous vein graft is sutured to the proximal aorta and the other end to the right coronary artery distal to a stenotic segment.

coronary arteries or their branches, especially if LV systolic contractile function is impaired.

Many patients with chronic, stable angina can be successfully managed with pharmacologic therapy alone. However, mechanical revascularization techniques are recommended for those individuals with refractory symptoms or those who experience intolerable side effects from antianginal medications. Percutaneous angioplasty is performed in such individuals who have suitable anatomy for the catheter-based procedures. For patients with stenoses that are not amenable to angioplasty, or for those in high-risk groups shown to demonstrate improved survival from surgical intervention (indicated in the previous paragraph), CABG is recommended instead. In addition, recent data has shown that diabetics with multivessel disease who are candidates for either angioplasty or CABG exhibit better long-term survival when the surgical bypass procedure is undertaken.

Treatment of Unstable Angina

Most patients with unstable angina have advanced atherosclerotic disease complicated by platelet thrombus formation that partially occludes a coronary artery, and/or superimposed vasoconstriction. Effective therapy is directed against these factors.

A patient with symptoms of unstable angina should be admitted to the hospital and placed at bed rest to reduce myocardial oxygen consumption. Serial electrocardiograms and serum markers of myocardial damage (see Chapter 7) are assessed to differentiate unstable angina from the irreversible necrosis of myocardial infarction. In order to help rebalance myocardial oxygen supply and demand, beta-blockers and nitrates are administered (often intravenously). In patients who have not received beta-blockers previously, the addition of a drug from this class decreases the likelihood of progression from unstable angina to myocardial infarction. Conversely, calcium channel blockers do not share this advantage; they do not prevent infarction or reduce mortality in unstable angina. Thus, calcium channel blockers should either not be used in unstable angina, or employed only as second-line drugs for pain control in individuals who do not respond to beta-blockers and nitrates.

Most important, since platelet aggregation and thrombus formation play a central role in the pathophysiology of unstable angina, antiplatelet (i.e., aspirin) and antocoagulant (i.e., intravenous heparin) therapies are standard treatment. Used alone or together, aspirin and heparin substantially reduce the progression from unstable angina to myocardial infarction. Conversely, thrombolytic agents, which are enormously beneficial in acute myocardial infarction (see Chapter 7) have *not* been shown to reduce mortality or complications in unstable angina and should not be administered in this setting. If a patient does not respond quickly to aspirin, heparin, beta-blocker and nitrate therapy, urgent coronary angiography is undertaken, often followed by revascularization procedures.

A dreaded complication of chronic ischemic heart disease or unstable angina is acute myocardial infarction, which is the subject of the next chapter.

SUMMARY

1. Cardiac ischemia results from an imbalance between myocardial oxygen supply and demand. Myocardial oxygen supply is determined by the oxygen-carrying capacity of the blood and coronary blood flow. The latter is dependent on the coronary perfusion pressure and coronary vascular resistance. Key regulators of myocardial oxygen demand include myocardial wall stress, heart rate, and contractility.

2. In the presence of atherosclerotic disease, myocardial oxygen supply is compromised. Atherosclerotic plaques cause vascular lumen narrowing and reduce epicardial coronary blood flow. In addition, atherosclerosis-associated endothelial cell dysfunction causes inappropriate vasoconstriction of the resistance coronary vessels.

3. Angina pectoris is the most frequent symptom of intermittent ischemia, and its diagnosis relies heavily on the patient's description of the discomfort. Angina may be accompanied by signs and symptoms of adrenergic stimulation, pulmonary congestion, and transient left ventricular systolic and diastolic dysfunction.

4. Laboratory studies useful in the diagnosis of angina include the electrocardiogram (ST segment depressions (subendocardial ischemia) or elevations (transmural ischemia)), exercise (or pharmacologic) stress testing, and coronary angiography.

5. Standard pharmacologic agents in the treatment of chronic angina include organic nitrates, β-blockers, and calcium channel antagonists, alone or in combination, as well as aspirin, and if indicated, anticholesterol therapy. Modifiable risk factors for atherosclerosis should be corrected. Angioplasty and coronary artery bypass graft surgery are reserved for selected patients.

ADDITIONAL READING

Anderson TJ, Meredith IT, Yeung AC, et al. The effect of cholesterol-lowering and antioxidant therapy on endothelium-dependent coronary vasomotion. N Engl J Med 1995;332:488–493.

Bittl JA. Advances in coronary angioplasty. N Engl J Med. 1996;335:1290–1302.

Bypass Angioplasty Revascularization Investigation (BARI) Investigators. Comparison of coronary bypass surgery with angioplasty in patients with multivessel disease. N Engl J Med. 1996;335:217–225.

Caracciolo EA, et al. Comparison of surgical and medical group survival in patients with left main coronary artery disease: long-term CASS experience. Circulation 1995;91:2325–2334.

CASS Principal Investigators and Their Associates. Coronary Artery Surgery Study (CASS): a randomized trial of coronary artery bypass surgery: survival data. Circulation 1983;68:939–950.

Fuster V, Badimon L, Badimon JJ, et al. The pathogenesis of coronary artery disease and the acute coronary syndromes. N Engl J Med 1992;326:242–250, 310–318.

Ganz P, Braunwald E. Coronary blood flow and myocardial ischemia. In: Braunwald E, ed. Heart Disease: A Textbook of Cardiovascular Medicine. Philadelphia: WB Saunders, 1997:1161–1183.

Gersh BJ, Braunwald E, Rutherford JD. Chronic coronary artery disease. In: Braunwald E, ed. Heart Disease: A Textbook of Cardiovascular Medicine. Philadelphia: WB Saunders, 1997:1289–1365.

Levine GN, Keaney JF Jr., Vita JA. Cholesterol reduction in cardiovascular disease: Clinical benefits and possible mechanisms. N Engl J Med 1995;332:512–521.

Mehta JL. Endothelium, coronary vasodilation, and organic nitrates. Am Heart J 1995;129:382–391.

Osborne JA, Stone PH. Recent advances in the understanding and management of stable and unstable angina pectoris and asymptomatic myocardial ischemia. Curr Opin Cardiol 1994;9:448–456.

Parisi AF, Folland ED, Hartigan P, on behalf of the Veterans Affairs ACME Investigators. A comparison of angioplasty with medical therapy in the treatment of single-vessel coronary artery disease. N Engl J Med 1992;326:10–16.

Post Coronary Artery Bypass Graft Trial Investigators. The effect of aggressive lowering of low-density lipoprotein cholesterol levels and low-dose anticoagulation on obstructive changes in saphenous-vein coronary artery bypass grafts. N Engl J Med. 1997;336:153–162.

RITA Trial Participants. Coronary angioplasty versus coronary artery bypass surgery: the randomised intervention treatment of angina (RITA) trial. Lancet 1993;341:573–580.

Treasure CB, Klein JL, Weintraub WS, et al. Beneficial effects of cholesterol-lowering therapy on the coronary endothelium in patients with coronary artery disease. N Engl J Med 1995;332:481–487.

Veterans Administration Coronary Artery Bypass Surgery Cooperative Study Group. Eleven-year survival in the Veterans Administration randomized trail of coronary bypass surgery for stable angina. N Engl J Med 1984;311:1333–1339.

Yusuf S, Zucker D, Peduzzi P, et al. Effect of coronary artery bypass graft surgery on survival: overview of 10-year results from randomised trials by the Coronary Artery Bypass Graft Surgery Trialists Collaboration. Lancet 1994;344:563–570.

Acknowledgments The previous edition of this chapter was written by Christopher P. Chiodo, MD, Carey Farquhar, MD, Rainu Kaushal, MD, William Carlson, MD, Michael E. Mendelsohn, MD, and Leonard S. Lilly, MD.

Acute Myocardial Infarction

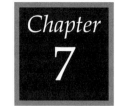

Chapter

7

Marc S. Sabatine, Patrick T. O'Gara, and Leonard S. Lilly

Myocardial infarction (MI) is the condition of irreversible necrosis of heart muscle that results from prolonged ischemia. Considering the physical stresses that our coronary arteries endure every minute—the pulling and compressing of a beating myocardium—and the wide variations in oxygen demand that they must supply, it may be surprising that severe myocardial ischemia does not occur more often. However, the autoregulatory mechanisms within the coronary arteries, described in the preceding chapter, usually preserve adequate oxygen delivery to the myocardium even in the presence of atherosclerotic plaques. It is when the usual defenses are circumvented that prolonged ischemia, or myocardial infarction, may result.

Nearly 1.5 million people in the United States sustain an MI each year, and this event proves fatal in approximately one-third of patients. Despite these daunting statistics, there has been a continuous decline in the mortality rate from myocardial infarction over the past three decades, due in part to a better understanding of the underlying pathophysiology, and to dramatic therapeutic advances.

Similar to other manifestations of ischemic heart disease, the complications of an MI often relate to the duration and magnitude of the imbalance between myocardial oxygen supply and demand, and the long-term outcome depends greatly on the extent of necrotic myocardium. In this chapter we consider the events that lead to myocardial infarction, the pathologic and functional changes that follow, and therapeutic approaches that ameliorate the aberrant pathophysiology.

ETIOLOGY AND PATHOGENESIS

Approximately 90% of myocardial infarctions result from formation of an acute thrombus that obstructs an atherosclerotic coronary artery. The thrombus transforms a region of plaque narrowing to one of complete vessel occlusion. The responsible thrombus appears to be generated by interactions between the atherosclerotic plaque, the coronary endothelium, circulating platelets, and the dynamic vasomotor tone of the vessel wall, all of which overwhelm natural protective mechanisms, as we will examine.

Normal Hemostasis

When a normal blood vessel is injured, the endothelial surface becomes disrupted and thrombogenic connective tissue is exposed. *Primary hemostasis* is the first line of defense against bleeding. This process begins within seconds of vessel injury and is mediated by circulating platelets, which adhere to collagen in the vascular subendothelium and aggregate to form a "platelet plug." While the primary hemostatic plug forms, the exposure of subendothelial tissue factor activates the plasma coagulation cascade, initiating the process of *secondary hemostasis*. The plasma coagulation proteins involved in secondary hemostasis are sequentially activated at the site of injury, and ultimately form a fibrin clot by the action of thrombin. The resulting clot stabilizes and strengthens the platelet plug.

The normal hemostatic system minimizes blood loss from injured vessels, but there is little difference between this physiologic response and the pathologic process of coronary thrombosis triggered by disruption of atherosclerotic plaques.

Endogenous Antithrombotic Mechanisms

Normal blood vessels, including the coronary arteries, are replete with safeguards that prevent spontaneous thrombosis and occlusion, some examples of which are shown in Figure 7.1.

Inactivation of Clotting Factors

Several natural inhibitors tightly regulate the coagulation process to oppose clot formation and maintain blood fluidity. The most important of these are antithrombin III, proteins C and S, and tissue factor pathway inhibitor.

Antithrombin III (ATIII) is a plasma protein that irreversibly binds to thrombin and other clotting factors, inactivating them and facilitating their clearance from the circulation (mechanism 1 in Fig. 7.1). The effectiveness of ATIII is increased a thousand-fold by binding to heparan sulfate, a heparin-like molecule normally present on the luminal surface of endothelial cells.

Protein C/Protein S/Thrombomodulin is a natural anticoagulant system that inactivates the "acceleration" factors of the coagulation pathway (i.e., factors Va and VIIIa). Protein C is synthesized in the liver and circulates in an inactivate form. Thrombomodulin is a thrombin-binding receptor normally present on endothelial cells. Thrombin that is bound to thrombomodulin cannot convert fibrinogen to fibrin (the final reaction in clot formation). Instead, the thrombin-thrombomodulin complex activates protein C. Activated protein C degrades factors Va and VIIIa (mechanism 2 in Fig. 7.1), thereby inhibiting coagulation. The presence of protein S in the circulation enhances the inhibitory function of protein C.

Tissue factor pathway inhibitor (TFPI) is a recently discovered plasma serine protease inhibitor that is activated by coagulation factor Xa. The factor Xa/TFPI complex binds to and inactivates the complex of tissue factor with factor VIIa that normally triggers the "extrinsic" coagulation pathway (mechanism 3 in Fig. 7.1). Thus TFPI serves as a negative feedback inhibitor that interferes with coagulation.

Lysis of Fibrin Clots

Tissue plasminogen activator (t-PA) is a protein secreted by endothelial cells in response to many triggers of clot formation. t-PA cleaves the protein plasminogen to form active plasmin, which in turn enzymatically degrades fibrin clots (mechanism 4 in Fig. 7.1). When t-PA binds to fibrin in a forming clot, its ability to convert plasminogen to plasmin is increased a hundred-fold.

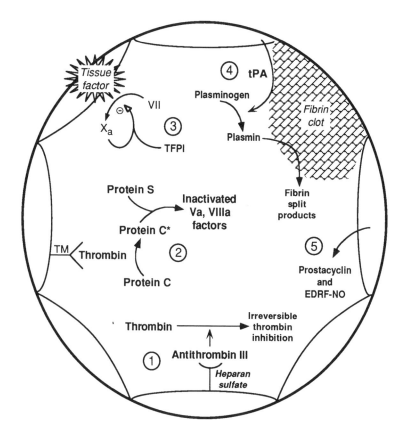

Figure 7.1. Endogenous protective mechanisms against thrombosis and vessel occlusion: 1. Inactivation of thrombin by antithrombin III (ATIII), the effectiveness of which is enhanced by binding of ATIII to heparan sulfate. **2.** Inactivation of clotting factors Va and VIIIa by activated protein C (protein C*), an action that is enhanced by protein S. Protein C is activated by the thrombomodulin (TM)-thrombin complex. **3.** Inactivation of factor VII/tissue factor complex by tissue factor pathway inhibitor (TFPI). **4.** Lysis of fibrin clots by tissue plasminogen activator (tPA). **5.** Inhibition of platelet activation by prostacyclin and EDRF-NO.

Endogenous Platelet Inhibition and Vasodilatation

Prostacyclin is synthecized and secreted by endothelial cells, as described in Chapter 6. It increases platelet levels of cyclic AMP, and thereby strongly inhibits platelet activation and aggregation (mechanism 5 in Fig. 7.1). Prostacyclin also *indirectly* inhibits coagulation via its potent vasodilating properties. Vasodilatation helps guard against thrombosis by augmenting blood flow (which minimizes contact between procoagulant factors) and by reducing shear stress (an inducer of platelet activation).

Endothelium-derived relaxing factor/ nitric oxide (EDRF-NO) is also secreted by endothelial cells as described in Chapter 6. It acts locally to inhibit platelet activation (mechanism 5 in Fig. 7.1), and it too serves as a potent vasodilator.

Pathogenesis of Coronary Thrombosis

Normally, the above mechanisms serve to prevent spontaneous intravascular thrombus formation. However, abnormalities associated with atherosclerotic lesions may overwhelm these defenses and result in coronary thrombosis and vessel occlusion (Fig. 7.2). Atherosclerosis contributes to thrombus formation by: 1) plaque rupture, which exposes the circulating blood el-

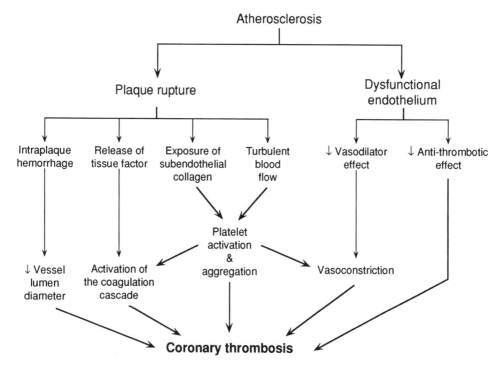

Figure 7.2.   Mechanisms of coronary thrombus formation. Factors that contribute to this process include plaque disruption (e.g. rupture), activation of platelets and the clotting cascade, and inappropriate vasoconstriction and loss of normal antithrombotic defenses because of a dysfunctional endothelium.

ements to thrombogenic substances, and 2) endothelial dysfunction with the loss of normal protective antithrombotic and vasodilatory properties.

Atherosclerotic **plaque rupture** is considered to be the major trigger of coronary thrombosis. The underlying causes of plaque disruption are likely multifactorial and include: 1) chemical factors that increase the vulnerability of plaque to rupture, and 2) physical stresses to which the atherosclerotic lesions are subjected. Plaques consist of a fibrous external cap that surrounds a lipid-laden and necrotic core. There is evidence that substances released from leukocytes within the plaque can compromise the integrity of the fibrous cap. For example, T lymphocytes elaborate gamma interferon, which inhibits collagen synthesis by smooth muscle cells, and thereby interferes with the usual strength of the fibrous cap. Additionally, cells within atherosclerotic lesions produce enzymes (e.g., collagenase and gelatinase) that degrade

the interstitial matrix, further compromising the stable structure of the plaque. A weakened, or thin-capped plaque is subject to rupture, particularly in its "shoulder" region (the border with the normal arterial wall that is subjected to high circumferential stress) either spontaneously or by physical forces, such as intraluminal blood pressure and torsion from the beating myocardium.

Myocardial infarctions sometimes occur in the setting of certain triggers, such as strenuous physical activity or emotional stress. The activation of the sympathetic nervous system in these situations increases the blood pressure, heart rate, and force of ventricular contraction, actions that may stress the atherosclerotic lesion, thereby causing the plaque to fissure or rupture. In addition, MIs are also most likely to occur in the early morning hours. This observation may relate to the fact that key physiologic stressors, such as systolic blood pressure, blood viscosity and plasma epinephrine levels tend to be most elevated at that time of day, and these factors subject vulnerable plaques to rupture.

Once plaque rupture occurs, the *exposure of subendothelial collagen* activates platelets, and *tissue factor* triggers the coagulation pathway, events that contribute to thrombus formation (Fig. 7.2). *Intraplaque hemorrhage* (see Chapter 5) can also occur during plaque rupture, which may further enlarge the volume of the atherosclerotic lesion, and thereby additionally compromise the coronary arterial lumen.

A fibrous plaque with a nonocclusive superimposed thrombus narrows the vessel lumen, and may therefore cause *turbulent blood flow* through the artery. This action may subject circulating platelets to substantial shear stress, thereby activating them, and promoting platelet aggregation. Furthermore, sudden changes in plaque geometry (e.g., by intraplaque hemorrhage) can additionally narrow the lumen and contribute to platelet shear stress and activation.

Activated platelets release the contents of their granules, which include facilitators of *platelet aggregation* (e.g., ADP, fibrinogen), *activators of the coagulation cascade* (e.g., factor Va), and *vasoconstrictors* (e.g., thromboxane and serotonin). The contribution of platelet aggregation to the forming thrombus further reduces the diameter of the vessel lumen.

During thrombus formation, vasoconstriction is promoted both by platelelet products (e.g., thromboxane and serotonin) and by thrombin within the developing clot. The *normal* platelet-associated vascular response is vasodilatation, because platelet products stimulate endothelial EDRF-NO and prostacyclin release, the influences of which predominate over direct platelet-derived vasoconstrictors (see Fig. 6.4). However, reduced secretion of endothelial vasodilators in atherosclerosis allows vasoconstriction to proceed unchecked. Similarly, thrombin in a forming clot is a potent vascular smooth muscle constrictor in the setting of dysfunctional endothelium. Vasoconstriction causes torsional stresses that can contribute to plaque rupture, or can

transiently occlude the stenotic vessel through heightened arterial tone. The reduction in coronary blood flow caused by vasoconstriction also reduces the washout of coagulation proteins, such that thrombogenicity is enhanced.

Dysfunctional endothelium, which is apparent even in mild atherosclerotic coronary disease, also increases the likelihood of thrombus formation. Dysfunctional endothelial cells secrete reduced amounts of vasodilators (i.e., EDRF-NO and prostacyclin), and therefore, relative vasoconstriction is manifest (Fig. 7.2). Moreover, endothelium-derived EDRF-NO and prostacyclin are normally inhibitors of platelet activation. Their reduced release from dysfunctional endothelium removes an important antithrombotic influence.

Significance of Coronary Thrombosis

The formation of an intracoronary thrombus results in one of several potential outcomes (Fig. 7.3). For example, plaque rupture is sometimes superficial, minor and self-limited, such that only a small, nonocclusive thrombus forms. In this case, the small thrombus may simply become incorporated into the growing atheromatous lesion through fibrotic organization, or lysed by natural fibrinolytic mechanisms. Recurrent asymptomatic plaque ruptures of this type may cause gradual progressive enlargement of the coronary stenosis.

However, deeper plaque rupture may result in greater exposure of subendothelial collagen and tissue factor, with formation of a larger thrombus that more substantially occludes the vessel's lumen. Such obstruction may cause prolonged severe ischemia and the development of an acute coronary syndrome, such as unstable angina or a myocardial infarction. If the intraluminal thrombus at the site of plaque disruption *totally* occludes the vessel, blood flow beyond the obstruction will cease, prolonged ischemia will occur and a myocardial infarction (usually a Q-wave MI) will likely result. Conversely, if the thrombus *partially* occludes the vessel (or if it totally occludes

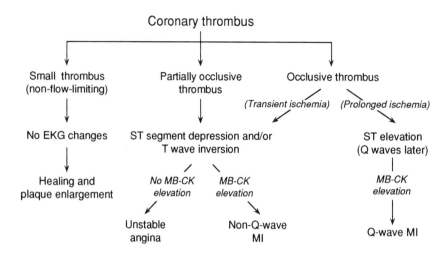

Figure 7.3. Consequences of coronary thrombosis. A small thrombus formed on superficial plaque rupture may not result in symptoms or EKG abnormalities, but healing and fibrous organization may incorporate the thrombus into the plaque, causing the atherosclerotic lesion to enlarge. A partially occlusive thrombus (with or without superimposed vasospasm) narrows the arterial lumen, restricts blood flow and can cause unstable angina or a non-Q-wave MI, either of which may result in ST depression or T wave inversion on the EKG. A totally occlusive thrombus with prolonged ischemia is the most common cause of Q-wave MI, and the EKG initially shows ST segment elevation (followed by Q wave development later). An occlusive thrombus that recanalizes, or one that develops in a region served by adequate collateral blood flow, may result in less prolonged ischemia and a non-Q-wave MI instead. CK-MB, creatine kinase MB isoenzyme (a serum marker of myocardial infarction).

the vessel, but only transiently, because of spontaneous recanalization, or by relief of superimposed vasospasm), the severity and duration of ischemia will be less, and a smaller non-Q-wave MI or unstable angina are the more likely outcomes (Fig. 7.3).

Occasionally, a non-Q-wave infarct may result from total, prolonged occlusion. In this case, it is likely that a substantial collateral blood supply limits the extent of necrosis, such that a larger Q-wave MI is prevented.

Nonatherosclerotic Causes of Acute MI

Rarely, mechanisms other than acute coronary thrombus formation can precipitate myocardial ischemia and infarction (Table 7.1). These should be suspected if ischemic syndromes develop in young individuals or those without coronary risk factors. For example, coronary emboli from mechanical or infected cardiac valves can lodge in the coronary circulation, or inflammation from acute vasculitis can initiate

TABLE 7.1. Causes of Myocardial Infarction

Atherosclerosis with Occlusive Thrombus
Vasculitic syndromes (Chapter 15)
Coronary emboli (e.g., from endocarditis, artificial valves)
Congenital anomalies of the coronary arteries
Coronary trauma or aneurysm
Severe coronary artery spasm (primary or cocaine-induced)
Increased blood viscosity (e.g., polycythemia vera, thrombocytosis)
Markedly increased myocardial oxygen demand (e.g., aortic stenosis)

coronary occlusion. Occasionally, intense transient coronary spasm can sufficiently reduce myocardial blood supply to result in infarction.

A very unfortunate cause of acute MI is cocaine abuse. Cocaine increases sympathetic tone by blocking the presynaptic reuptake of norepinephrine and by enhancing the release of adrenal catecholamines, which can lead to vasospasm and therefore decreased myocardial oxygen supply. Infarction may ensue as a result of increased myocardial oxygen demand associated with cocaine-associated sympathetic my-ocardial stimulation (increased heart rate and blood pressure), in the face of the de-creased oxygen supply.

PATHOLOGY AND PATHOPHYSIOLOGY

Infarcts can be described pathologically by the extent of necrosis within the myocar-dial wall. **Transmural infarcts** are most common and span the thickness of the my-ocardium and result from total, prolonged occlusion of an epicardial coronary artery. Conversely, **subendocardial infarcts** exclu-sively involve the innermost layers of the myocardium. This subendocardium is par-ticularly susceptible to ischemia because it is the zone subjected to the highest pressure from the ventricular chamber, has few col-lateral vessels that supply it, and is perfused by vessels that must pass through layers of contracting myocardium.

Infarction is not a single event but a process of intensifying ischemia that results in cell death. Myocardium that is supplied directly by an occluded vessel may die quickly. The adjacent tissue may not necrose immediately, because it may also be perfused by nearby vessels. The neighbor-ing cells may become increasingly ischemic over time, however, as demand for oxygen continues in the face of decreased oxygen supply. Thus, the region of infarction may subsequently extend outward. The extent of tissue that ultimately succumbs to infarc-tion therefore relates to: 1) the mass of my-ocardium perfused by the occluded vessel, 2) the oxygen demand of the affected re-gion, 3) the adequacy of collateral vessels that provide blood flow from neighboring nonoccluded coronary arteries, and 4) the degree of tissue response that modifies the ischemic process.

The pathophysiologic events that tran-spire during myocardial infarction predict efficacious therapies and possible complica-tions. Generally, these events occur in two stages: early changes at the time of acute in-farction and late changes during myocar-dial reconstruction.

Early Changes

Early changes include the histologic evo-lution of the infarct and the functional im-pact of oxygen deprivation on myocardial contractility. These changes culminate in coagulative necrosis of the myocardium in 2 to 4 days (Fig. 7.4)

Cellular Changes

As oxygen levels fall in the myocardium supplied by an abruptly occluded coronary vessel, there is a rapid shift from aerobic to anaerobic, glycolytic metabolism. Because mitochondria can no longer oxidize fats or products of glycolysis, high-energy phos-phate production drops dramatically and anaerobic glycolysis leads to the accumu-lation of lactic acid. The lowered pH de-creases myocardial compliance and con-tractility as early as 2 min following occlusive thrombosis. Without interven-tion, irreversible cell injury ensues in 20 min and becomes apparent with mitochondrial swelling, margination of nuclear chro-matin, membrane defects, and glycogen de-pletion.

Intracellular ATP levels decrease within minutes because glycolytic production lags far behind myocardial ATP consumption. The paucity of ATP slows the transmem-brane Na^+/K^+ ATPase, with resultant ele-vation in intracellular $[Na^+]$ and extracellu-lar $[K^+]$. Rising $[Na^+]$ contributes to cellular edema. Membrane leak and rising extracel-lular K^+ concentration contributes to alter-ations in the transmembrane electrical po-tential, predisposing the myocardium to lethal arrhythmias (see Chapter 11).

Intracellular Ca^{++} accumulates during acute ischemia by a variety of mechanisms, including: 1) activation of the Na^+/Ca^{++} exchange pump owing to the rising intra-cellular $[Na^+]$, 2) Ca^{++} leakage from the sarcoplasmic reticulum into the cytosol, and 3) alterations in voltage-regulated Ca^{++} channels and the Ca^{++}-ATPase efflux system. With progressive disruption of the cell membrane, Ca^{++} entry from the extra-cellular space cannot be removed by normal

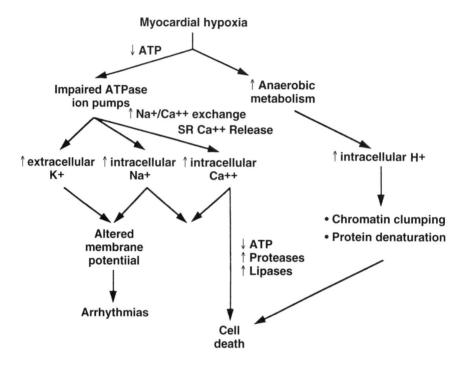

Figure 7.4.   Mechanisms of cell death in myocardial infarction. Acute ischemia rapidly depletes the intracellular supply of ATP as aerobic metabolism fails. Subsequent intracellular acidosis and impairment of ATP-dependent processes culminate in intracellular calcium accumulation, edema, and cell death.

energy-dependent mechanisms, which marks the transition from reversible to irreversible cell damage. High intracellular concentrations of Ca^+ are thought to be the final, common pathway to cell destruction through the activation of degradative lipases and proteases.

Severe membrane injury results from lack of high-energy phosphates, loss of endogenous antioxidants, and the production of oxygen-free radicals by infiltrating neutrophils. As proteolytic enzymes leak from the myocytes, they damage adjacent myocardium; the release of specific macromolecules into the circulation serves as a marker of acute infarction (see below).

Edema of the myocardium develops within 4 to 12 hours, as vascular permeability increases (because of the release of inflammatory mediators) and interstitial oncotic pressure rises (because of the leak of intracellular proteins). The earliest histologic changes of irreversible injury are **wavy myofibers,** which appear as intercel-

lular edema separates the myocardial cells that are tugged about by the surrounding, functional myocardium (Fig. 7.5). **Contraction bands** can often be seen near the borders of the infarct: sarcomeres are contracted and consolidated and appear as bright eosinophilic belts.

An acute inflammatory response, with infiltration of neutrophils, begins after approximately 4 hours and releases toxic oxygen-derived free radicals, inciting further tissue damage. Within 18 to 24 hours, **coagulation necrosis** is evident with pyknotic nuclei and bland eosinophilic cytoplasm, seen by light microscopy. These early changes are demonstrated in Figure 7.5 and summarized in Table 7.2.

Gross Changes

Gross morphologic changes do not appear until 18 to 24 hours after coronary occlusion, although certain staining techniques (e.g., tetrazolium) permit the

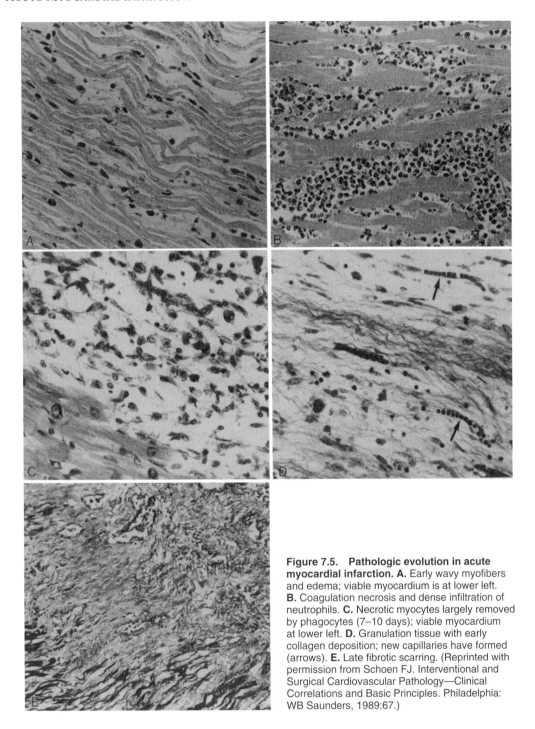

Figure 7.5. Pathologic evolution in acute myocardial infarction. A. Early wavy myofibers and edema; viable myocardium is at lower left. **B.** Coagulation necrosis and dense infiltration of neutrophils. **C.** Necrotic myocytes largely removed by phagocytes (7–10 days); viable myocardium at lower left. **D.** Granulation tissue with early collagen deposition; new capillaries have formed (arrows). **E.** Late fibrotic scarring. (Reprinted with permission from Schoen FJ. Interventional and Surgical Cardiovascular Pathology—Clinical Correlations and Basic Principles. Philadelphia: WB Saunders, 1989:67.)

pathologist to identify regions of infarction earlier. Most often, ischemia and infarction begin in the subendocardium, and then extend laterally and outward toward the epicardium.

Late Changes

Late pathologic changes in the course of acute MI (Table 7.2) include: 1) the clearing of necrotic myocardium by macrophages,

TABLE 7.2. Pathologic Timecourse in Transmural Infarction

Time	Event
Early changes	
1–2 min	ATP levels fall; cessation of contractility
10 min	50% depletion of ATP; cellular edema, decreased membrane potential and susceptibility to arrhythmias
20–24 min	Irreversible cell injury
1–3 hours	Wavy myofibers
4–12 hours	Hemorrhage, edema, PMN infiltration
18–24 hours	Coagulation necrosis (pyknotic nuclei with eosinophilic cytoplasm), edema
2–4 days	Total coagulation necrosis (no nuclei or striations, rimmed by hyperemic tissue); monocytes appear
Late Changes	
5–7 days	Yellow-softening from resorption of dead tissue by macrophages
7 days +	Ventricular remodeling
7 weeks	Fibrosis and scarring complete

and 2) the deposition of collagen to form scar tissue.

Irreversibly injured myocytes do not regenerate; rather, the cells are removed and replaced by fibrous tissue. Macrophages invade the inflamed myocardium shortly after neutrophil infiltration to remove the necrotic tissue. This period of tissue resorption is termed **yellow-softening,** as connective tissue elements are destroyed and removed along with dead myocardial cells. This phagocytic clearing, combined with thinning and dilation of the infarcted zone, results in structural weakness of the ventricular wall, and the possibility of myocardial wall rupture at this stage. **Fibrosis** subsequently ensues, and scarring is complete by 7 weeks after infarction (Fig. 7.5).

Functional Changes

Impaired Contractility

Infarction quickly leads to impaired contractile function of the ventricle, and often to decreased cardiac output. Ventricular output is further compromised because *synchronous* contraction of myocytes is lost: When infarction results in an area of decreased contractility, that region is termed "hypokinetic," segments that do not contract at all are called "akinetic," and "dyskinetic" regions are those that bulge *outward* during systolic ventricular contraction.

Stunning and Hibernation

It was previously thought that ischemic cardiac injury resulted in either irreversible myocardial necrosis or rapid full recovery of myocyte function. It is now known that ischemic insults can sometimes result in a period of *prolonged* contractile dysfunction *without* myocyte necrosis, and recovery of normal function may ultimately follow.

For example, **stunned myocardium** refers to tissue that, after suffering a period of severe ischemia (but not necrosis), demonstrates prolonged systolic dysfunction, even after the return of normal myocardial blood flow. In this setting, the functional, biochemical, and ultrastructural abnormalities following ischemia are temporary and reversible, and contractile strength gradually recovers. The mechanism responsible for this delayed recovery of function is not known, but may involve myocyte calcium overload, the accumulation of oxygen-derived free radicals, or disruption of excitation-contraction coupling because of transiently dysfunctional sarcoplasmic reticulum. In general, the magnitude of stunning is proportional to the degree of the preceding ischemia. Thus, "stunning" is likely the pathophysiologic response to an ischemic insult that just falls short of causing irreversible necrosis.

Hibernating myocardium is a state that differs from stunned myocardium. It refers to tissue that manifests *chronic* contractile dysfunction in the face of a persistently reduced blood supply, usually because of multivessel coronary artery disease. In this situation, irreversible damage has not been done and contractility can *promptly* improve if appropriate blood flow is restored. In essence, in the face of chronic hypoperfusion, the myocardium demonstrates reduced activity (i.e., acts as if it is "sleeping"), so as to bring oxygen supply and demand into balance.

The concepts of stunned and hibernating myocardium are clinically relevant. For example, if a patient with an acute MI or chronic ischemic heart disease demonstrates regions of impaired ventricular contractile function that are *potentially reversible,* then this knowledge may influence decision-making regarding revascularization procedures such as coronary artery bypass surgery. Currently, the ability to detect stunned and hibernating myocardium is limited, but certain radionuclide techniques (e.g., PET scanning described in Chapter 3) are useful in this regard.

Ventricular Remodeling

Following an MI, changes occur in the geometry of both the infarcted and noninfarcted ventricular walls. Alterations in chamber size and wall thickness affect long-term ventricular function as well as prognosis.

In the early post-MI period, infarct *expansion* may occur, in which the affected ventricular segment enlarges without additonal myocyte necrosis. Infarct expansion represents thinning and dilatation of the necrotic zone of tissue, likely because of "slippage" between the muscle fibers, resulting in a decreased volume of myocytes in the region of the infarct. Infarct expansion can be detrimental because it increases ventricular size, which: 1) augments wall stress, 2) impairs systolic contractile function, and 3) increases the likelihood of aneurysm formation.

In addition to early expansion of the infarcted territory, remodeling of the ventricle may also involve dilatation of the overworked *noninfarcted* segments, which are subjected to increased wall stress. This dilatation begins in the early postinfarct period, and continues over the ensuing weeks and months. Initially, chamber dilatation serves a compensatory role (it increases cardiac output via the Frank Starling mecha-

nism), but progressive enlargement may ultimately lead to heart failure and also predisposes to ventricular arrhythmias.

Adverse ventricular remodeling can be beneficially modified by certain interventions. At the time of infarction, for example, reperfusion therapies limit infarct size and therefore decrease the likelihood of infarct expansion. In addition, the use of angiotensin converting-enzyme inhibitors has been shown to attenuate progressive remodeling, and reduces short- and long-term post-MI mortality (see below).

Q-WAVE AND NON-Q-WAVE INFARCTIONS

Pathologically, MIs can be divided into transmural infarcts and subendocardial infarcts, as described above. Previous dogma was that transmural infarcts produced Q waves after initial ST elevations on the EKG, and that subendocardial infarcts generated ST depressions without Q wave development. It is now known that these EKG findings do not reliably correlate with the pathologic findings and that there is much overlap between the two types of infarction. That is, some patients with pathologic evidence of transmural infarction do not demonstrate Q waves, whereas others with subendocardial infarcts *do* have Q waves on the EKG. In general, however, non-Q-wave infarctions tend to be smaller, and may represent less occlusive thrombi (or briefer periods of severe ischemia) than those of Q-wave MIs.

In terms of clinical course, a distinction between Q-wave and a non-Q-wave MIs is still valuable. Initial hospital mortality is lower in patients with non-Q-wave infarction than those with Q-wave MI. However, during subsequent months of follow up, patients with non-Q-wave infarcts have high rates of reinfarction and mortality, because these patients often have severe multivessel coronary disease, and neighboring viable tissue is subject to recurrent ischemia. Therefore, aggressive evaluation is particularly important in this group for therapeutic planning.

CLINICAL PRESENTATION

The symptoms and physical findings of acute MI (Table 7.3) arise directly from the pathophysiology described earlier in this chapter.

The **pain of MI** resembles anginal pain qualitatively (see Chapter 6) but is usually more severe, lasts longer, and may radiate more widely. Like angina, the pain may result from the release of mediators such as adenosine and lactate from ischemic myocardial cells onto local nerve endings. Because ischemia persists and proceeds to necrosis, these provocative substances continue to accumulate and activate afferent nerves for longer periods. The pain of infarction is often referred to other regions of the C7–T4 dermatomes, including the neck, shoulders, and arms. The pain of myocardial infarction is rapid in onset and often briskly crescendos to leave its victims discomfited with profound "feelings of doom." Unlike a transient attack of angina, the pain does not wane with rest, and there may be little response to the administration of nitroglycerin.

Not all myocardial infarcts are accompanied by such forms of discomfort, however. Up to 25% of patients who sustain an MI are *asymptomatic* during the acute event, and the diagnosis is made only in retrospect through a routine electrocardiogram or when complications ensue. This is particularly common among diabetic patients who may not experience pain because of peripheral neuropathy. In addition, occasional patients who present with MI complicated by acute pericarditis may feel more of a sharp, pleuritic-type pain (see Chapter 14), rather than the typical MI symptoms.

The combination of pain and baroreceptor unloading (if hypotension is present) may trigger a dramatic **sympathetic nervous system response.** Systemic signs of catecholamine release include diaphoresis (sweating), tachycardia, and cool and clammy skin due to vasoconstriction.

As reduced LV contractility decreases the stroke volume, the diastolic volume and pressure within that chamber rise. The increase in LV pressure, compounded by the ischemia-induced stiffness of the chamber, is conveyed to the left atrium and pulmonary veins. The resultant pulmonary congestion decreases lung compliance and stimulates juxtacapillary receptors. These "J receptors" effect a reflex that results in rapid, shallow breathing and evokes the subjective feeling of **dyspnea.** Transudation of fluid into the alveoli exacerbates this symptom.

Physical findings can be apparent on auscultation during an acute MI but depend on the location and extent of the infarct. The S_4 sound, indicative of atrial contraction into a noncompliant left ventricle, can be heard shortly after infarction. An S_3 sound (rapid ventricular filling) is heard in many post-MI patients and signifies the presence of failing left ventricular systolic function. Pericardial friction rubs may be present over the heart if inflammation has extended to the pericardium. Finally, systolic murmurs appear when papillary muscle dysfunction or infarction causes

---

TABLE 7.3. Signs and Symptoms of Myocardial Infarction

1. **Characteristic pain**
2. **Sympathetic effect**
   - Diaphoresis
   - Cool and clammy skin
3. **Parasympathetic (vagal effect)**
   - Nausea, vomiting
   - Weakness
4. **Inflammatory response**
   - Mild fever
5. **Cardiac findings**
   - S_4 (and S_3 if CHF present) gallop
   - Dyskinetic bulge (in anterior wall MI)
   - Pericardial friction rub (if pericarditis present)
   - Systolic murmur (if mitral regurgitation or VSD)
6. **Other**
   - Pulmonary rales (if CHF present)
   - Jugular venous distension (if right ventricular MI)

mitral valvular insufficiency or when infarcts rupture through the interventricular septum to create a ventricular septal defect.

Myocardial necrosis also activates **systemic responses to inflammation.** Cytokines such as interleukin-1 and tumor necrosis factor are released from macrophages and vascular endothelium in response to tissue injury. These mediators evoke an array of clinical responses including low-grade fever and leukocytosis.

DIAGNOSIS

The diagnosis of acute myocardial infarction is made on the basis of 1) a characteristic history and presentation, 2) typical EKG changes, and 3) detection of specific myocardial macromolecules in the serum. Table 7.4 lists other common causes of acute chest pain that may resemble that of myocardial infarction.

EKG Abnormalities

EKG changes occur during myocardial infarction in a characteristic, temporal sequence, as described in Chapter 4. In Q-wave myocardial infarction, *ST segment elevation, T wave inversion, and Q waves* evolve over the injured regions (Fig. 7.6), whereas *ST depression and T wave inversions* develop during non-Q-wave infarcts (Fig. 7.7).

Serum Markers of Infarction

Necrosis of myocardial tissue causes disruption of the sarcolemma, and intracellular macromolecules are released into the cardiac interstitium, and ultimately into the bloodstream (Fig. 7.8). Laboratory detection of these molecules in the serum serves an important diagnostic role in myocardial infarction.

Creatine kinase. The enzyme creatine kinase (CK) reversibly transfers a phosphate

TABLE 7.4. Conditions That May Be Confused With Acute MI

Condition	Differentiating Features
Cardiac	
Myocardial infarction	• Retrosternal pressure, radiating to neck, jaw, or left shoulder and arm; more severe and lasts longer than previous anginal attacks
	• EKG: localized ST elevations or depressions
Pericarditis	• Sharp pleuritic pain (worsens with inspiration)
	• Pain varies with position (relieved by sitting)
	• Friction rub auscultated over precordium
	• EKG: diffuse ST elevations (see Chapter 14)
Aortic dissection	• Tearing, ripping pain that migrates over time (chest and back)
	• Asymmetry of arm blood pressures
	• Widened mediastinum on chest radiograph
Pulmonary	
Pulmonary embolism	• Localized pleuritic pain, accompanied by dyspnea
	• Pleural friction rub may be present
	• Predisposing conditions for venous thrmobosis
Pneumonia	• Pleuritic chest pain
	• Cough and sputum production
	• Abnormal lung auscultation and percussion (i.e., consolidation)
	• Infiltrate on chest radiograph
Pneumothorax	• Sudden sharp, pleuritic unilateral chest pain
	• Decreased breath sounds and hyperresonance of affected side
	• Chest radiograph: ↑lucency and absence of pulmonary markings
Gastrointestinal	
Esophageal spasm	• Retrosternal pain, worsened by swallowing
	• History of dysphagia
Acute cholecystitis	• Right upper quadrant abdominal tenderness
	• Often accompanied by nausea
	• History of fatty food intolerance

Q-wave Myocardial Infarction

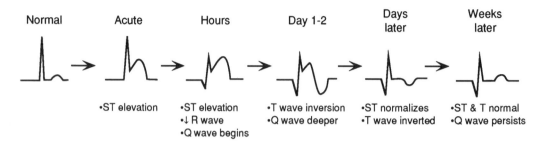

Figure 7.6.   EKG evolution during acute Q-wave myocardial infarction.

group from creatine phosphate, the endogenous storage form of high-energy phosphate bonds, to ADP, thus producing ATP. Because creatine kinase is found in heart, skeletal muscle, brain, and many other organs, serum concentrations of this enzyme may become elevated following injury to any of these tissues.

There are, however, three *isoenzymes* of CK that improve diagnostic specificity for a myocardial source: CK-MM (found mainly in skeletal muscle), CK-BB (located predominantly in the brain), and **CK-MB** (localized mainly in the heart). Sequential measurements of the serum CK-MB level is

currently the "gold standard" for the chemical diagnosis of an MI, and modern monoclonal assays for this isoenzyme are highly sensitive and specific. It is important to note that the heart also contains CK-MM; therefore, that isoenzyme level rises during an acute MI, as well. Furthermore, small amounts of CK-MB are found in other tissues, including the uterus, prostate, gut, diaphragm, and tongue. In the absence of trauma to these other organs, elevation of CK-MB is highly suggestive of myocardial injury. Since CK-MB makes up 1%–3% of the CK in skeletal muscle, muscle trauma or intramuscular injections could also cause

Non-Q-wave Myocardial Infarction

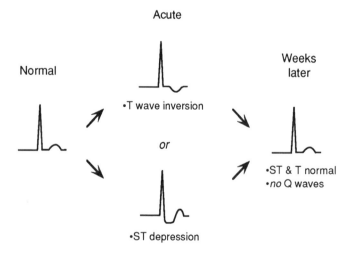

Figure 7.7.   EKG evolution during non-Q-wave myocardial infarction.

the appearance of this isoenzyme in the circulation. Therefore, to facilitate the diagnosis of myocardial infarction, it is common to calculate the ratio of CK-MB/total CK. When using the sensitive monoclonal ("mass") assay for CK-MB, this ratio is usually $> 2.5\%$ in the setting of myocardial injury, and less than that when due to pure skeletal muscle injury.

The serum level of CK-MB starts to rise 4 to 8 hours following infarction, peaks at 24 hours and returns to normal within 48 to 72 hours (Fig. 7.8). This temporal sequence is important because other potential sources of CK-MB (e.g., skeletal muscle injury), or other non-MI cardiac conditions that raise serum levels of the isoenzyme (e.g., myocarditis) do not usually show this pattern. Reperfusion procedures (such as thrombolytic therapy) during an MI result in a washout effect with an *earlier* than usual peak of the CK and CK-MB serum levels.

Since CK-MB levels do not become significantly elevated in the serum until several hours after the onset of symptoms of an MI, a single normal value drawn in a hospital emergency department does not rule out an acute infarction. Therefore, CK-MB levels cannot be used to help decide which patients with chest pain to admit to the hospital for observation and which to send home. That decision must currently be made on the basis of the patient's history, physical findings, and EKG.

In an attempt to more conclusively diagnose myocardial infarction in the critical early hours of presentation, several other serum markers have been evaluated. For example, **CK-MB isoforms** have been characterized. $CK-MB_2$ is released from infarcted myocardial tissue and is enzymatically converted in the circulation to $CK-MB_1$. Recent studies have shown that within just a few hours after the onset of symptoms, an elevated absolute level of $CK-MB_2$ (or an elevated ratio of MB_2/MB_1) was twice as sensitive for the diagnosis of acute MI as the standard CK-MB test. **Myoglobin,** a heme protein, is released into the circulation after myocardial injury and can be detected in the serum within 2 hours after the onset of an MI, much earlier than elevation of serum CK-MB. However, the rapid renal clearance of this molecule and its low specificity for myocardial damage limits its diagnostic value. Most promising are recently developed assays for serum levels of the cardiac-specific isoenzymes of **troponin T** and **troponin I.** Each of these

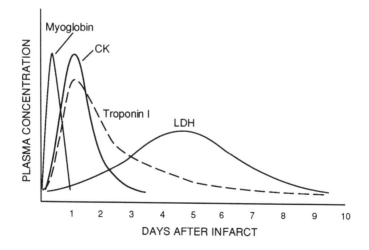

Figure 7.8. Evolution of serum markers in acute MI. The CK (and CK-MB isoenzyme) rises several hours after the acute infarct and peaks at 24 hours; myoglobin is detected in the serum earlier, but is less specific for myocardial injury. Cardiac specific troponins are highly sensitive and specific for myocardial injury, and remain detectable in the serum for several days after an acute MI. LDH serum levels rise more gradually and peak at 3–5 days after the acute event.

markers is highly specific for myocardial infarction, and they can be detected in the serum by 3 hours after the onset of MI-associated chest pain. As a result of their sensitivity and specificity, the use of the troponin serum markers in the diagnosis of acute MI is rapid expanding.

Lactate dehydrogenase (LDH) catalyzes the reversible formation of lactate from pyruvate. LDH is present in many tissues, and five isoenzymes have been identified. The isoenzyme most specific for the heart is LDH_1, and an LDH_1/LDH_2 ratio $>$ 1.0 is indicative of myocardial necrosis. (LDH_2 is found in erythrocytes; LDH_4 and LDH_5 are derived from liver and skeletal muscle.) As serum levels of LDH peak 3 to 5 days after an acute MI, the measurement of this enzyme is diagnostically useful in patients who present 2 to 3 days following symptoms of an acute MI, because the elevation of serum CK will have already passed.

If the symptoms and standard laboratory testing are equivocal for the diagnosis of an acute MI, certain other laboratory tests may be helpful. *Echocardiography* may demonstrate new abnormalities of ventricular contraction in the region of the infarct. It may also demonstrate mechanical complications arising from infarction, such as ventricular septal defect or mitral regurgitation. *Nuclear scans* using technetium-99m pyrophosphate may document infarcted tissue: Pyrophosphate collects within regions of high calcium concentration such as necrotic myocardium, and infarction can be visualized as zones of increased intensity if imaged more than 12 hours after the acute event (see Chapter 3).

ACUTE TREATMENT

The initial treatment of myocardial infarction focuses on the salvage of jeopardized ischemic myocardium. Contemporary practice has witnessed an enormous innovation in MI management in the form of reperfusion therapies, which have been shown to reduce the extent of myocardial necrosis and improve survival.

Thrombolytic Therapy

Since the vast majority of acute Q-wave MIs occur as a result of occlusive thrombus formation within a coronary artery, agents capable of lysing that clot can restore blood flow and limit myocardial damage. Current thrombolytic agents include streptokinase, anisoylated plasminogen-streptokinase activator complex (APSAC), and recombinant tissue plasminogen acivator (t-PA). Although their mechanisms of action differ (Fig. 7.9), all function by activating the protease plasmin, which lyses fibrin clots. Administration within several hours of acute MI restores blood flow in the majority of coronary occlusions and significantly reduces the extent of tissue damage. Early thrombolytic therapy yields the greatest benefit. For example, administration within the first hour of a Q-wave MI results in reperfusion rates of up to 80%, and is accompanied by a marked reduction in mortality.

Large-scale comparisons of thrombolytic agents have been conducted. Although initial studies found no difference in survival among the available drugs, a recent large trial (the "GUSTO" trial) showed t-PA to be somewhat superior to streptokinase, at the price of a slightly higher stroke rate. Our current understanding, however, is that it matters less which thrombolytic is given, compared with how soon it is administered: Patients who receive thrombolytics within 2 hours of the onset of chest pain have mortality rates *half* that of patients receiving therapy after 6 hours of symptoms.

Contraindications to thrombolytic therapy include situations in which hemorrhage would likely be precipitated by lysis of *necessary* fibrin clots within the circulation (e.g., active peptic ulcer disease, an underlying bleeding disorder, patients who are recovering from recent surgery).

When coronary flow is successfully reestablished by thrombolytic therapy, ST segment elevations return to baseline and any rise in the serum CK-MB peaks earlier than usual, as tissue is salvaged and the en-

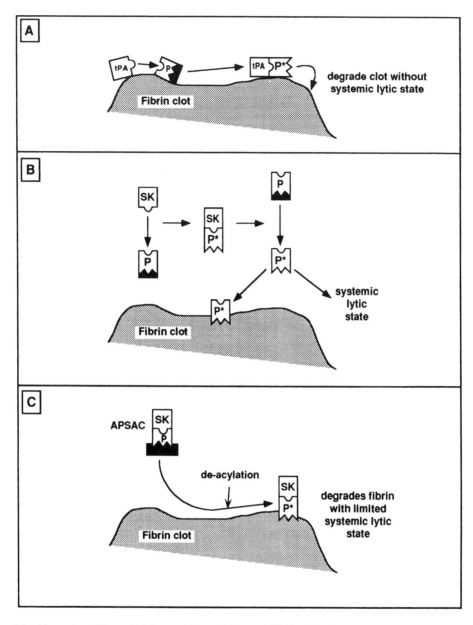

Figure 7.9. Examples of thrombolytic agents used in acute MI. A. t-PA cleaves fibrin-bound plasminogen (P) to form active plasmin (P*), which degrades the fibrin clot. The selectivity of t-PA for fibrin-bound P results in localized thrombolysis and minimizes generalized systemic fibrinolysis. **B.** Streptokinase (SK) combines with fibrin-bound and circulating plasminogen to form an active complex, which in turn activates additional plasminogen molecules. The lack of selectivity for fibrin-bound plasminogen results in more of a systemic lytic state. **C.** Anisoylated plasminogen-streptokinase activator complex (APSAC) is inactive when administered, as the enzymatic site is blocked. However, upon binding to fibrin, deacylation frees the enzymatic site, allowing it to degrade thrombus. Relative fibrin selectivity exists at low dosage, but a systemic lytic state is often produced at conventional doses.

zyme is "washed-out" by restored blood flow. Thrombolytic therapy is generally followed by a course of intravenous heparin anticoagulation to prevent immediate vessel reocclusion.

Primary PTCA

An alternative to thrombolytic therapy in acute MI is immediate cardiac catheterization and percutaneous angioplasty of the coronary lesion responsible for the infarction (termed "primary PTCA"). It is a particularly attractive option for patients with contraindications to thrombolytic drugs. Studies suggest that immediate angioplasty can restore coronary artery patency in more than 90% of patients and reduce the rates of recurrent ischemia, reinfarction, and mortality. However, primary PTCA is currently limited to centers that are extremely experienced in angioplasty and are equipped to perform it on an emergency basis.

Hospital Management

Whether acute thrombolytic therapy or primary PTCA is performed, the early treatment of MI is directed toward: 1) the restoration of the balance between myocardial oxygen supply and demand so that further ischemia does not occur, 2) pain relief, and 3) prevention and treatment of the complications that may arise from the infarcted myocardium. These goals are best met by admitting the patient to a coronary care unit (CCU), a specialized hospital unit that is dedicated to the management of acute MI and its complications. Standard treatment includes:

1. **Bed rest** in a quiet setting, where continuous EKG monitoring for arrhythmias can be achieved.
2. **Oxygen** administration by face mask or nasal cannula to help maximize oxygen supply.
3. **Aspirin** decreases platelet adhesiveness and has been shown to decrease mortality and reinfarction after MI. Aspirin therapy should be started immediately upon presentation of acute MI and continued indefinitely unless a contraindication to its use exists (e.g., an underlying bleeding disorder or allergy).
4. **β-blockers.** In the absence of contraindications (asthma, bronchospasm, hypotension), β-blockers are administered because they have been shown to reduce the rate of reinfarction and recurrent ischemia. By decreasing the sympathetic drive to the myocardium, they reduce myocardial work and contribute to electrical stability.
5. **Nitrates** bring about anginal relief through venodilatation, which lowers myocardial oxygen demand by diminishing venous return to the heart (↓ preload and therefore ↓ wall stress). Although nitrates have been a mainstay for the treatment of chronic ischemic heart disease, their utility in acute MI appears limited to symptomatic relief (and as a vasodilator agent in some patients with heart failure or severe hypertension during early infarction), with no apparent impact on mortality. Thus, in the setting of an acute MI, nitroglycerin is often administered by the sublingual route, or sometimes intravenously, until the patient is free of pain and it is then discontinued.
6. **Morphine** is a potent analgesic that can eliminate the patient's pain and decrease anxiety, thereby reducing sympathetic drive and myocardial oxygen demand. Morphine is also a venodilator and thus decreases preload, thereby further reducing myocardial oxygen requirements.
7. **Anticoagulants.** In addition to its role as adjuvant therapy following thrombolytic therapy, intravenous heparin is also indicated to prevent intracardiac thrombus formation in patients with large anterior MIs, low cardiac output, or atrial fibrillation. All other patients hospitalized for acute MI should receive low-dose subcutaneous heparin while bedridden to prevent deep venous thrombosis in the lower extremities and pelvis.
8. **Angiotensin converting enzyme (ACE) inhibitors** (described further in Chapter 17) have been shown to limit postinfarct ventricular remodeling, to reduce the incidence of heart failure and recurrent ischemic events following an MI, and to improve survival. Their benefit is additive to that of aspirin and beta-blocker therapies, and they have shown the greatest long-term benefit in patients with ventricular dysfunction following the MI (i.e., a lower than normal LV ejection fraction). Thus, oral ACE inhibitors

are begun early in the course of an MI, and are continued indefinitely after hospital discharge in patients with impaired LV contractile function.

COMPLICATIONS

Complications of an acute MI result from the inflammatory, mechanical, and electrical abnormalities induced by regions of necrosing myocardium (Fig. 7.10). Immediate complications result from myocardial necrosis itself. Those that develop several days to weeks later may be due to the inflammation and healing of necrotic tissue.

Recurrent Ischemia and Reinfarction

Postinfarction angina occurs in 20%–30% of patients. Indicative of inadequate residual coronary blood flow, it is a poor omen and correlates with an increased risk for reinfarction. Such patients are referred for immediate cardiac catheterization, often followed by mechanical revascularization by PTCA or CABG.

Recurrent myocardial infarction occurs in 5%–20% of patients within the first 6 weeks following an MI. Reinfarction can involve the zone of the original MI (if viable tissue had survived in that region) or may involve a previously uninfarcted segment.

Arrhythmias

Arrhythmias are extremely common during acute MI (Table 7.5) and are a major source of mortality. Modern CCUs are highly attuned to the detection and treatment of rhythm disturbances, so that once a patient is hospitalized, arrhythmia-associated mortality is fairly uncommon. Mechanisms that contribute to arrhythmogenesis after MI include the following:

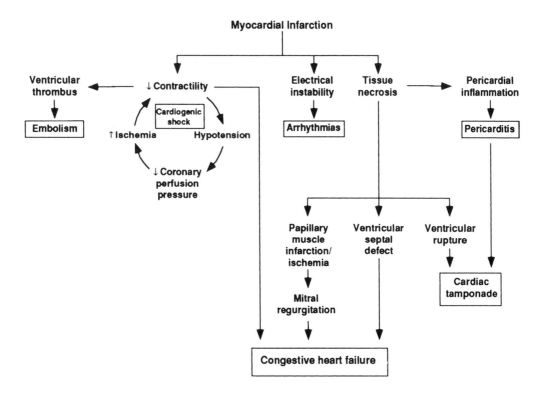

Figure 7.10. Complications of MI. Infarction results in decreased contractility, electrical instability, and tissue necrosis, which lead to these important complications.

TABLE 7.5. Arrhythmias in Acute Myocardial Infarction

Rhythm	Cause
Sinus bradycardia	• ↑vagal tone • ↓SA nodal artery perfusion
Sinus tachycardia	• Pain and anxiety • CHF • Volume depletion • Pericarditis • Chronotrophic drugs (e.g., dopamine)
APBs, atrial fibrillation	• CHF • Atrial ischemia
VPBs, VT, VF	• Ventricular ischemia • CHF
AV block (1°, 2°, 3°)	• IMI: ↑vagal tone and ↓AV nodal artery flow • AMI: extensive destruction of conduction tissue

IMI, inferior myocardial infarction; AMI, anterior myocardial infarction; VPB, ventricular premature beat; VT, ventricular tachycardia; VF, ventricular fibrillation; APB, atrial premature beat

1. Anatomic interruption of perfusion to structures of the conduction pathway (e.g., SA node, AV node, bundle branches); the normal perfusion of pertinent components of the conduction system are shown in Table 7.6.
2. Accumulation of local metabolic factors (e.g., cellular acidosis) and abnormal transcellular ion concentrations due to membrane leaks.
3. Autonomic stimulation (sympathetic and parasympathetic).
4. Administration of potentially arrhythmogenic drugs (e.g., digitalis, dopamine).

Ventricular Fibrillation

Ventricular fibrillation (rapid, disorganized electrical activity of the ventricles) is largely responsible for episodes of sudden cardiac death during the course of acute MI. Unfortunately, most fatal episodes occur prior to the arrival of medical assistance and hospitalization. Episodes of ventricular fibrillation that occur during the first 48 hours of MI are often related to transient electrical instability, and the long-term

mortality of survivors of such events is not affected. However, ventricular fibrillation occurring later than 48 hours after the acute MI usually reflects severe left ventricular dysfunction and is associated with a high subsequent mortality.

Ventricular ectopic beats, ventricular tachycardia, and ventricular fibrillation during an acute MI arise from either re-entrant circuits or enhanced automaticity of ventricular cells (see Chapter 11). Ventricular ectopy is common, but usually is not treated unless the abnormal beats become consecutive, multifocal, or frequent. Intravenous lidocaine (a class I antiarrhythmic drug described in Chapter 17) is effective in preventing ventricular fibrillation in the ischemic setting, but is not indicated in the routine management of acute MI patients because of its potential side effects and because CCU personnel are proficient at arrhythmia detection and effective treatment when they occur.

Supraventricular Arrhythmias

Supraventricular arrhythmias are also common in acute MI. *Sinus bradycardia* results from either excessive vagal stimulation or SA nodal ischemia, usually in the setting of an inferior wall MI. *Sinus tachycardia* is also common and may result from many causes, especially pain and anxiety, congestive heart failure (CHF), drug ad-

TABLE 7.6. Blood Supply of the Conduction System

Conduction Pathway	Primary Arterial Supply
SA node	• RCA (70% of patients)
AV node	• RCA (85% of patients)
Bundle of His	• LAD (septal branches)
RBB	• Proximal portion by LAD • Distal portion by RCA
LBB:	
Left anterior fascicle	• LAD
Left posterior fascicle	• LAD and PDA

SA, sinoatrial; AV, atrioventricular; RBB, right bundle branch; LBB, left bundle branch; RCA, right coronary; LAD, left anterior descending coronary artery; PDA, posterior descending artery

ministration (e.g., dopamine, nitrates), or intravascular volume depletion. Differentiating between CHF and volume depletion may require the placement of a transvenous pulmonary artery catheter: The pulmonary capillary wedge pressure is low in volume depletion, whereas it is elevated in CHF. Because sinus tachycardia increases myocardial oxygen demand and could exacerbate ischemia, identifying and treating its cause is important. *Atrial premature beats* and *atrial fibrillation* (see Chapter 12) may result from atrial ischemia or atrial distention secondary to left ventricular failure.

Conduction Blocks

Conduction blocks (AV nodal block and bundle branch blocks) develop frequently in acute MI. They may result from ischemia or necrosis of conduction tracts (Table 7.6), or in the case of AV blocks, may develop transiently because of increased vagal tone (discussed in Chapter 11). Vagal activity may be increased because of stimulation of afferent fibers by the inflamed myocardium, or as a result of generalized autonomic activation in association with the pain of an acute MI.

Myocardial Dysfunction

Congestive Heart Failure

Acute cardiac ischemia results in impaired ventricular contractility (decreased systolic function), as well as increased myocardial stiffness (decreased diastolic function), both of which may lead to symptoms of heart failure. In addition, arrhythmias and acute mechanical complications of MI (described below) may culminate in heart failure (Fig. 7.10). Signs and symptoms of such decompensation include dyspnea, pulmonary rales, and a third heart sound (S_3). Treatment consists of standard CHF therapy (discussed in Chapter 9) and includes diuresis and vasodilator therapy.

Cardiogenic Shock

Cardiogenic shock is a condition of severely decreased cardiac output and hypotension (systolic BP < 90 mm Hg) with inadequate perfusion of peripheral tissues, that develops when more than 40% of the left ventricular mass has infarcted. It may also follow the severe mechanical complications described below. Demise in cardiogenic shock is self-perpetuating because (Fig. 7.10): 1) hypotension leads to decreased coronary perfusion, which exacerbates ischemic damage, and 2) decreased stroke volume increases LV size and therefore augments myocardial oxygen demand. Despite aggressive treatment, the mortality rate of cardiogenic shock is greater than 70%.

Patients in cardiogenic shock require intravenous inotropic agents (e.g., dobutamine) to increase cardiac output, as well as arterial vasodilators, to reduce the resistance to LV contraction. Such patients are often stabilized by the insertion of an **intra-aortic balloon pump.** This device is inserted into the aorta via a femoral artery and consists of an inflatable, flexible chamber that expands during diastole to increase intra-aortic pressure, thus augmenting perfusion of the coronary arteries and the peripheral tissues. During systole it deflates to create a vacuum that aids in the ejection of blood from the left ventricle into the aorta. It can be left in place for only a few days, lest thrombosis or infection supervene.

Right Ventricular Infarction

Approximately one-third of patients with infarction of the left ventricular inferior wall also develop necrosis of portions of the RV, because the same coronary artery (usually the right coronary) perfuses both regions in most individuals. The resulting abnormal contraction and decreased compliance of the RV leads to signs of right-sided heart failure (e.g., jugular venous distention) out of proportion to signs of left-sided failure. In addition, profound hypotension may result because right ventricular dysfunction impairs blood flow through the lungs, so that the left ventricle becomes underfilled. In this setting, intravenous volume infusion often serves to correct hypotension, guided by hemodynamic measurements by a transvenous pulmonary artery catheter.

Mechanical Complications

Mechanical complications following MI result from tissue ischemia and necrosis.

Papillary Muscle Rupture

Ischemic necrosis and rupture of a left ventricular papillary muscle may be rapidly fatal because of acute severe mitral regurgitation, as the valve leaflets lose their anchoring attachments. *Partial* rupture, with more moderate regurgitation, is not immediately lethal but may result in symptoms of heart failure or pulmonary edema. The posteromedial LV papillary muscle is more susceptible to infarction than the anterolateral one, because it has a more precarious blood supply; therefore this complication is more common following an inferoposterior MI.

Ventricular Free Wall Rupture

An infrequent but deadly complication, rupture of the LV free wall through a tear in the necrotic myocardium, may occur within the first 2 weeks following MI. It is more common among women and individuals with a history of hypertension. Hemorrhage into the pericardial space owing to such rupture results in rapid cardiac tamponade, in which blood fills the pericardial space and severely restricts ventricular filling (see Chapter 14). Survival is rare.

On occasion, a **pseudoaneurysm** results if rupture of the free wall is incomplete and held in check by thrombus formation that "plugs" the hole in the myocardium. This situation is the cardiac equivalent of a time bomb, because subsequent complete rupture into the pericardium and tamponade

could follow. If detected (usually by echocardiography), surgical correction may prevent an otherwise disastrous outcome.

Ventricular Septal Rupture

This complication is analogous to LV free wall rupture, but the abnormal flow of blood is not directed across the left ventricular wall into the pericardium. Rather, blood is shunted across the ventricular septum from the LV to the RV, usually precipitating CHF because of subsequent volume overload of the pulmonary capillaries. A loud systolic murmur at the left sternal border, representing trans-septal flow, is common in this situation. The murmur of ventricular septal rupture can be differentiated from that of acute mitral regurgitation by Doppler echocardiography, or by measuring the O_2 saturation of blood in the right-sided heart chambers through a transvenous catheter: The O_2 content in the RV is abnormally higher than that in the RA if there is shunting of oxygenated blood from the LV across the septal defect.

True Ventricular Aneurysm

This is a late complication of MI, occurring weeks to months after the acute event. It develops as the ventricular wall is *weakened,* but not perforated by the phagocytic clearance of necrotic tissue and results in a localized outward bulge when the residual viable heart muscle contracts. Unlike the pseudoaneurysm described above, there is no communication between the LV cavity and the pericardium, so that rupture and tamponade do not develop. Complications of LV aneurysm include: 1) thrombus formation within this region of stagnant blood flow, serving as a potential source of emboli to peripheral organs, 2) ventricular arrhythmias associated with the stretched myofibers, and 3) heart failure due to reduced forward cardiac output, because some of the LV stroke volume is "wasted" by filling the aneurysm cavity during systole.

Clues to the presence of an LV aneurysm

include persistent ST segment elevation over the site of infarction on EKG (weeks after an acute Q-wave MI), and a bulge of the LV border on chest radiograph. The presence of an aneurysm (and thrombus within it) can usually be confirmed by echocardiography.

Pericarditis

Acute pericarditis may occur in the early postinfarction period as necrosis and neutrophilic infiltrates extend to the epicardium and pericardial layers (see Chapter 14). Sharp pain, fever, and pericardial friction rubs may develop and help distinguish pericarditis from the pain of recurrent myocardial ischemia. Anticoagulants are relatively contraindicated in MI complicated by pericarditis, to avoid hemorrhage from the inflamed pericardial lining. The frequency of MI-associated pericarditis has declined since the introduction of thrombolytic therapy, since that modality limits the extent of myocardial damage and inflammation.

Thromboembolism

Turbulence and stasis of blood flow in regions of impaired left ventricular contraction post-MI may incite intracavity thrombus formation, especially when an infarction involves the LV apex, or when a true aneurysm has formed. Subsequent thromboemboli can result in devastating infarction of peripheral organs (e.g., an embolism to the brain may cause a stroke).

POST-MI RISK STRATIFICATION AND MANAGEMENT

Most patients can be safely discharged 5 to 7 days following acute MI. Reinfarction can occur, and it is important to identify patients at high risk for this complication. The most important predictor of post-MI outcome is the *extent of left ventricular dysfunction*. Other features that portend adverse outcomes include: early recurrence of

ischemia, a large volume of residual myocardium still at ischemic risk by atherosclerotoc disease, and high-grade ventricular arrhythmias.

To identify those patients at highest risk, an exercise treadmill test is performed (low-level at time of discharge, with more rigorous testing 4 to 6 weeks later). Patients with significantly abnormal results or those who demonstrate an early spontaneous recurrence of angina are referred for cardiac catheterization in order to define their coronary anatomy.

Standard postdischarge therapy includes: 1) aspirin, 2) a β-blocker, and 3) an ACE inhibitor (especially if LV dysfunction is demonstrated). Cholesterol-lowering therapy (often an HMG CoA reductase inhibitor) is prescribed as needed to achieve the target LDL value of < 100 mg/dl. Rigorous attention to other cardiac risk factors, such as smoking, hypertension, and diabetes is also mandatory, and a formal exercise rehabilitation program often speeds convalescence.

SUMMARY

1. Myocardial infarction (MI) is the condition of myocyte necrosis that results from prolonged ischemia. Most infarcts are due to the formation of an occlusive coronary artery thrombus at the site of atherosclerotic plaque. Plaque rupture is the usual trigger for thrombus formation through activation of platelets and the coagulation cascade. Atherosclerosis-induced endothelium dysfunction contributes to the process by producing decreased amounts of vasodilators and antithrombotic agents.

2. Acute MI results in biochemical and mechanical changes that impair systolic contraction, decrease myocardial compliance (decrease "diastolic function"), and predispose to dangerous arrhythmias. The infarction initiates an inflammatory response that clears necrotic tissue and leads to scar formation. Transient severe ischemia without infarction can lead to stunned myocardium, a con-

dition of contractile dysfunction that persists beyond the period of ischemia, with subsequent gradual recovery.

3. The diagnosis of acute MI rests on a characteristic history, typical EKG changes, and temporal evolution of specific serum markers. Echocardiography, nuclear scans, and other imaging techniques can help localize infarcted portions of the ventricular wall.

4. Acute treatment for MI includes attempts at limiting myocardial damage through reperfusion therapy with thrombolytic agents or immediate percutaneous angioplasty. Other agents commonly administered include aspirin, a beta-blocker, an ACE inhibitor, and when appropriate, heparin. Morphine and nitrates are used to alleviate pain. Arrhythmias are carefully monitored in the CCU setting.

5. Immediate complications of MI include arrhythmias such as ventricular tachycardia and fibrillation, AV blocks, bundle branch blocks, and supraventricular arrhythmias. Cardiogenic shock or congestive heart failure may develop because of ventricular dysfunction or mechanical complications including ventricular rupture, mitral regurgitation, and formation of a ventricular septal defect. In addition, wall motion abnormalities of the infarcted segment may predispose to thrombus formation.

6. Standard pharmacologic therapy following discharge from the hospital includes aspirin and a β-blocker, and when appropriate, an ACE inhibitor (if LV dysfunction present), systemic anticoagulation (if intraventricular thrombus or a large akinetic segment are present) and anticholesterol drug therapy.

7. Post-MI risk stratification seeks to identify those patients with a high risk of reinfarction or death. Impaired left ventricular function, electrical instability (high-grade ventricular arrhythmias), and ischemic changes during exercise testing all portend unfavorable outcomes and warrant further investigations and treatment.

ADDITIONAL READING

Ambrose JA, Weinrauch M. Thrombosis in ischemic heart disease. Arch Intern Med. 1996;156:1382–1394.

Anderson HV, Willerson JT. Thrombolysis in acute myocardial infarction. N Engl J Med 1993;329:703–709.

Antman EM, Braunwald E. Acute myocardial infarction. In: Braunwald E, ed. Heart Disease: A Textbook of Cardiovascular Medicine. 5th ed. Philadelphia: WB Saunders, 1997:1184–1288.

Califf RM, Bengtson JR. Cardiogenic shock. N Engl J Med 1994;330:1724–1730.

Committee on Management of Acute Myocardial Infarction. ACC/AHA guidelines for the management of patients with acute myocardial infarction. J Am Coll Cardiol 1996;28:1328–1428.

Fuster V, Badimon L, Badimon JJ, et al. The pathogenesis of coronary artery disease and the acute coronary syndromes. N Engl J Med 1992;326:242–250, 310–318.

Fuster V, Verstraete M. Hemostasis, thrombosis, fibrinolysis, and cardiovascular disease. In: Braunwald E, ed. Heart Disease: A Textbook of Cardiovascular Medicine. 5th ed. Philadelphia: WB Saunders, 1997:1809–1842.

Gruppo Italiano per lo Studio della Sopravvivenza nell'Infarto Miocardico. GISSI-3: effects of lisinopril and transdermal glyceryl trinitrate singly and together on 6-week mortality and ventricular function after acute myocardial infarction. Lancet 1994;343:1115–1122.

GUSTO Investigators. An international randomized trial comparing four thrombolytic strategies for acute myocardial infarction. N Engl J Med 1993;329:673–682.

Hennekens CH, Albert CM, Godfried SL, et al. Adjunctive drug therapy of acute myocardial infarction: evidence from clinical trials. N Engl J Med 1996;335:1660–1667.

Huber K, Maurer G. Thrombolytic therapy in acute myocardial infarction. Semin Thromb Hemost 1996;22:15–26.

ISIS-4 (Fourth International Study of Infarct Survival) Collaborative Group. ISIS-4: a randomised factorial trial assessing early oral captopril, oral mononitrate, and intravenous magnesium sulphate in 58,050 patients with suspected acute myocardial infarction. Lancet 1995;345:669–685.

Kawai C. Pathogenesis of acute myocardial infarction: novel regulatory systems of bioactive substances in the vessel wall. Circulation. 1994;90:1033–1043.

Kloner RA, Przyklenk K, Patel B. Altered myocardial states: the stunned and hibernating myocardium. Am J Med 1989;86(Suppl 1A):14–22.

McGovern PG, Pankow JS, Shahar E, et al. Recent trends in acute coronary heart disease—mortality, morbidity, medical care, and risk factors. N Engl J Med 1996;334:884–890.

Mitchell G, Pfeffer MA. Left ventricular remodeling after myocardial infarction. In: Kloner RA, ed. The Guide to Cardiology. 3rd ed. Greenwich, CT: Le Jacq Communications, Inc., 1995:317–328.

Pfeffer MA. ACE inhibition in acute myocardial infarction. N Engl J Med 1995;332:118–120.

Phibbs B. "Transmural" versus "subendocardial" myocardial infarction: an electrocardiographic myth. J Am Coll Cardiol 1983;1:561.

Puleo PR, Meyer D, Wathen C, et al. Use of a rapid assay of subforms of creatine kinase MB to diagnose or rule out acute myocardial infarction. N Engl J Med 1994;331:561–566.

Sacks FM, Pfeffer MA, Moye LA, et al. The effect of pravastatin on coronary events after myocardial infarction in patients with average cholesterol levels. Cholesterol and Recurrent Events Trial investigators. N Engl J Med 1996;335:1001–1009.

Van de Werf F. Cardiac troponins in acute coronary syndromes. N Engl J Med. 1996;335:1388–389.

Acknowledgments The authors thank Dr. Robert Handin for his helpful suggestions. The previous edition of this chapter was written by J. G. Fletcher, MD, William Carlson, MD, and Leonard S. Lilly, MD.

Valvular Heart Disease

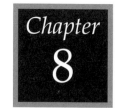

Stephen K. Frankel, Leonard S. Lilly, and John A. Bittl

This chapter reviews the pathophysiology and clinical assessment of patients with valvular heart disease. Each of the common valvular abnormalities will be discussed separately, because unifying pathophysiologic principles do not govern the behavior of all stenotic or regurgitant valves.

The evaluation of valvular heart disease begins at the bedside with a careful history and physical examination, from which the trained clinician can usually identify the type of valvular abnormalities that are present. Accurate assessment of the severity of the valve lesion often requires additional information from the electrocardiogram, chest radiograph, and echocardiography. In selected patients, further investigation by exercise testing or cardiac catheterization may be necessary to fully define the severity of the condition and guide therapy. Thus, effective management of patients with valvular disease requires accurate identification of the lesion, an evaluation of its severity, and a clear understanding of the pathophysiologic consequences and natural history of the condition.

RHEUMATIC FEVER

Acute rheumatic fever (ARF) was once among the most common causes of valvular heart disease, but its incidence has waned considerably in the past half-century in in-dustrialized society. In the 1940s, the yearly incidence of ARF exceeded 200,000 cases in the United States, whereas the disease is now rare. The decline of this condition immediately preceded or coincided with the introduction of penicillin, as well as with improvement of general health care and relief from overcrowding. Recent reports have identified occasional local outbreaks in the United States, but a major resurgence has not been seen. Nevertheless, in developing countries of the Middle East, Southeast Asia, and Indian subcontinent, ARF continues to be a scourge with fulminant consequences.

ARF is an inflammatory condition primarily involving the heart, skin, and connective tissues. It is a complication of upper respiratory tract infections caused by Group A Streptococci, and mainly occurs in childhood and young adulthood. During epidemics, approximately 3% of patients with acute streptococcal pharyngitis develop ARF 2 to 3 weeks after the initial throat infection. The pathogenesis of ARF remains unknown, but does not involve direct bacterial infection of the heart. Some proposed mechanisms include the elaboration of a toxin by the streptococci, or autoimmune cross-reactivity between bacterial antigens and those on the endocardium. The most common presenting symptoms are chills, fever, migratory arthralgias, and fatigue. The cardinal symptoms and clinical manifestation of the disease that establish the diagnosis are known as the *Jones' criteria* (Table 8.1).

Pathologically, rheumatic carditis (i.e., cardiac inflammation) may affect all three layers of the heart. The pathognomonic finding is the "Aschoff body," an area of focal fibrinoid necrosis surrounded by inflammatory cells including lymphocytes, plasma cells, and macrophages that later resolve to form fibrous scar tissue. The most devastating sequelae result from inflammatory involvement of the valvular endocardium, which leads to chronic rheumatic heart disease, characterized by permanent deformity and impairment of one or more cardiac valves. Symptoms of valvular dysfunction, however, generally do not become manifest until *10 to 30 years* after ARF has subsided, though this latency period may be considerably shorter with more aggressive disease observed in developing countries.

During the acute episode, carditis may be associated with decreased left ventricular contractility and transient murmurs of mitral regurgitation, aortic regurgitation, or a mid-diastolic murmur at the cardiac apex (termed the "Carey-Coombs" murmur), which are most likely related to turbulent flow across inflamed valve leaflets. Treatment of ARF includes the use of high-dose aspirin to reduce inflammation, penicillin to

eliminate residual streptococcal infection, and therapy of complications such as congestive heart failure and pericarditis.

During the chronic phase, regurgitation or stenosis of the mitral valve is common. Forty percent of patients with rheumatic heart disease will develop mitral stenosis. An additional 25% will develop aortic regurgitation or stenosis in addition to the mitral abnormality. Infrequently, the tricuspid valve is affected, as well.

Acute rheumatic fever recurs in 10% of patients, and such recurrences can incite further cardiac damage. Therefore, patients who have experienced ARF should receive low-dose penicillin prophylaxis until young adulthood (i.e., approximately age 30), by which time exposure and susceptibility to the streptococcal infection has sufficiently diminished.

MITRAL VALVE DISEASE

Mitral Stenosis

Etiology

Mitral stenosis (MS) is almost always a sequella of rheumatic fever, and therefore, virtually all adults with MS have typical rheumatic deformity of the valve on pathologic examination. About 50% of patients with symptomatic MS provide a history of ARF that had occurred, on average, 20 years before presentation. Other rare causes of MS (less than 1%) include congenital stenosis of the valve, prominent calcification extending from the mitral annulus in elderly patients, or endocarditis with very large vegetations that obstruct the valve orifice.

Pathology

Acute and recurrent inflammation produce the typical pathologic features of rheumatic MS. These include fibrous thickening and calcification of the valve leaflets, fusion of the commissures (the borders where the leaflets meet), and thickening and shortening of the chordae tendineae.

TABLE 8.1. Jones' Criteria for Diagnosis of Rheumatic Fever[a]

Major criteria
  Carditis
  Polyarthritis
  Chorea
  Erythema marginatum (skin rash with advancing
    edge and clearing center)
  Subcutaneous nodules
Minor criteria
  Previous episode of rheumatic fever
  Migratory arthralgias
  Fever
  Increased acute phase reactants (ESR, leukocytosis)
  Prolonged PR interval on electrocardiogram
Evidence of streptococcal infection
  Antistreptolysin O antibodies
  Positive throat culture for Streptococci Group A
  Recent scarlet fever

[a]Diagnosis requires evidence of streptococcal infection and
  either: 2 major criteria, or 1 major plus 2 minor criteria

Pathophysiology

At the onset of diastole in the normal heart, the mitral valve opens and blood flows freely from the left atrium (LA) into the left ventricle (LV), and there is a negligible pressure difference between the two chambers. In mitral stenosis, however, there is obstruction to blood flow across the valve such that emptying of the LA is impeded and there is an abnormal pressure gradient between the LA and LV (Figs. 8.1, 8.2). As a result, the left atrial pressure is higher than normal, a necessary feature in order for blood to be propelled forward across the obstructed valve. The normal cross-sectional area of the mitral valve orifice is 4 to 6 cm². Hemodynamically significant mitral stenosis becomes apparent when the valve area is reduced to less than approximately 2 cm². Although the left ventricular pressures are usually normal in MS, the increased resistance across the mitral valve decreases ventricular filling, which may result in decreased LV stroke volume and cardiac output.

The high left atrial pressure in MS is transmitted to the pulmonary circulation, resulting in increased pulmonary venous and capillary pressures (Fig. 8.1). This elevation of hydrostatic pressure in the pulmonary vasculature may cause transudation of plasma into the lung interstitium and alveoli, producing dyspnea and other symptoms of congestive heart failure. In severe cases, marked elevation of pulmonary venous pressure leads to the opening of collateral channels between the pulmonary and bronchial veins. Subsequently, the high pulmonary vascular pressures may cause rupture of a bronchial vein into the lung parenchyma, resulting in hemoptysis (coughing blood).

The elevation of left atrial pressure in MS can result in two distinct forms of pulmonary hypertension: passive and reactive. Most patients with MS exhibit *passive* pulmonary hypertension. This is actually an "obligatory" increase in pulmonary artery pressure that develops in order to preserve forward flow in the setting of increased left atrial and pulmonary venous pressures. Additionally, approximately 40% of patients with MS demonstrate *reactive* pulmonary hypertension with medial hypertrophy and intimal fibrosis of the pulmonary arterioles. Reactive pulmonary hypertension is "beneficial" because the higher arteriolar resistance impedes blood flow into the engorged pulmonary capillary bed and thereby reduces capillary hydrostatic pressure. Thus, reactive pulmonary hypertension "protects" the pulmonary capillaries from even higher pressures and lessens pulmonary congestion. However, this benefit is at the cost of decreased blood

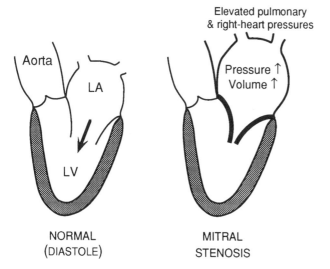

Figure 8.1. Pathophysiology of mitral stenosis. In the normal heart, blood flows freely from the left atrium (LA) into the left ventricle (LV) during diastole. In mitral stenosis, there is obstruction to LA emptying. Thus, LA pressure increases, which in turn results in elevated pulmonary and right-heart pressures.

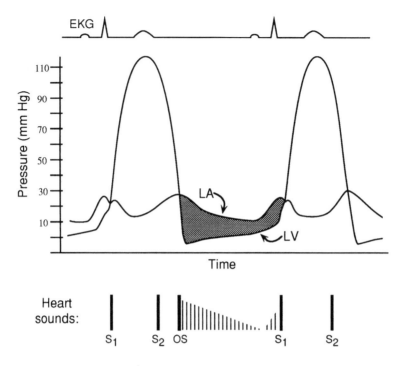

Figure 8.2.   Hemodynamic profile of mitral stenosis. The left atrial (LA) pressure is elevated, and there is a pressure gradient (shaded area) between the LA and left ventricle (LV) during diastole. Compare with schematic of normal tracing (Fig. 2.1). Abnormal heart sounds are present: there is a diastolic opening snap (OS) that corresponds to opening of the mitral valve, followed by a decrescendo murmur. There is accentuation of the murmur just before S_1, due to the increased pressure gradient when the LA contracts. EKG, electrocardiogram.

flow through the pulmonary vasculature with resultant elevation of the *right*-sided heart pressures. Chronic elevation of the right ventricular pressure leads to hypertrophy of that chamber and ultimately to right-sided heart failure.

Chronic pressure overload of the left atrium in MS causes that chamber to enlarge, stretches the atrial conduction fibers and may lead to *atrial fibrillation* (a rapid irregular heart rhythm described in Chapter 12). Atrial fibrillation causes the cardiac output to fall in MS because the increased heart rate shortens diastole, which in turn reduces the time available for blood to flow across the obstructed mitral valve.

The relative stagnation of blood flow in the dilated left atrium in MS, especially when combined with the development of atrial fibrillation, predisposes to intra-atrial thrombus formation. Thromboemboli to peripheral organs may follow, leading to devastating complications such as cerebrovascular occlusion (a stroke).

The turbulent blood flow across the obstructed mitral valve in MS predisposes to *infective endocarditis* (see below); however that complication occurs less frequently in MS than in other forms of acquired valvular disease.

Clinical Manifestations and Evaluation

The natural history of MS without intervention leads to a markedly reduced lifespan with a median survival of 7 years after the onset of symptoms. Patients with even mild symptoms are likely to succumb within 10 years if repair of the mitral valve is not performed (Table 8.2).

The clinical presentation of MS depends in large part on the degree of reduction in valve area. The more severe the stenosis, the greater the symptoms related to elevation of left atrial and pulmonary venous pressures. The earliest manifestations are those of dyspnea and reduced exercise capacity. In mild

TABLE 8.2. Follow-up of Mitral Stenosis Patients Treated Without Surgery

	Status 10 years later (%)		
Status at Diagnosis	No change	Worse	Deceased
Asymptomatic	59	25	16
Mild symptoms	21	21	58
Moderate symptoms	4	11	85

Adapted from Rowe JC, et al. The course of mitral stenosis without surgery. Ann Intern Med 1960;52:741.

MS, dyspnea may be absent at rest; however, it develops upon exertion as LA pressure rises with the exercise-induced increase in blood flow through the heart and faster heart rate (i.e., decreased diastolic filling time). Other conditions that increase heart rate and cardiac blood flow and therefore exacerbate symptoms of MS include fever, anemia, hyperthyroidism, pregnancy, and rapid arrhythmias such as atrial fibrillation.

With more severe MS (i.e., a smaller valve area) dyspnea occurs even at rest. Increasing fatigue and more severe signs of pulmonary congestion, such as orthopnea and paroxysmal nocturnal dyspnea, occur. With advanced MS and pulmonary hypertension, signs of right-sided heart failure ensue, including engorged jugular veins, hepatomegaly, ascites, and peripheral edema. Compression of the recurrent laryngeal nerve by the enlarged pulmonary artery or left atrium may cause hoarseness.

Less often, the diagnosis of mitral stenosis is heralded by one of its complications—atrial fibrillation, thromboemboli, infective endocarditis, or hemoptysis, as described in the pathophysiology section above.

On examination, there are several typical findings. Palpation of the precordium often reveals a right ventricular "tap" due to the increased right ventricular pressures. Auscultation discloses a loud S_1 (the heart sound associated with mitral valve closure) in almost all cases. This is so because the high atrial-ventricular pressure gradient keeps the mobile portions of the mitral valve leaflets widely separated throughout diastole; at the onset of systole, ventricular contraction abruptly slams the leaflets together from the relatively wide-open position, increasing the intensity of the valve closure sound (see Chapter 2).

A main feature of auscultation in MS is a high-pitched "opening snap" (OS) that follows S_2. The OS is thought to be due to the sudden tensing of the chordae tendineae and stenotic leaflets upon opening. The interval between S_2 and the OS relates inversely to the severity of MS: The more severe the MS, the higher the LA pressure, and the earlier the valve is forced open during LV relaxation in diastole. The OS is followed by a low-frequency decrescendo murmur (termed a diastolic "rumble") due to turbulent flow across the stenotic valve during diastole (Fig. 8.2). The duration, but not the intensity of the diastolic murmur, relates to the severity of mitral stenosis: The more severe the stenosis, the longer it takes for the LA to empty and for the gradient between the LA and LV to dissipate. Near the end of diastole, contraction of the left atrium causes the pressure gradient between the LA and LV to transiently rise (Fig. 8.2), and therefore, the murmur briefly becomes louder. This final accentuation of the murmur does not occur if atrial fibrillation has developed, as there is no effective atrial contraction in that situation.

Murmurs due to other valvular lesions are often found concurrently in patients with MS. For example, mitral regurgitation (see below) frequently coexists with MS. Additionally, right-sided heart failure caused by severe MS may induce tricuspid regurgitation. A diastolic decrescendo murmur along the left sternal border may be due to coexistent aortic regurgitation (because of rheumatic involvement of the aortic leaflets) or pulmonic regurgitation (because of mitral stenosis induced pulmonary hypertension).

The *electrocardiogram* in MS routinely shows left atrial enlargement and, if pulmonary hypertension has developed, right ventricular hypertrophy. Atrial fibrillation may be present. The *chest radiograph* reveals left atrial enlargement, pulmonary vascular redistribution, interstitial edema, and Kerley B lines due to edema within the pulmonary septae (see Chapter 3). With the development of pulmonary hypertension, right ventricular enlargement and prominence of the pulmonary arteries also appear.

Echocardiography is of major diagnostic value in mitral stenosis. It reveals thickened mitral leaflets and abnormal fusion of their commissures with restricted separation during diastole. Left atrial enlargement can be assessed, and if present, intra-atrial thrombus may be visualized. The mitral valve area can be measured directly on cross-sectional views or calculated from Doppler-echocardiographic velocity measurements.

While *cardiac catheterization* is not necessary to confirm the diagnosis of MS, it is often performed to accurately assess the valve area and to identify whether mitral regurgitation, pulmonary hypertension, or coronary artery disease is present.

Treatment

Therapy of MS includes prophylaxis against recurrent ARF in young individuals, and against infective endocarditis in all patients (see below). Diuretics are used to treat symptoms of vascular congestion. Digoxin is useful if mitral stenosis is accompanied by impaired left ventricular contractile function or if atrial fibrillation has developed, in which case it is used to slow the rapid ventricular rate (see Chapter 17). Beta-blockers or the calcium channel antagonists verapamil or diltiazem may also be used to slow the heart rate. Anticoagulant therapy (to prevent thromboembolism) is recommended for patients with mitral stenosis with atrial fibrillation or concurrent congestive heart failure, or if previous embolic episodes have occurred.

If symptoms of MS persist despite diuretic therapy and control of rapid heart rates, mechanical correction of the stenosis is warranted. *Percutaneous transvenous mitral valvuloplasty* was first introduced in 1985, and is a "non-surgical" approach performed via cardiac catheterization. During this procedure, a balloon catheter is ad-

vanced from the femoral vein into the right atrium, across the atrial septum (by creating a small hole there), and advanced through the narrowed mitral valve orifice. The balloon is then rapidly inflated, thereby "cracking" open the fused commissures. The procedure is most effective in the absence of complicating features, such as mitral regurgitation, extensive valve calcification, or atrial thrombus. The results of this procedure in randomized trials compare favorably with those of surgical treatment.

Surgical options for correcting MS include *open mitral commissurotomy* (an operation in which the stenotic commissures are separated under direct visualization), and in severe disease, *mitral valve replacement* (MVR). Perioperative mortality for MVR is approximately 1%–2%, and 10-year survival exceeds 80%, a marked improvement over the natural history of this disease (Table 8.2).

Mitral Regurgitation

Etiology

Normal closure of the mitral valve during systole requires the coordinated action of each component of the valve apparatus. Therefore, mitral regurgitation (MR) may result from structural abnormalities of the mitral annulus, the valve leaflets, the chordae tendineae or the papillary muscles (Table 8.3). Myxomatous degeneration of the valve (termed "mitral valve prolapse") causes MR because enlarged, redundant leaflets bow excessively into the LA during systole rather than opposing each other normally. Ischemic heart disease may scar or cause transient dysfunction of a papillary muscle, interfering with valve closure. Infective endocarditis can result in mitral regurgitation because of leaflet perforation or rupture of infected chordae. Primary (idiopathic) rupture of chordae tendineae is associated with acute, severe valvular incompetence. Rheumatic fever may lead to MS, as already discussed, or primarily mitral regurgitation if excessive shortening of the chordae tendineae and retraction of the leaflets occur. Hypertrophic cardiomyopathy (described in Chapter 10) is associated with abnormal systolic motion of the anterior mitral leaflet, which prevents normal valve closure, causing significant MR in 50% of patients. Marked left ventricular enlargement of any cause results in MR because of two mechanisms that interfere with mitral leaflet closure: 1) the spatial separation between the papillary muscles is augmented, and 2) the mitral annulus is stretched to a increased diameter. Calcification of the mitral annulus can occur with

normal aging, but is more common among patients with hypertension or aortic stenosis. Such calcification immobilizes the basal portion of the valve leaflets, interfering with their excursion and systolic coaptation.

Pathophysiology

In MR, a portion of the left ventricular stroke volume is ejected backward into the low-pressure LA (Fig. 8.3). As a result, the forward cardiac output (into the aorta) is less than the left ventricle's total (forward flow + backward leak) output. Therefore, the direct consequences of MR include: 1) elevation of the left atrial volume and pressure, 2) a reduction of forward cardiac output into the aorta, and 3) a volume-related stress on the left ventricle when the regurgutated volume returns to the LV in diastole along with normal pulmonary venous return. In order to meet normal circulatory needs and to eject the additional volume, the LV stroke volume must increase. This is accomplished by the Frank-Starling mechanism (see Chapter 9)

TABLE 8.3. Common Causes of Mitral Regurgitation

Myxomatous degeneration (e.g., mitral valve prolapse)
Ischemic heart disease with papillary muscle dysfunction
Infective endocarditis
Idiopathic ruptured chordae
Rheumatic deformity
Hypertrophic cardiomyopathy (Chapter 10)
Marked left ventricular enlargement from any cause
Mitral annulus abnormalities (calcification or dilatation)

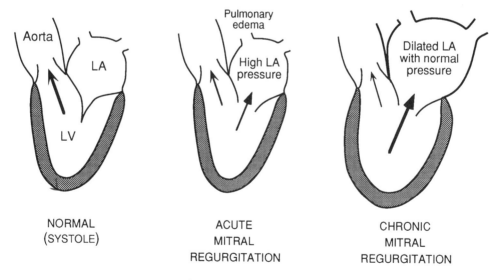

NORMAL (SYSTOLE)   ACUTE MITRAL REGURGITATION   CHRONIC MITRAL REGURGITATION

Figure 8.3. Pathophysiology of mitral regurgitation. In the normal heart, left ventricular (LV) contraction during systole forces blood exclusively through the aortic valve into the aorta; the closed mitral valve prevents regurgitation into the left atrium (LA). In mitral regurgitation (MR), a portion of the LV output is forced retrograde into the LA, so that forward cardiac output into the aorta is reduced. In *acute* MR, the LA is of normal size and is noncompliant, such that the LA pressure rises markedly and pulmonary edema may result. In *chronic* MR, the LA has enlarged and is more compliant, such that LA pressure is less elevated and pulmonary congestive symptoms are less common if LV contractile function is intact. There is LV enlargement and eccentric hypertrophy due to the chronic increased volume load.

whereby the elevated LV diastolic volume (i.e., increased preload) causes increased myofiber stretch and an augmented stroke volume with each contraction. The subsequent hemodynamic consequences of MR vary depending on the severity of the regurgitation and how long it has been present.

The severity of MR and the ratio of forward cardiac output to backward flow are dictated by five factors: 1) the size of the mitral orifice during regurgitation, 2) the systolic pressure gradient between the LV and LA, 3) the systemic vascular resistance opposing forward LV blood flow, 4) the left atrial compliance, and 5) the duration of regurgitation with each systolic contraction. The *regurgitant fraction* in MR is defined as

$$\frac{\text{Volume of MR}}{\text{Total LV stroke volume}}$$

and this ratio rises whenever the resistance to aortic outflow is increased (i.e., the blood follows the path of least resistance). For example, high systemic blood pressure or the presence of aortic stenosis will increase the regurgitant fraction. Left atrial compliance (a measure of the chamber's distensibility expressed as the change in volume per change in unit pressure) is important because it governs how much the left atrial pressure will rise in response to the regurgitated volume. For example, when atrial compliance is low, as in *acute* MR, the LA is relatively stiff and a small increase in left atrial volume produces a large increase in left atrial pressure such that further regurgitation is prevented. When there is greater LA compliance (e.g., due to gradual stretching of the chamber in *chronic* MR), a larger regurgitant volume can be accommodated before left atrial pressure rises substantially and inhibits further regurgitation.

In *acute MR* (e.g., due to papillary muscle ischemia or rupture of chordae tendineae), left atrial compliance is normal (i.e., a relatively stiff chamber) and when it is suddenly exposed to the regurgitant volume, the LA pressure rises sharply (Fig. 8.3). This increase in LA pressure is quickly transmitted to the pulmonary circulation resulting

in pulmonary congestion and edema, a medical emergency. In acute MR, measurements of the LA pressure or the pulmonary capillary wedge pressure (an indirect measurement of LA pressure described in Chapter 3), demonstrate a prominent "v" wave, reflecting increased LA pressure during systole (Fig. 8.4). Additionally, as in MS, pulmonary artery and right heart pressures passively rise such that forward flow through the heart is maintained.

In acute MR, the LV accommodates the increased volume load from the LA according to the Frank-Starling relationship. Thus, the increased LV volume results in: 1) an obligatory increase in LV diastolic pressure, and 2) a compensatory increase in the LV stroke volume, such that at the end of each systolic contraction, LV volume is normal in the nonfailing heart. Systolic emptying of the ventricle is facilitated in MR by the fact that the total impedance to LV contraction is reduced (i.e., the afterload is lower than normal), since a portion of the LV output is

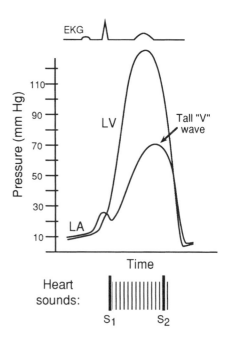

Figure 8.4. Hemodynamic profile of acute mitral regurgitation. A large systolic "v" wave is noted in the left atrial (LA) pressure tracing. A holosystolic murmur is present, beginning at the first heart sound (S₁) and continuing through the second heart sound (S₂). EKG, electrocardiogram; LV, left ventricle.

directed into the relatively low-pressure left atrium, compared with normal outflow into the higher-pressure aorta.

In contrast to the acute situation, the more gradual development of *chronic MR* (e.g., due to rheumatic deformity or chronic myxomatous thickening) permits the LA to undergo compensatory changes that lessen the effects of regurgitation on the pulmonary circulation (Fig. 8.3). In particular, the LA dilates and its compliance increases such that the chamber is able to accommodate large volumes without a substantial increase in pressure. Left atrial dilatation is therefore adaptive in that it prevents marked increases in pulmonary vascular pressures. However, this adaptation occurs at the cost of inadequate forward cardiac output, because the compliant LA becomes a preferred low-pressure "sink" for left ventricular ejection, compared with the greater impedance of the aorta. Consequently, as progressively larger fractions of blood regurgitate into the LA, the main symptoms of chronic MR become those of low forward cardiac output (e.g., fatigue). In addition, chronic left atrial dilatation predisposes to the development of atrial fibrillation.

In chronic MR, the LV also undergoes gradual compensatory dilatation (eccentric hypertrophy, described in Chapter 9) in response to the volume load. Compared with acute MR, the increased ventricular compliance accommodates the increased filling volume with a relatively normal filling pressure. Forward output in chronic MR is preserved to near-normal levels by maintaining a high stroke volume via the Frank-Starling mechanism. Over time (usually several years), however, the chronic volume overload results in deterioration of left ventricular systolic function and leads to declining forward output and symptoms of heart failure.

In summary, the main differences between acute and chronic mitral regurgitation relate to left atrial size and compliance (Fig. 8.3):

1. Acute mitral regurgitation: normal LA size and compliance, high LA pressure, high pulmonary venous pressures and pulmonary congestion.
2. Chronic mitral regurgitation: increased LA size and compliance, more normal LA and pulmonary venous pressures, and symptoms of fatigue due to low cardiac output.

Clinical Manifestations and Evaluation

As should be clear from the pathophysiology discussion above, patients with *acute* MR usually present with symptoms of pulmonary edema (Chapter 9). The symptoms of *chronic* MR are predominantly due to low cardiac output, especially during exertion, and consist of fatigue and weakness. Patients with severe MR or the development of LV contractile dysfunction often complain of dyspnea and may describe orthopnea or paroxysmal nocturnal dyspnea. In severe chronic MR, symptoms of right heart failure (increased abdominal girth, peripheral edema) may be present, as well.

The physical examination of a patient with MR reveals an apical holosystolic murmur that radiates to the axilla (Fig. 8.4). This description, accurate for rheumatic MR has some exceptions. For example, when ischemic papillary muscle dysfunction interferes with normal mitral valve closure, the regurgitant jet may be directed toward the anterior left atrial wall immediately posterior to the aorta. In this setting, the murmur may be best heard in the "aortic" area (Chapter 2) and may not be holosystolic. Fortunately, the distinction between the systolic murmur of MR and that of aortic stenosis (AS) can be made on dynamic auscultation. If the patient is instructed to clench the fists, systemic vascular resistance will increase, and the severity of MR and its murmur will intensify, whereas the murmur of AS will not. Even more helpful in this distinction is to note the effect of varying cardiac cycle length (time between consecutive heart beats) on the intensity of the systolic murmur. In a patient with atrial fibrillation or frequent premature beats, the LV fills to a degree that directly depends on the preceding cycle length (e.g., long cycle lengths permit greater left ventricular filling). The systolic murmur of AS becomes very loud after long cycle lengths because even small pressure gradients are amplified as more blood is ejected across the reduced aortic orifice. In MR, however, the murmur does not vary significantly from short to long cardiac cycle lengths because the relative change in the LV to LA pressure gradient is altered very little.

In addition to the systolic murmur, a common finding in chronic MR is the presence of an S_3, which reflects increased volume returning to the LV in early diastole. In chronic MR, the palpated cardiac apical impulse is often laterally displaced toward the axilla, because of LV enlargement.

The *chest radiograph* in chronic MR demonstrates left ventricular and atrial enlargement. Calcification of the mitral annulus may be seen if that is the cause of the MR. The *electrocardiogram* typically demonstrates left atrial enlargement and signs of left ventricular hypertrophy. *Echocardiography* can often identify the structural cause of MR, and grade its severity by color Doppler interrogation. Left ventricular size and function (usually vigorous in the "compensated" heart because of the increased stroke volume) can be observed. *Cardiac catheterization* is useful for identifying a coronary ischemic cause (i.e., papillary muscle dysfunction) and for grading the severity of mitral regurgitation. The characteristic hemodynamic abnormality is a large "v" wave on the pulmonary capillary wedge pressure (reflecting LA pressure) tracing (Fig. 8.4).

Natural History and Treatment

The natural history of chronic MR is related to its underlying cause. For example, in rheumatic heart disease, the course is one of very slow progression with a 15-year survival rate of 70%. On the other hand, abrupt worsening of chronic MR of any cause can occur with superimposed complications such as rupture of chordae tendineae or endocarditis, and result in an immediate life-threatening situation.

Medical therapy of MR involves augmenting forward cardiac output while reducing regurgitation into the LA, and relieving pulmonary congestion. In acute MR with heart failure, treatment includes intravenous diuretics in order to relieve pulmonary edema, and vasodilators (e.g., intravenous sodium nitroprusside) to reduce the resistance to forward flow and augment forward cardiac output. In chronic MR, improvement in forward flow can be accomplished by oral arteriolar vasodilators such as angiotensin converting-enzyme inhibitors or hydralazine.

Because chronic MR produces continuous left ventricular volume overload, it can slowly result in left ventricular contractile impairment and, ultimately, heart failure. Mitral valve surgery should be performed before such impairment occurs, but the operative mortality and the drawbacks associated with prosthetic valves are motivations for delaying surgery as long as possible. After more than 30 years' experience, the timing of surgery for a patient with chronic MR remains one of the most difficult decisions in the practice of cardiology. This is so because survival after *mitral valve replacement* is not clearly better than the natural history of the disease (because of potential complications of implanted artificial heart valves), even though symptomatic improvement is the rule. Fortunately, recent refinements in mitral valve surgery are allowing many patients to undergo *mitral valve repair* rather than replacement, eliminating many of the problems due to artificial valves. Mitral valve repair involves the surgical reconstruction of parts of the valve responsible for the regurgitation. For example, a perforated leaflet may be patched with transplanted autologous pericardium, or a ruptured chord may be reattached to a papillary muscle. In such patients, the postoperative survival rate appears to be *better* than the natural history of MR and has provided impetus toward earlier surgical intervention.

The operative mortality rate is approximately 2% to 4% for mitral valve repair and 8% to 10% for mitral replacement. The 10-

year survival rate is about 80% for mitral repair and 50% for mitral replacement. In general, mitral valve repair is more often appropriate for younger patients with myxomatous involvement of the mitral valve, and mitral replacement is more often employed for older patients with more extensive valve pathology.

Mitral Valve Prolapse

Mitral valve prolapse (MVP) is a common and usually asymptomatic billowing of the mitral leaflets into the LA during ventricular systole, sometimes accompanied by mitral regurgitation. Other names for this condition include "floppy" mitral valve, myxomatous mitral valve, or Barlow's syndrome. Pathologically, the valve leaflets, particularly the posterior leaflet, are enlarged, and the normal dense collagen and elastin matrix of the valvular fibrosa is fragmented and replaced with loose, "myxomatous" connective tissue. Additionally, in more severe lesions, elongated or ruptured chordae, annular enlargement, or thickened leaflets may be present. Mitral valve prolapse occurs in about 3% to 5% of the normal population and is more common among women. This condition may be inherited as a primary autosomal dominant disorder, or may occur as a part of other connective tissue diseases such as the Marfan or Ehlers-Danlos syndromes.

Mitral prolapse is often asymptomatic, but affected people may describe chest pains, or palpitations because of associated arrhythmias. Most often, it is found on routine physical examination, identified by the presence of a midsystolic "click" and late systolic murmur heard best at the cardiac apex. The systolic click is thought to correspond to the sudden tensing of the involved mitral leaflet or chordae tendineae as the leaflet is forced back toward the left atrium, while the murmur corresponds to regurgitant flow through the incompetent valve. The click and murmur are characteristically altered during dynamic auscultation: Maneuvers that increase the volume of the LV

(e.g., sudden squatting) delay the timing of the leaflet prolapse and cause the click and murmur to occur later in systole (i.e., further from S_1). Conversely, if the volume of blood in the LV is decreased (e.g., upon sudden standing), then the click and murmur should occur earlier in systole (closer to S_1). Confirmation of the diagnosis is obtained by echocardiography, which demonstrates posterior displacement of one or both mitral leaflets during systole. The *electrocardiogram* and chest radiograph are usually normal unless chronic MR has resulted in left atrial and left ventricular enlargement.

The clinical course of mitral prolapse is most often benign, and treatment consists of reassurance about the usually good prognosis, and antibiotic prophylaxis for endocarditis if substantial valve thickening or MR are present. Of the potential complications, the most common is the development of gradually progressive MR. Occasionally, rupture of a myxomatous chord can cause sudden severe regurgitation and pulmonary edema. Other rare complications include infective endocarditis, peripheral emboli due to microthrombus formation behind the redundant valve tissue and atrial or ventricular arrhythmias.

AORTIC VALVE DISEASE

Aortic Stenosis

Etiology

Previously attributed to rheumatic heart disease in almost all cases, aortic stenosis (AS) is now most frequently caused by either deterioration of a congenitally bicuspid aortic valve or "senile" calcific degeneration. Most patients who present with AS over the age of 65 years have "senile" degeneration, whereas the majority of those under the age of 65 have calcification of a congenitally bicuspid valve. Approximately 95% of patients who do have rheumatic AS also have coexisting rheumatic disease of the mitral valve.

Pathology

The pathologic appearance in AS is derived from its etiology:

1. In *senile* AS, cumulative "wear-and-tear" leads to endothelial and fibrous damage, resulting in calcification of an otherwise normal valve. Therefore, symptoms associated with this pathology do not generally appear until the seventh or eighth decade.
2. In the case of a congenitally deformed *bicuspid* aortic valve, years of abnormal hemodynamic flow through the valve disrupts the endothelium and collagen matrix of the leaflets, resulting in gradual calcium deposition similar to that of the senile form, but usually decades earlier.
3. In *rheumatic* aortic valve stenosis, endocardial inflammation leads to organization and fibrosis of the valve, resulting in fusion of the commissures, as well as the formation of calcified masses within the aortic cusps.

Irrespective of cause, the final pathologic findings in advanced aortic stenosis are similar. Calcification is seen deep within the fibrosa of the valve cusps, extending toward the surface, resulting in heaped up or nodular deposition extending into the sinuses of Valsalva of the aortic root.

Pathophysiology

In AS, blood flow across the aortic valve is obstructed during systole (Fig. 8.5). When the valve orifice area is reduced by more than 50% of its normal size, significant elevation of left ventricular pressure is necessary to drive blood into the aorta (Fig. 8.6). In advanced aortic stenosis, it is common to measure pressure gradients greater than 100 mmHg between the LV and the aorta.

Over time, the LV undergoes concentric hypertrophy in response to the high systolic pressure it must generate. Such hypertrophy serves an important compensatory role in reducing ventricular wall stress (Chapter 6); however, it also reduces the compliance

of the ventricle. The resulting elevation in diastolic LV pressure also causes the LA to hypertrophy in order to fill the "stiff" LV. Whereas left atrial contraction contributes only a small portion of the left ventricular stroke volume in normal individuals, it may contribute more than 25% of the stroke volume to the stiffened LV in AS patients. Thus, left atrial hypertrophy is beneficial, and the loss of effective atrial contraction (e.g., the development of atrial fibrillation) can cause marked clinical deterioration.

Three major symptoms occur in patients with advanced AS, as described below: 1) congestive heart failure, 2) angina, and 3) syncope, all of which can be explained on the basis of the underlying pathophysiology. Early in the course of AS, the abnormal increase in left atrial pressure occurs mostly at the end of diastole, when the LA contracts into the thickened noncompliant LV. As a result, the *mean* left atrial pressure and the pulmonary venous pressure are not greatly affected early in the disease. However, with progression of the stenosis, the LV develops contractile dysfunction due to the insurmountably high afterload, leading to increased left ventricular end diastolic volume and pressure. The accompanying marked elevation of LA and pulmonary venous pressures produces pulmonary alveo-

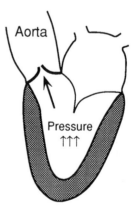

Figure 8.5. Pathophysiology of aortic stenosis (AS). Obstruction to systolic left ventricular (LV) outflow in AS results in elevation of the intraventricular pressures and secondary LV hypertrophy.

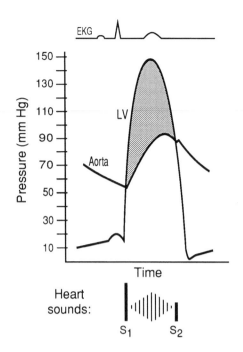

Figure 8.6. Hemodynamic profile of aortic stenosis. A large systolic pressure gradient (shaded area) is present between the left ventricle (LV) and aorta. The second heart sound (S_2) is diminished in intensity, and there is a crescendo-decrescendo systolic murmur that does not extend beyond S_2. EKG, electrocardiogram.

lar congestion and the symptoms of *congestive heart failure*.

Aortic stenosis may result in *angina* because it creates a substantial imbalance between myocardial oxygen supply and demand. Myocardial oxygen *demand* is increased in two ways. First, the muscle mass of the LV is increased, requiring greater than normal perfusion. Second, wall stress is increased because of the elevated systolic ventricular pressure. In addition, AS reduces myocardial oxygen *supply* as the elevated left ventricular diastolic pressure reduces the coronary perfusion pressure gradient between the aorta and the myocardium (particularly in the subendocardium where intramural pressure is greatest).

Finally, AS may cause *syncope*. Although left ventricular hypertrophy allows the ventricle to generate a high pressure and maintain a normal cardiac output at rest, the ventricle cannot significantly increase its

cardiac output during exercise because of the fixed stenotic aortic orifice. In addition, exercise leads to vasodilatation of the peripheral muscle beds. Thus, the combination of peripheral vasodilatation and the inability to augment cardiac output contribute to decreased cerebral perfusion pressure, and potentially, syncope upon exertion.

The normal aortic valve area is greater than 3.0 cm². When the valve area is reduced to less than 1.2 cm², a significant pressure gradient between the LV and aorta first appears (mild AS). If the aortic valve area is reduced to less than 0.7 cm², critical obstruction is said to be present.

Clinical Manifestations and Evaluation

Angina, syncope, and congestive heart failure may appear after many asymptomatic years of slowly progressive valve stenosis. Once these symptoms develop, they confer a markedly decreased survival if surgical relief of AS is not undertaken (Table 8.4).

Physical examination often permits accurate detection and estimation of the severity of aortic stenosis. The key features are: 1) a coarse late-peaking systolic ejection murmur (Fig. 8.6), and 2) a weakened ("parvus") and delayed ("tardus") upstroke of the carotid artery pulsations due to the obstructed LV outflow. Other common findings on cardiac examination include the presence of an S_4 (because of atrial contraction into the "stiff" LV) and reduced intensity or complete absence of the aortic component of the second heart sound (Fig. 8.6).

TABLE 8.4. Median Survival in Symptomatic Aortic Stenosis

Clinical Symptoms	Median Survival
Angina	5 years
Syncope	3 years
Congestive heart failure	2 years
Atrial fibrillation	6 months

Reprinted with permission from Ross J Jr, Braunwald E. Aortic stenosis. Circ Suppl 1968; 38:v–61.

On the *electrocardiogram*, left ventricular hypertrophy is common in advanced AS, but *echocardiography* is a more sensitive technique to assess LV wall thickness. The transvalvular gradient can be measured by Doppler echocardiographic velocity measurements. *Cardiac catheterization* is useful for clarifying the severity of AS and for defining coronary anatomy, because concurrent coronary artery bypass surgery is often necessary at the time of aortic valve replacement in patients with coexisting coronary disease.

Treatment

The natural history of severe, symptomatic, uncorrected AS is very poor. Data from the Mayo Clinic indicate that the 1-year survival rate is 57% for patients with severe AS who do not undergo surgery. The only effective treatment for advanced AS is surgical replacement of the valve.

Aortic valve replacement (AVR) is indicated for patients with symptomatic or severe AS. The left ventricular ejection fraction almost always increases after valve replacement, even in patients with impaired left ventricular function. The effect of AVR on the natural history of AS is dramatic, with the 10-year survival rate exceeding 75%.

Unlike mitral stenosis, the results of percutaneous balloon valvuloplasty in aortic stenosis have been disappointing, and therefore, that procedure is not performed routinely. Occasionally, it is undertaken for temporary palliation of symptoms in severely symptomatic, elderly patients with AS who are considered to be at very high surgical risk.

Mild, asymptomatic AS has a slow rate of progression such that over a 20-year period, only 20% of patients will progress to severe or symptomatic AS. Medical therapy for asymptomatic AS includes close clinical follow-up, endocarditis antibiotic prophylaxis, and avoidance of medications that could result in hypotension in this setting (e.g., vasodilators, diuretics, nitroglycerin).

Aortic Regurgitation

Etiology

Aortic regurgitation (AR), also termed aortic insufficiency, may result from: 1) diseases of the aortic leaflets, or 2) dilatation of the aortic root. The most common causes of AR are listed in Table 8.5.

Pathophysiology

In AR, abnormal regurgitation of blood from the aorta into the LV occurs during diastole. Therefore, with each contraction, the LV must pump the regurgitant volume *plus* the normal volume of blood returning from the LA, and hemodynamic compensation relies on the Frank-Starling mechanism to augment the LV stroke volume during systole. The factors influencing the severity of AR are analogous to those of mitral regurgitation: 1) the size of the regurgitant aortic orifice, 2) the pressure gradient across the aortic valve during diastole, and 3) the duration of diastole.

As is the case with mitral regurgitation, the hemodynamic abnormalities and symptoms differ in acute and chronic AR (Fig. 8.7). In *acute* AR, the LV is of normal size and is relatively noncompliant. Thus, the volume load of regurgitation causes the LV diastolic pressure to rise substantially. The sudden high diastolic LV pressure is transmitted to the LA and pulmonary circulation, often producing dyspnea and pulmonary edema. Thus, acute severe AR is usually a surgical emergency, requiring immediate valve replacement.

In *chronic* AR, the LV undergoes com-

TABLE 8.5. Examples of Aortic Insufficiency

Abnormalities of valve leaflets
1. Rheumatic
2. Endocarditis
3. Congenital (bicuspid valve)

Dilatation of aortic root
1. Aortic aneurysm/dissection
2. Annulo-aortic ectasia
3. Marfan syndrome
4. Syphilis

pensatory adaptation in response to the long-standing regurgitation. AR subjects the LV primarily to volume overload, but also to excessive pressure; therefore, the ventricle compensates through dilatation and, to a lesser degree, hypertrophy. Over time, the dilatation increases the compliance of the LV and allows it to accommodate a large regurgitant volume with less of an increase in diastolic pressure, reducing the pressure transmitted into the LA and pulmonary circulation. However, by allowing the aorta to regurgitate a huge volume of blood during diastole, LV dilatation also causes the aortic (and therefore systemic arterial) diastolic pressure to drop substantially. The combination of a high LV stroke volume (and therefore high systolic arterial pressure) with a reduced aortic diastolic pressure produces a widened *pulse pressure* (the difference between arterial systolic and diastolic pressures), a hallmark of chronic AR (Fig. 8.8). As a result of the decreased aortic diastolic pressure, the coronary artery perfusion pressure falls, resulting in decreased myocardial oxygen supply. This, coupled with the increase in LV size (which causes increased wall stress and myocardial oxygen demand) sometimes produces angina, even in the absence of atherosclerotic coronary disease.

Because left ventricular dilatation and hypertrophy are generally adequate to meet the demands of chronic AR, the patient is usually asymptomatic for many years. Gradually, however, progressive remodeling of the LV occurs, resulting in myocardial systolic dysfunction. This in turn results in decreased forward cardiac output, and an increase in left atrial and pulmonary pressures. At that point, the patient develops the symptoms of heart failure.

Clinical Manifestations and Assessment

Common symptoms of chronic AR include dyspnea on exertion, fatigue, decreased exercise tolerance, and the uncomfortable sensation of a forceful heartbeat associated with the high pulse pressure. Physical examination may show bounding pulses due to the wide pulse pressure, a hyperdynamic LV impulse, and the blowing murmur of AR in early diastole along the left sternal border (Fig. 8.8). It is best heard with the patient leaning forward, after exhaling.

In chronic AR, the *chest radiograph* shows an enlarged left ventricular silhouette. This is usually absent in acute AR in which pulmonary vascular congestion is the more likely finding. *Doppler echocardiography* can identify and quantify the degree of AR and often identify its cause. *Cardiac catheterization* is also useful for evaluation of left ven-

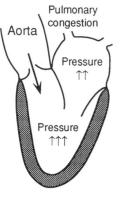

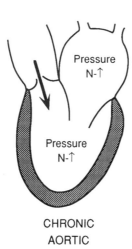

ACUTE AORTIC REGURGITATION

CHRONIC AORTIC REGURGITATION

Figure 8.7. Pathophysiology of acute and chronic aortic regurgitation (AR). Abnormal regurgitation of blood from the aorta into the left ventricle (LV) is shown in each schematic drawing (large arrows). In acute AR, the LV is of normal size and relatively low compliance, such that its diastolic pressure rises markedly; this is reflected back to the left atrium (LA) and pulmonary vasculature, resulting in pulmonary congestion or edema. In chronic AR, adaptive LV and LA enlargement have occurred, such that a greater volume of regurgitation can be accommodated with less of an increase in diastolic LV pressure, so that pulmonary congestion is less likely. N, normal.

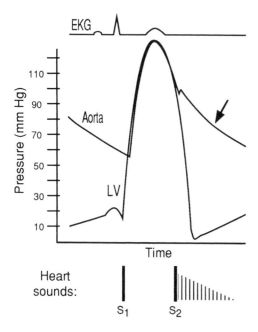

Figure 8.8. Hemodynamic profile of aortic regurgitation. During diastole, the aortic pressure falls rapidly (arrow), and left ventricular (LV) pressure rises as blood regurgitates from the aorta into the LV. A diastolic decrescendo murmur, beginning at the second heart sound (S₂) corresponds with the abnormal regurgitant flow.

tricular function, quantification of the degree of AR, and for assessment of coexisting coronary artery disease.

Treatment

Data from the National Institutes of Health suggests that 60% of patients with asymptomatic chronic AR and normal LV contractile function will remain asymptomatic at 10 years of follow-up. Therefore, asymptomatic patients simply need regular clinical evaluation, periodic assessment of LV function (usually by echocardiography), and endocarditis antibiotic prophylaxis. Symptomatic patients with preserved LV function may respond to therapy with diuretics and afterload reducing vasodilators (e.g., angiotensin converting-enzyme inhibitors or hydralazine). Recently, the calcium-channel blocker nifedipine has been shown to reduce LV enlargement, increase the LV ejection fraction, and delay the need

for valve surgery in patients with severe AR who have normal LV contractile function.

The onset of symptoms in a patient with chronic AR usually heralds the development of LV contractile dysfunction. Symptomatic patients with severe chronic AR or asymptomatic patients with evidence of impaired LV systolic function as a result of regurgitation should undergo surgical valve replacement, in order to prevent further deterioration of LV function.

TRICUSPID VALVE DISEASE

Tricuspid Stenosis

Tricuspid stenosis (TS) is usually due to rheumatic heart disease. The opening snap and diastolic murmur of tricuspid stenosis are similar to MS, but the murmur is heard closer to the sternum and it intensifies upon inspiration because of increased right-heart blood flow. In TS, the neck veins are distended and show a large "a" wave due to right atrial contraction against the stenotic tricuspid valve orifice. Surgical therapy is usually required (valvuloplasty or valve replacement).

Tricuspid Regurgitation

Tricuspid regurgitation (TR) is usually "functional" rather than structural; that is, it develops because of right ventricular enlargement due to pressure or volume overload, rather than primary valve disease. In patients with rheumatic mitral stenosis, 20% have significant TR (of whom 80% have "functional" TR because of pulmonary hypertension with RV enlargement and 20% have "organic" TR due to rheumatic involvement of the tricuspid valve). The most sensitive physical signs are prominent "v" waves in the jugular veins and a pulsatile liver because of regurgitation of right ventricular blood into the systemic veins. The systolic murmur of TR is heard at the lower left sternal border. It is often soft, but becomes louder upon inspiration. Doppler echocardiography is sensitive for the detection and quantification of TR. The primary therapy of functional TR is directed at the conditions responsible for the elevated right ventricular size or pressure, as well as diuretic therapy; surgical repair of the valve is indicated in severe cases.

PULMONIC VALVE DISEASE

Pulmonic Stenosis

The cause of pulmonic stenosis (PS) is almost always congenital deformity of the valve. Severe cases are associated with a pressure gradient of greater than 80 mmHg, moderate cases with a gradient of 40 to 80 mmHg, and mild cases with a gradient of less than 40 mmHg. Only those with moderate to severe gradients are symptomatic. Transcatheter balloon valvuloplasty is usually effective therapy for patients with severe or symptomatic PS.

Pulmonic Regurgitation

Pulmonic regurgitation often develops in the setting of severe pulmonary hypertension, because of dilatation of the valve ring by the enlarged pulmonary artery. Auscultation reveals a high-pitched decrescendo murmur along the left sternal border that is often indistinguishable from AR (the two conditions are easily differentiated by Doppler echocardiography). Treatment of the underlying cause of pulmonary hypertension is the usual therapy.

PROSTHETIC VALVES

The patient who undergoes valve replacement surgery often benefits dramatically from hemodynamic and symptomatic improvement, but also acquires a new set of potential complications related to the intracardiac prosthesis itself. Because all available valve substitutes have certain limitations, valve replacement surgery is not a true "cure."

Currently available valve substitutes are either mechanical or bioprosthetic (derived from animal or human tissue) in construction. Older mechanical valves include a ball-in-cage design, the bulky shape of which often left a significant valvular gradient and occasionally produced intravascular hemolysis from mechanical red blood cell trauma. This valve, however, also has an impressive record for valve durability, with some models functioning well for more than 30 years. Newer mechanical valves, such as the St. Jude bileaflet prosthesis, provide a lower profile and superior hemodynamics (smaller transvalvular gradients) without an apparent sacrifice of durability. The St. Jude valve is a hinged bi-leaflet valve consisting of two pyrolyte carbon discs. The discs open opposite each other like the doors of a saloon in the Old West.

Mechanical valves, while extremely durable, present foreign thrombogenic surfaces to the circulating blood and require chronic systemic anticoagulation (usually with warfarin) to prevent thromboembolism.

The most commonly used bioprostheses are made from glutaraldehyde fixed porcine valves secured in a support frame. In recent years, bovine pericardium and human homograft (cryopreserved from human cadavers) prostheses have also been introduced. Bioprosthetic valves have limited durability compared with mechanical valves, and structural failure occurs in up to 50% of valves at 10 years, with failure rates accelerating thereafter. Structural failure rates vary greatly depending on the position of the valve. Bioprosthetic valves in the mitral position deteriorate more rapidly than those in the aortic position, probably because valve closure occurs during systolic contraction in the mitral position and is therefore associated with higher leaflet stresses than those experienced by leaflets in the aortic position that close under diastolic pressures. The principal causes of bioprosthetic valve failure include leaflet tears and calcification. Despite their increased rate of deterioration, bioprosthetic valves have a very low rate of thromboembolism and do not require long-term anticoagulation.

Common to all types of valve replacements is the risk of infective endocarditis, which occurs at an incidence of 1% to 2% per patient per year (see below). If endocarditis occurs in the first 60 days after surgery, the mortality rate is exceedingly high (50% to 80%). If endocarditis occurs later, mortality rates range from 20% to 50%. Reoperation is usually required if endocarditis involves a mechanical prosthesis because an adjacent abscess is almost always present (the organism cannot infect the prosthetic material itself). Some cases of bioprosthetic valve endocarditis can be treated with antibiotic therapy alone.

Given their respective advantages and disadvantages, the mortality and complication rates of mechanical and bioprosthetic valves are similar for the first 10 years following replacement.

INFECTIVE ENDOCARDITIS

Infection of the endocardial surface of the heart, including the cardiac valves, by microbial organisms is a serious condition that can lead to extensive tissue damage and is often fatal. It carries a 10% to 30% mortality rate even with appropriate therapy, and 100% mortality if it is not recognized and treated correctly.

There are three clinically useful ways to classify infective endocarditis (IE): 1) by clinical course, 2) by host substrate, or 3) by the specific infecting microorganism. In the first classification scheme, IE is termed **acute bacterial endocarditis** (ABE) when the syndrome presents as an acute, fulminant infection, and a highly virulent and invasive organism such as *Staphylococcus aureus* is implicated. Because of the aggressiveness of the responsible microorganism, ABE may occur on previously healthy heart valves. When IE presents with a more insidious clinical course, it is termed **subacute bacterial endocarditis** (SBE), and less virulent organisms such as *Streptococcus viridans* are involved. SBE most frequently occurs in individuals with previous underlying valvular damage.

The second means of classification of IE is according to the host substrate: 1) native valve endocarditis (NVE), 2) prosthetic valve endocarditis (PVE), or 3) endocarditis in the setting of intravenous drug abuse (IVDA). Of these, NVE accounts for 60% to 80% of patients with endocarditis. Different microorganisms and clinical courses are associated with each of these categories. For example, the skin contaminant *Staphylococcus epidermidis* is a common cause of prosthetic valve endocarditis, but that is rarely the case when endocarditis occurs on a native heart valve.

The third classification of IE is according to the specific infecting microorganism (e.g., "*Staphylococcus aureus* endocarditis"). While the remainder of this discussion will focus on the endocarditis syndromes based on clinical course, it is important to recognize that all three classifications of IE are used.

Pathogenesis

The pathogenesis of endocarditis requires several conditions: 1) endocardial surface injury, 2) thrombus formation at the site of injury, 3) bacterial entry into the circulation, and 4) bacterial adherence to the injured endocardial surface. The first two conditions provide an environment favorable to infection, whereas the latter two permit implantation of the organism on the endocardial surface. The most common cause of endothelial injury is turbulent blood flow resulting from underlying valvular abnormalities that lead to high-velocity jets that mechanically injure the endothelial surface. About 70% of patients with endocarditis have evidence of underlying structural or hemodynamic abnormalities (Table 8.6). Endothelial injury may also be induced by the presence of foreign material within the circulation, such as in-dwelling intravenous catheters or prosthetic heart valves.

Once the endocardial surface of a valve is injured, platelets adhere to the exposed subendocardial connective tissue and initiate the formation of a sterile thrombus (termed a "vegetation") through fibrin deposition. This process is referred to as nonbacterial thrombotic endocarditis (NBTE) or "marantic" endocarditis. NBTE makes

TABLE 8.6. Cardiac Lesions that Predispose to Endocarditis

- Rheumatic valvular disease
- Other acquired valvular lesions
  Calcific aortic stenosis
  Aortic regurgitation
  Mitral regurgitation
  Mitral valve prolapse (if murmur auscultated or detected by Doppler)
- Hypertrophic obstructive cardiomyopathy
- Congenital heart disease, including:
  Ventricular septal defect
  Patent ductus arteriosus
  Tetralogy of Fallot
  Aortic coarctation
  Bicuspid aortic valve
  Pulmonic stenosis
- Surgically implanted intravascular hardware, including:
  Prosthetic heart valves
  Pulmonary-systemic vascular shunts
  Ventriculo-atrial shunts for hydrocephalus
- Previous episode of endocarditis

the endocardium more hospitable to microbes in two ways. First, the fibrin-platelet deposits provide a surface for adherence by bacteria. Second, the fibrin covers adherent organisms and protects them from host defenses by inhibiting chemotaxis and migration of phagocytes.

When NBTE is present, the delivery of microorganisms in the blood stream to the injured surface can lead to infective endocarditis. Table 8.7 lists the infectious agents that most commonly cause endocarditis, and their relative frequencies of involvement. Three factors determine the ability of an organism to induce IE: 1) access to the bloodstream, 2) survival of the organism in the circulation, and 3) adherence of the bacteria to the endocardium. Bacteria can be introduced into the bloodstream whenever a mucosal or skin surface harboring an organism is traumatized, such as from the mouth during dental procedures, or from the skin during intravenous drug use. However, while transient bacteremia is a relatively common event, only those microorganisms that are suited for survival in the circulation and are able to adhere to the vegetation will result in infective endocarditis. For example, Gram-positive organisms account for approximately 90% of cases of endocarditis, in large part because

of their resistance to destruction in the circulation by complement. Furthermore, the production by certain streptococcal species of dextran, a bacterial cell wall component that adheres to thrombus, correlates with their ability to incite endocarditis.

Once organisms adhere to the injured surface, they may be protected from phagocytic activity by the overlying fibrin. The organisms are then free to multiply, which further enlarges the infected vegetation. The presence of an infected vegetation provides a source for continuous bacteremia and can lead to several complications. These complications may occur secondary to: 1) mechanical cardiac injury, 2) thrombotic or septic emboli, or 3) immune injury, mediated by antigen-antibody deposition. For example, local extension of the infection within the heart can result in progressive valvular damage (leading to heart failure), abscess formation, or erosion into the cardiac conduction system. Portions of a vegetation may embolize peripherally, often to the central nervous system, kidneys or spleen, and incite infection or infarction of the target organs. Immune-complex deposition can result in glomerulonephritis, arthritis, or vasculitis. Each of these is a potentially fatal complication.

Clinical Manifestations

Acute IE is an explosive and rapidly progressive illness that presents with high

TABLE 8.7. Common Causes of Infective Endocarditis

Organism	Incidence (%)
Streptococci	70
Viridans	35
Enterococci	10
Other streptococci	25
Staphylococci	20
S. aureus	18
Coagulase-negative	2
Other organisms	10
(e.g., gram-negative, haemophilus, fungi)	

Reprinted with permission from Freeman R, Hall R. Infective endocarditis. In: Julian DG, et al. Diseases of the Heart. London: Baillière Tindall 1989:855.

fever and shaking chills. In contrast, subacute IE presents less dramatically with lower grade fever often accompanied by nonspecific constitutional symptoms such as fatigue, anorexia, weakness, myalgias, or night sweats. Subacute IE often mimics other illnesses such as influenza or an upper respiratory tract infection, and the diagnosis requires a high-degree of suspicion. A history of a valvular lesion or other condition known to predispose to endocarditis is helpful.

The systemic inflammatory response produced by the infection is responsible for fever and splenomegaly, as well as for a number of laboratory findings including an elevated white blood cell count with a leftward shift (increase in proportion of neutrophils and immature granulocytes due to acute inflammation), an elevated erythrocyte sedimentation rate, and in about 50% of cases, an elevated serum rheumatoid factor.

Cardiac examination may reveal a murmur representing the underlying valvular pathology that predisposed the patient to IE. Alternatively, auscultation may also reveal a new murmur of valvular insufficiency due to IE-induced damage of one or more cardiac valves. Right-sided valvular lesions, while rare in normal hosts, are particularly common in IVDA-related endocarditis. Overall, murmurs are found more commonly in SBE than ABE. However, serial examination in ABE may be especially useful as changes in a particular murmur (i.e., worsening regurgitation) over time may correspond with rapidly evolving valvular damage specific to ABE. During the course of endocarditis, valvular damage may result in signs of congestive heart failure.

Infected emboli may travel to any end-organ including the skin, brain, kidney, viscera, or spleen. Central nervous system emboli are seen in up to 33% of patients with endocarditis. Injury to the kidneys, of immunologic or embolic origin, may be manifest as hematuria, flank pain, or renal failure. Lung infarction (pulmonary embolism) or infection (pneumonia) are particularly common in endocarditis involving the right-sided heart valves. Embolic infarction and seeding of the vasa vasora of arteries can cause localized aneurym formation (termed a "mycotic aneurysm") that weakens the vessel wall and may rupture. Mycotic aneurysms may be found in the aorta, viscera, or peripheral organs, but are particularly dangerous in cerebral vessels, as rupture can result in a fatal intracranial hemorrhage.

Other physical findings that may appear in IE are associated with septic embolism or immune-complex mediated vasculitis at distal sites. For example, petechiae appear as tiny, circular, red-brown discolorations on mucosal surfaces or skin. "Splinter hemorrhages," the result of subungual micro-emboli, are small, longitudinal hemorrhages found under the nails. Painless, slightly nodular discolorations found on the palms and soles are called "Janeway lesions." Tender, pea-sized, erythematous nodules found primarily in the pulp space of the fingers and toes are termed "Osler's nodes." Emboli to the retina produce "Roth spots," which are micro-infarctions that appear as white dots surrounded by hemorrhage.

The diagnosis and appropriate treatment of endocarditis rely on the identification of the responsible microorganism by *blood cultures*. Treatment can then be tailored to the specific microorganism according to its antibiotic sensitivities. A specific etiologic agent will be identified by culture approximately 95% of the time. Blood cultures may fail to grow the responsible organism if antibiotics have been recently administered or if the organism has unusual growth requirements.

Other laboratory techniques may also be helpful. The *electrocardiogram* may identify extension of the infection into the cardiac conduction system, which may appear as

---

TABLE 8.8. Procedures Warranting Endocarditis Prophylaxis

Dental manipulations that produce gingival bleeding
Rigid bronchoscopy and surgery of the upper respiratory tract
Genitourinary procedures, including:
    Indwelling bladder catheter
    Cystoscopy
    Prostatecomy
    Vaginal delivery (if peripartum infection present)
Gastrointestinal surgery, including cholecystectomy

TABLE 8.9. Summary of Major Valvular Lesions

Valve Lesion	Causes	Symptoms	Physical Findings	Compensatory Mechanisms
Mitral stenosis	Sequella of rheumatic fever	• Symptoms of left-sided (and later right-sided) heart failure[a]	• Loud S_1 • Opening snap • Diastolic rumble	• Pulmonary arteriolar constriction "protects" pulmonary vasculature
Mitral regurgitation	*Acute:* • Endocarditis • Ruptured chordae • Papillary muscle dysfunction *Chronic:* • Rheumatic • Mitral prolapse • Calcified annulus • LV dilatation	*Acute:* • Pulmonary edema *Chronic:* • Symptoms of left-sided heart failure[a] and low cardiac output (e.g., fatigue)	• Widely split S_2 • Holosystolic murmur at apex	*Acute:* • Frank-Starling mechanism increases stroke volume and maintains normal end-systolic volume *Chronic:* • Left atrial dilatation serves as volume "sink"
Aortic stenosis	• Congenital • Rheumatic • Senile calcific	• Chest pain • Syncope • Dyspnea on exertion	*Carotids:* delayed upstroke and decreased volume *Palpation:* Suprasternal thrill *Auscultation:* • Soft A_2 • Late-peaking systolic ejection-type murmur	• Compensatory left ventricular hypertrophy
Aortic regurgitation	• Congenital (e.g., bicuspid valve) • Endocarditis • Rheumatic • Aortic root dilatation	• Dyspnea on exertion • Chest pain (sometimes)	• Wide pulse pressure • Bounding pulses • Early diastolic decrescendo murmur	• Frank-Starling mechanism increases stroke volume and maintains normal end-systolic volume • (Chronic) Left ventricular hypertrophy

[a]Symptoms of left-sided heart failure include exertional dyspnea, orthopnea, paroxysmal nocturnal dyspnea; symptoms of right-sided heart failure include peripheral edema, abdominal bloating, and right upper quadrant tenderness (hepatic enlargement).

various degrees of heart block or new ar-rhythmias. *Echocardiography* is diagnostically useful when vegetations are directly visual-ized. It is often even more helpful in the iden-tification of complications of IE such as valvular dysfunction or abscess formation. *Transesophageal echocardiography* is much more sensitive for imaging vegetations that the standard transthoracic technique.

Treatment of endocarditis entails pro-longed (4–6 weeks), high-dose intravenous antibiotic therapy tailored to the impli-cated microorganism. Surgical interven-tion, usually with valve replacement is undertaken only if antibiotic therapy fails to erradicate the infection or life-threaten-ing complications ensue, such as severe valvular dysfunction with heart failure, recurrent emboli or formation of a myocar-dial abscess.

Perhaps the most important aspect of therapy is *prevention* of endocarditis by ad-ministering antibiotics prior to procedures that result in bacteremia in susceptible indi-viduals (Table 8.8).

SUMMARY

Valvular heart disease is a significant source of disability and mortality. From simple bedside observations to complex physiologic measurements, much has been learned about the pathophysiology of these conditions. A summary of the important findings associated with the major valve le-sions is presented in Table 8.9.

ADDITIONAL READING

Carabello BA, Crawford FA. Valvular heart disease. N Engl J Med 1997;337:32–41.

Carroll JD, Feldman T. Percutaneous mitral balloon valvotomy and the new demographics of mitral stenosis. JAMA 1993;270:1731–1736.

Cheitlin MD, Douglas PS, Parmley WW. Task Force 2: acquired valvular heart disease. J Amer Coll Cardiol 1994;24:874–880.

Cohen DJ, Kuntz RE, et. al. Predictors of long-term out-come after percutaneous balloon mitral valvulo-plasty. N Engl J Med 1992;327:1329–1334.

Dajani AS, Ayoub E, Bierman FZ, et al. Guidelines for the diagnosis of rheumatic fever: Jones criteria, up-dated 1992. Circulation 1993;87:302–307.

Durack DT. Prevention of infective endocarditis. N Engl J Med 1995;332:38–44.

Hammermeister KE, Sethi C K, et. al. A comparison of outcomes in men 11 years after heart-valve re-placement with a mechanical valve or bioprosthe-sis. N Engl J Med 1993;328:1289–1296.

Jones EL. Mitral valve replacement: indications, choice of valve prosthesis, results, and long-term morbid-ity of porcine and mechanical valves. J Card Surg 1994;9(Suppl):218–221.

Pellikka PA, Nishimura RA, Bailey KR, et al. The nat-ural history of adults with asymptomatic, hemody-namically significant AS. J Am Coll Cardiol 1990; 15:1012–1017.

Scognamiglio R, Rahimtoola SH, Fasoli G, et al. Nifedipine in asymptomatic patients with severe AR and normal left ventricular function. N Engl J Med 1994;331:689–694.

Vongpatanasin W, Hillis LD, Lange RA. Medical progress: prosthetic heart valves. N Engl J Med 1996;335:407–416.

Waller BF, Howard J, Fess S. Pathology of mitral valve stenosis and pure mitral regurgitation—Part I. Clin Cardiol 1994;17:330–336,395–402.

Wisenbaugh T. Mitral valve disease. Curr Opin Car-diol 1994;9:146–151.

Acknowledgments The previous edition of this chapter was written by Edward Chan, MD; Elia Duh, MD; Brian Stidham, MD; John A. Bittl, MD; and Leonard S. Lilly, MD.

Heart Failure

Stephen K. Frankel
and Michael A. Fifer

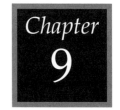

Chapter
9

The heart normally accepts blood at low filling pressures during diastole and then propels it forward at higher pressures in systole. Heart failure is defined as *the inability of the heart to pump blood forward at a sufficient rate to meet the metabolic demands of the body ("forward failure"), or the ability to do so only if the cardiac filling pressures are abnormally high ("backward failure"), or both.* Although conditions outside of the heart may cause this definition to be met through inadequate tissue perfusion (e.g., severe hemorrhage) or increased metabolic demands (e.g., hyperthyroidism), in this chapter only *cardiac* causes of heart failure are considered.

Heart failure may be the principal manifestation of nearly every form of cardiac disease, including coronary atherosclerosis, myocardial infarction, valvular diseases, hypertension, congenital heart disease, and the cardiomyopathies. More than 400,000 new cases of heart failure develop in the United States each year, and its incidence is *increasing*, in part because of the aging population, and also because of interventions that now significantly prolong survival after acute cardiac insults such as myocardial infarction.

Because heart failure most commonly results from conditions of impaired left ven-tricular function, we begin by reviewing the physiology of normal myocardial contraction and relaxation.

PHYSIOLOGY

Experimental studies of isolated cardiac muscle segments have demonstrated several important physiologic principles that can be applied to the intact heart.

As an experimental muscle segment is stretched apart, the relation between its length and the tension it passively develops is curvilinear, reflecting its intrinsic elastic properties (Fig. 9.1A, lower curve). If the muscle is first passively stretched and then stimulated to contract while its ends are held at fixed positions (an isometric contraction), the total tension (active + passive tension) generated by the fibers is proportional to the length of the muscle at the time of stimulation (Fig. 9.1A, upper curve). That is, stretching the muscle prior to stimulation optimizes the overlap of myosin and actin filaments, increasing the number of cross bridges and the force of contraction. Stretching cardiac muscle fibers also increases the sensitivity of the myofilaments to calcium, which further augments force development.

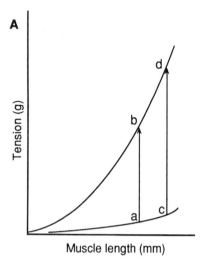

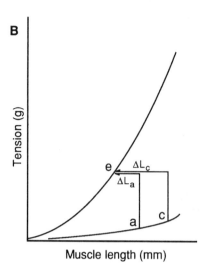

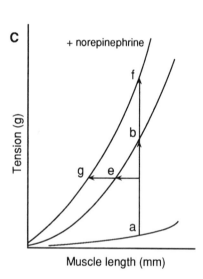

Figure 9.1. **A.** Passive (lower curve) and total (upper curve) length-tension relations for isolated cat papillary muscle. Lines ab and cd represent the force developed during isometric contractions. Initial passive muscle length c is longer (i.e., has been stretched more) than length a, and therefore has a greater passive tension. When the muscle segments are stimulated to contract, the muscle with the longer initial length generates greater total tension (point d versus point b). **B.** If the muscle fiber preparation is allowed to shorten against a fixed load, the length at the end of the contraction is dependent on the load, but not the initial fiber length: stimulation at point a or c results in the same final fiber length (e). Thus, the muscle that starts at length c shortens a greater distance (ΔL_c) than the muscle at length a (ΔL_a). **C.** The uppermost curve is the length-tension relation in the presence of the positive inotropic agent norepinephrine. For any given initial length, an isometric contraction in the presence of norepinephrine generates greater force (point f) than one in the absence of norepinephrine (point b). When contracting against a fixed load, the presence of norepinephrine causes greater muscle fiber shortening and a smaller final muscle length (point g) compared with contraction in the absence of the inotropic agent (point e). (Adapted from Downing SE, Sonnenblick EH. Cardiac muscle mechanics and ventricular performance: force and time parameters. Am J Physiol 1964;207:705–715.)

The relationship between the initial fiber length and force development is of great importance in the intact heart: Within a physiologic range, the larger the ventricular volume during diastole, the more the fibers are stretched prior to stimulation, and the greater will be the force of the next contraction. This is the basis of the Frank-Starling relationship, the observation that ventricular output increases in relation to the **preload** (the stretch on the myocardial fibers prior to contraction).

A second observation from the isolated muscle experiments arises when the fibers are not tethered at a fixed length, but are allowed to *shorten* during stimulation against a fixed load (termed the **afterload**). In this situation (an isotonic contraction), the final length of the muscle at the end of contraction is directly related to the magnitude of the load, but is *independent* of the length of the muscle prior to stimulation (Fig. 9.1B). That is, 1) the tension generated by the fiber is equal to the fixed load; 2) the greater the load opposing contraction, the less the muscle fiber can shorten; 3) if the fiber is stretched to a longer length prior to stimulation but the afterload is kept constant, the muscle shortens a greater distance and attains the same final length at the end of contraction; and 4) the maximum tension that a fiber can produce during isotonic contraction (i.e., such that the fiber is just unable to shorten) is the same as the force produced by an isometric contraction for the applied preload. The concept of afterload is relevant to the intact normal heart: The pressure generated by the ventricle and the size of the chamber at the end of each contraction depend upon the load against which the ventricle contracts (i.e., largely the arterial pressure), but are independent of the stretch on the myocardial fibers prior to contraction.

A third key experimental observation relates to myocardial **contractility** (also termed the **inotropic state**), which accounts for changes in the force of contraction independent of the initial fiber length and afterload. Contractility generally reflects chemical and hormonal influences on cardiac contraction, such as exposure to catecholamines. When contractility is enhanced pharmacologically (e.g., by a norepinephrine infusion), the relation between initial fiber length and force developed during contraction is shifted upward (Fig. 9.1C) such that a greater total tension develops with isometric contraction at any given preload. Similarly, when contractility is augmented and the cardiac muscle is allowed to shorten against a fixed afterload, the fiber will contract to a greater extent and achieve a shorter final fiber length, compared with the normal state. Enhanced contractility is likely induced by an increase in the cycling rate of actin-myosin cross-bridge formation.

Determinants of Ventricular Contractile Function and Cardiac Output

In a normal individual, the cardiac output is matched to the body's total metabolic need. Cardiac output (CO) is equal to the product of stroke volume (SV, the volume of blood ejected with each contraction) and the heart rate (HR):

$$CO = SV \times HR$$

The three major determinants of stroke volume are preload, afterload, and myocardial contractility, as shown in Figure 9.2.

Preload

The concept of preload (Table 9.1) in the intact heart was described by physiologists Frank and Starling a century ago. In experimental preparations, they showed that within physiologic limits, the more a normal ventricle is distended (i.e., filled with blood) during diastole, the greater the volume of blood ejected during the next systolic contraction. This relationship is illustrated graphically by the Frank-Starling curve, also known as the ventricular function curve (Fig. 9.3). The graph relates a measurement of cardiac performance (such as cardiac output or stroke volume) on the vertical axis as a function of preload on the horizontal axis. As described above, the preload can be thought of as the amount of myocardial stretch at the end of diastole, just prior to contraction. Measurements that correlate with myocardial stretch, and which are often used to indicate the preload on the horizontal axis, are the ventricular end-diastolic volume (EDV) or end-diastolic pressure (EDP). Conditions that decrease intravascular volume, and thereby

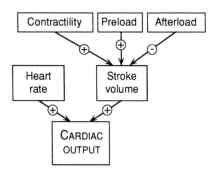

Figure 9.2. Key mediators of cardiac output. Determinants of the stroke volume include contractility, preload, and afterload. Cardiac output = Heart rate × Stroke volume.

TABLE 9.1. Terms Related to Cardiac Performance

Term	Definition
Preload	The ventricular wall tension at the end of diastole. In clinical terms, it is the stretch on the ventricular fibers just prior to contraction, often approximated by the end-diastolic volume or end-diastolic pressure.
Afterload	The ventricular wall tension during contraction; the resistance that must be overcome in order for the ventricle to eject its contents. It is often approximated by the systolic ventricular (or arterial) pressure
Contractility (Inotropic State)	Property of heart muscle that accounts for changes in the strength of contraction, independent of the preload and afterload. Often reflects chemical or hormonal influences (e.g., catecholamines) on the force of contraction.
Stroke Volume	Volume of blood ejected from the ventricle during systole. (= end-diastolic volume − end-systolic volume)
Ejection Fraction (EF)	The fraction of end-diastolic volume ejected from the ventricle during each systolic contraction. (Normal range = 55%–75%) $$EF = \frac{\text{stroke volume}}{\text{end-diastolic volume}}$$
Cardiac Output	Volume of blood ejected from the ventricle per minute (= stroke volume × heart rate)
Compliance	Intrinsic property of a chamber that describes its pressure-volume relationship during filling. Reflects the ease or difficulty with which the chamber can be filled. Strictly defined, $$\text{Compliance} = \frac{\Delta \text{ Volume}}{\Delta \text{ Pressure}}$$

reduce ventricular preload (e.g., dehydration or severe hemorrhage), result in a smaller end-diastolic volume, and hence, a reduced stroke volume during contraction. Conversely, an increased volume within the left ventricle during diastole (e.g., a large intravenous infusion) results in a greater than normal stroke volume.

Afterload

Afterload (Table 9.1) in the intact heart reflects the resistance that the ventricle must overcome in order to empty its contents. It is more formally defined as the ventricular wall stress that develops during systolic ejection. Wall stress (σ), like pressure, is expressed as force per unit area, and for the left ventricle, may be estimated from the LaPlace relation for a hollow sphere:

$$\sigma = \frac{P \cdot r}{2h}$$

in which P is ventricular pressure, r is ventricular chamber radius, and h is ventricular wall thickness. In general, a useful measurement to estimate the afterload is the ar-

terial systolic pressure (which is the same as ventricular systolic pressure in the absence of an obstruction between the ventricle and the great artery). Ventricular wall stress increases in response to a higher pressure load (e.g., hypertension) or an increased chamber size (e.g., a dilated left ventricle seen in many types of heart failure). As discussed below, an increase in wall thickness serves a compensatory role in reducing wall stress, as the force is distributed over a greater mass per unit surface area of ventricular muscle.

Contractility

In the intact heart, as in the isolated muscle preparation, contractility accounts for changes in the force generated by the myocardium for a given set of preload and afterload. By relating a measure of ventricular performance (stroke volume or cardiac output) to preload (left ventricular end-diastolic pressure or volume), each Frank-Starling curve is a reflection of the heart's current inotropic state (Fig. 9.3). The effect on stroke volume by an alteration in pre-

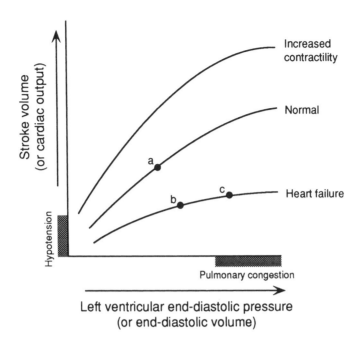

Figure 9.3. **Left ventricular (LV) performance (Frank-Starling) curves relate preload, measured as LV end-diastolic volume (EDV) or pressure (EDP), to cardiac performance, measured as ventricular stroke volume or cardiac output.** On the curve of a normal individual (middle line), cardiac performance continuously increases as a function of preload. States of increased contractility (e.g., norepinephrine infusion) are characterized by an augmented stroke volume at any level of preload (upper line). Conversely, decreased LV contractility (commonly associated with heart failure) is characterized by a curve that is shifted downward (lower line). Point a is an example of a normal individual at rest. Point b represents the same individual after developing systolic dysfunction and heart failure (e.g., after a large MI): stroke volume has fallen, and the decreased LV emptying results in elevation of the EDV. Because point b is on the ascending portion of the curve, the increased EDV serves a compensatory role because it results in an increase in subsequent stroke volume, albeit much less so than if operating on the normal curve. Further augmentation of LV filling (e.g., increased circulating volume) in the heart failure patient is represented by point c, which resides on the relatively flat part of the curve: Stroke volume is only slightly augmented, but the markedly increased EDP results in pulmonary congestion.

load is reflected by a change in position along a particular Frank-Starling curve. Conversely, a change in contractility actually shifts the entire curve in an upward or downward direction. Thus, when contractility is enhanced pharmacologically (e.g., by an infusion of norepinephrine), the ventricular performance curve is displaced upward such that at any given preload, the stroke volume is increased. Conversely, when a drug that reduces contractility (e.g., a β-blocker) is administered or the ventricle's contractile function is impaired (as in many types of heart failure), the curve shifts in a downward direction, so that at any given preload, the stroke volume and cardiac output are reduced.

Pressure-Volume Loops

Another useful graphic display to illustrate the determinants of cardiac function is the ventricular pressure-volume loop, which relates changes in ventricular volume to corresponding changes in pressure throughout the cardiac cycle (Fig. 9.4). In the left ventricle, filling of the chamber begins after the mitral valve opens in early diastole (point a). The curve between points a and b represents diastolic filling. As the volume increases during diastole, it is associated with a small rise in pressure, in accordance with the passive length tension properties or **compliance** (Table 9.1) of the myocardium, analogous to the lower curve in Fig. 9.1A for an isolated

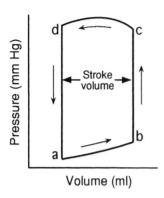

Figure 9.4. Example of a normal left ventricular (LV) pressure-volume loop. At point a the mitral valve opens. During diastolic filling of the LV (line ab), the volume increases in association with a gradual rise in pressure. When ventricular contraction commences, and its pressure exceeds that of the left atrium, the mitral valve (MV) close (point b), and isovolumetric contraction of the LV ensues (the aortic valve is not yet open, and no blood leaves the chamber), as shown by line bc. When LV pressure rises to that in the aorta, the aortic valve (AV) opens (point c) and ejection begins. The volume within the LV declines during ejection (line cd), but LV pressure continues to rise until ventricular relaxation commences. At point d, the LV pressure during relaxation falls below that in the aorta, and the AV closes, leading to isovolumetric relaxation (line da). As the LV pressure falls further, the mitral valve reopens (point a). Point b represents the end-diastolic volume (EDV) and pressure, and point d is the end-systolic volume (ESV) and pressure. Stroke volume is the difference between the EDV and ESV.

muscle preparation. Next, the onset of left ventricular systolic contraction causes the ventricular pressure to rise. When the LV pressure exceeds that of the left atrium (point b), the mitral valve closes. As the pressure increases, the ventricular volume does not change at first, because the aortic valve has not yet opened, and therefore this phase is called isovolumetric contraction. When the ventricular pressure reaches the aortic diastolic pressure, the aortic valve opens (point c), and ejection of blood into the aorta commences. During ejection, the volume within the ventricle decreases, but its pressure continues to rise until ventricular relaxation begins. The pressures against which the ventricle ejects (afterload) is represented by the curve cd. Ejection ends during ventricular relaxation, when the pressure falls below that of the aorta and the aortic valve closes (point d). As the ventricle continues to relax, its

pressure declines while its volume remains constant since the mitral valve has not yet opened (this phase is known as isovolumetric relaxation). When the ventricular pressure falls below that of the left atrium, the mitral valve opens (point a), and the cycle repeats. Note that point b represents the pressure and volume at the end of diastole, whereas point d represents the pressure and volume at the end of systole. The difference between the end-diastolic and end-systolic volumes represents the quantity of blood ejected during contraction (the stroke volume).

Changes in any of the determinants of cardiac function are reflected by alterations in the pressure-volume loop. By analyzing the effects of a change in an individual parameter (preload, afterload, or contractility) on the pressure-volume loop, the resulting alterations in ventricular pressure and stroke volume can be predicted (Fig. 9.5).

Preload

If afterload and contractility are held constant, but preload is caused to increase (e.g., by administration of intravenous fluids), left ventricular end-diastolic volume will rise. This increase in preload augments the stroke volume via the Frank-Starling mechanism such that the end-systolic volume achieved is the same as it was prior to increasing the preload. This means that the normal LV is able to adjust its stroke volume and effectively empty its contents to match its diastolic filling volume, as long as contractility and afterload are kept constant.

Note that while end-diastolic volume and end-diastolic pressure are often used interchangeably as markers for preload, the relationship between filling volume and pressure (known as ventricular compliance (Table 9.1)) largely governs the extent of ventricular filling. If ventricular compliance is reduced (e.g., in severe left ventricular hypertrophy), then the slope of the diastolic filling curve (segment ab in Figure 9.4) becomes steeper, as discussed below. A "stiff" or poorly compliant ventricle reduces the ability of the chamber to fill during diastole resulting in a lower than normal ventricular end-diastolic volume. In this circumstance, if afterload and

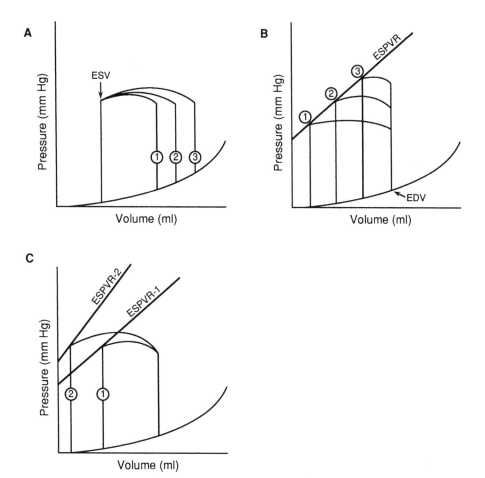

Figure 9.5.   The effect of varying preload, afterload, and contractility on the pressure-volume loop. A.
When arterial pressure (afterload) and contractility are held constant, sequential increases (lines 1, 2, 3) in preload
(measured in this case as end-diastolic volume (EDV)) are associated with loops that have progressively higher
stroke volumes but a constant end-systolic volume (ESV). **B.** When the preload (EDV) and contractility are held
constant, sequential increases (points 1, 2, 3) in arterial pressure (afterload) are associated with loops that have
progressively lower stroke volumes and higher end-systolic volumes. There is a nearly linear relationship between
the afterload and ESV, termed the end-systolic pressure-volume relation (ESPVR). **C.** A positive inotropic
intervention shifts the end-systolic pressure-volume relation upward and leftward from ESPVR-1 to ESPVR-2,
resulting in loop 2, which has a larger stroke volume, and smaller end-systolic volume than the original loop 1.

contractility remain unaltered, then the *end-systolic* volume is unchanged, and therefore the stroke volume will be reduced.

Afterload

If preload and contractility are held constant and afterload is augmented (e.g., high-impedance states such as hypertension or aortic stenosis), then the pressure generated by the LV during ejection is caused to increase. In this situation, more ventricular work is expended in overcoming the resistance to ejection, and less fiber shortening takes place. As shown in Figure 9–5B, an in-

crease in afterload results in a higher ventricular systolic pressure and a higher than normal LV end-systolic volume. Thus, in the setting of increased afterload, the ventricular stroke volume (EDV–ESV) is reduced.

The dependence of the end-systolic volume on afterload is approximately linear: The greater the afterload, the higher the end-systolic volume will be. This relationship is depicted in Figure 9.5 as the end-systolic pressure volume relation (ESPVR) and is analogous to the total tension curve in the isolated muscle experiments described above.

Contractility

The slope of the ESPVR line on the pressure-volume loop graph is a function of cardiac contractility. In conditions of increased contractility (e.g., an infusion of norepinephrine), the ESPVR slope becomes more steep; that is, it shifts upward and toward the left. Hence, at any given preload or afterload, the ventricle empties more completely (the stroke volume increases) and results in a smaller than normal end-systolic volume (Fig. 9.5C). Conversely, in situations of reduced contractility (e.g., during high-dose β-blocker therapy or in the presence of a dilated cardiomyopathy), the ESPVR line is shifted downward, consistent with a decline in stroke volume and a higher end-systolic volume. Thus, the end-systolic volume is *dependent* upon the afterload against which the ventricle contracts and the inotropic state of the ventricle, but is *independent* of the end-diastolic volume of the ventricle prior to contraction.

To summarize the important concepts of physiology presented in this section:

1. Ventricular stroke volume (SV) is a function of preload, afterload, and contractility. SV rises when there is an increase in preload, a decrease in afterload, or augmented contractility.
2. Ventricular end-diastolic volume (or end-diastolic pressure) is often used as a representation of preload. The end-diastolic volume is influenced by the chamber's compliance.
3. Ventricular end-systolic volume depends upon the afterload and contractility, but not the preload.

PATHOPHYSIOLOGY

As indicated in the introduction to this chapter, heart failure may result from any of a wide array of cardiovascular insults. The etiologies can be grouped into those that cause heart failure because of: 1) impaired contractility, 2) increased afterload, or 3) impaired ventricular filling. Heart failure that results from an abnormality of ventricular emptying (due to impaired contractility or excessive afterload) is termed *systolic dysfunction,* while that due to abnormalities of diastolic relaxation or ventricular filling is termed *diastolic dysfunction.* Approximately two-thirds of patients with heart failure have systolic dysfunction, while the remainder suffer primarily from diastolic dysfunction. Figure 9.6 presents a general schema of cardiac conditions that may result in heart failure.

Systolic Dysfunction

In systolic dysfunction, there is a diminished capacity to eject blood from the affected ventricle due to impaired myocardial contractility or pressure overload (i.e., high afterload). Loss of contractility may be the result of destruction of myocytes, impaired myocyte function, or fibrosis. Pressure overload impairs ventricular ejection by markedly increasing resistance to flow. Figure 9.7A depicts the effects of systolic dysfunction due to impaired contractility on the pressure-volume loop: The ESPVR is shifted downward such that systolic emptying ceases at a higher end-systolic volume than normal. As a result, the stroke volume falls. When normal pulmonary venous return is added to the increased end-systolic volume that has remained in the ventricle because of incomplete emptying, the diastolic chamber volume increases, resulting in a higher than normal end-diastolic volume and pressure. While the increase in preload that results induces a compensatory rise in stroke volume (via the Frank-Starling mechanism), impaired contractility and the reduced ejection fraction cause the end-systolic volume to remain elevated.

During diastole, the persistently elevated left ventricular pressure is transmitted retrograde to the left atrium (through the open mitral valve) and then to the pulmonary veins and capillaries. An elevated pulmonary capillary hydrostatic pressure, when sufficiently high (usually > 20 mmHg), results in the transudation of fluid into the pulmonary interstitium and leads to symptoms of pulmonary congestion.

Diastolic Dysfunction

Approximately one-third of patients with heart failure have normal ventricular contractile (systolic) function. Many of these individuals demonstrate abnormalities of *diastolic* function: either impaired early diastolic relaxation (an active, energy dependent process), increased stiffness of the ventricular wall (a passive property), or both. Acute myocardial ischemia is an example of a condition that transiently in-hibits energy delivery and can impair dias-tolic relaxation, whereas LV hypertrophy, fibrosis, or restrictive cardiomyopathy (see Chapter 10) cause the LV walls to become chronically stiffened. The effect of impaired diastolic function is reflected in the pres-sure-volume loop (Fig. 9.7B): In diastole, filling of the ventricle occurs at higher than normal diastolic pressures because the lower part of the loop (the diastolic filling curve) is shifted upward, due to the re-duced chamber compliance. Patients with

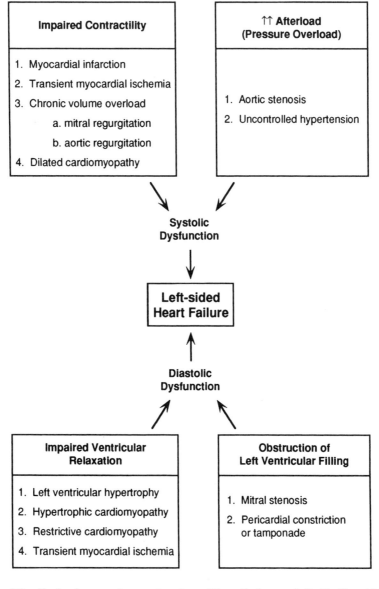

Figure 9.6.   Mechanisms and examples of conditions that cause left-sided heart failure.

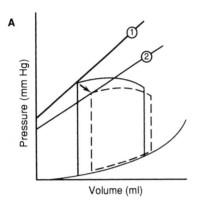
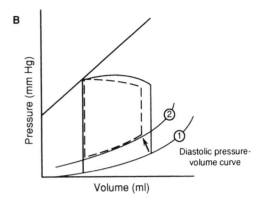

Figure 9.7. **A.** The normal pressure-volume loop (solid line) is compared with one demonstrating systolic dysfunction (dashed line). In systolic dysfunction due to decreased cardiac contractility, the end-systolic pressure-volume relation is shifted downward and rightward (from line 1 to line 2). As a result, the end-systolic volume (ESV) is increased (arrow). As normal venous return is added to the greater than normal ESV remaining in the ventricle, there is an obligatory increase in the end-diastolic volume (EDV) and pressure (preload), which serves a compensatory function by partially elevating stroke volume towards normal via the Frank-Starling mechanism. **B.** The pressure-volume loop of diastolic dysfunction due to increased stiffness (decreased compliance) of the ventricle (dashed line). The passive diastolic pressure-volume curve is shifted upward (from line 1 to line 2) such that at any diastolic volume, the ventricular pressure is greater than normal. The result is a decreased EDV (arrow) because of reduced filling of the stiffened ventricle, at a higher than normal end-diastolic pressure.

diastolic dysfunction often present with signs of vascular congestion because of the elevated diastolic pressures that are transmitted retrograde to the pulmonary and systemic veins.

Right-sided Heart Failure

While the physiologic principles developed earlier in this chapter may be applied to right-sided, as well as left-sided heart failure, distinct differences are found between right and left ventricular (LV) function. Compared with the LV, the right ventricle is a thin-walled, highly compliant chamber that accepts its blood volume at very low pressures, and ejects against a low pulmonary vascular resistance. As a result of its high compliance, the RV demonstrates little difficulty accepting a wide range of filling volumes (i.e., venous return), without marked changes in its filling pressures. Conversely, the RV is quite susceptible to failure in situations that present a sudden increase in afterload (i.e., states of increased resistance to ejection), such as acute pulmonary embolism or advanced pulmonary disease.

The most common cause of right-sided failure is actually left-sided heart failure (Table 9.2). In this situation, excessive afterload confronts the right ventricle because of the elevation of pulmonary vascular pressures due to LV dysfunction. Isolated right heart failure (i.e., in the setting of normal left ventricular function) is less common, and most often reflects increased RV afterload due to diseases of the lung parenchyma or pulmonary vasculature (e.g., pulmonary embolism). Right-sided heart disease that occurs as a result of a primary pulmonary process is known as *cor*

TABLE 9.2. Examples of Conditions that Cause Right Heart Failure

Cardiac causes
  Left-sided heart failure
  Pulmonic valve stenosis
  Right ventricular infarction
Parenchymal pulmonary disease
  Chronic obstructive pulmonary disease
  Interstitial lung disease (e.g., sarcoidosis)
  Adult respiratory distress syndrome
  Chronic lung infection or bronchiectasis
Pulmonary vascular disease
  Pulmonary embolism
  Primary pulmonary hypertension

pulmonale, and often leads to right heart failure.

When the right ventricle fails, the elevated diastolic pressure is transmitted retrograde to the right atrium with subsequent congestion of the systemic veins, accompanied by signs of right-sided heart failure (see below). Indirectly, isolated right heart failure may also influence left heart function: The decreased right ventricular output results in reduced LV filling (preload) and therefore a fall in left ventricular stroke volume and output.

COMPENSATORY MECHANISMS

Several natural compensatory mechanisms are called into action in heart failure, which serve to buffer the fall in cardiac output and help to maintain sufficient blood pressure in order to perfuse the vital organs. These include: 1) the Frank-Starling mechanism, 2) the development of myocardial hypertrophy, and 3) neurohormonal activation.

Frank-Starling Mechanism

As shown in Figure 9.3, heart failure due to impaired left ventricular contractile function results in a downward shift of the ventricular performance curve. Therefore, at a given preload, stroke volume is decreased compared with normal. The reduced stroke volume results in incomplete chamber emptying during contraction; as a result, the volume of blood accumulating in the ventricle during diastole is higher than normal (Fig. 9.3, point b). This increased stretch on the myofibers (i.e., increased preload), acting via the Frank-Starling mechanism induces a greater stroke volume on subsequent contraction, which helps to empty the enlarged LV and preserve forward cardiac output. There are limits to this beneficial compensatory mechanism, however. In the case of severe heart failure and marked depression of contractility, the curve may be flat at higher diastolic volumes, such that little augmentation of cardiac output is achieved by increased filling.

However, in such a circumstance, marked elevation of end-diastolic volume and pressure (which is transmitted retrograde to the left atrium, pulmonary veins, and capillaries) may result in pulmonary congestion and edema (Fig. 9.3, point c).

Ventricular Hypertrophy

Ventricular wall stress (σ) may be increased in heart failure, either because of LV dilatation (increased chamber radius) or the need to generate high systolic pressures to overcome excessive afterload (e.g., in heart failure due to aortic stenosis or hypertension). A sustained increase in wall stress (along with neurohormonal activation, as described below) stimulates the development of myocardial hypertrophy (i.e., an increase in ventricular mass) by the addition of myocytes and deposition of extracellular matrix. The increased mass of muscle fibers serves as a compensatory mechanism that helps to maintain contractile force and *reduces* ventricular wall stress (wall thickness is in the denominator of the wall stress formula). However, because of the increased stiffness (reduced compliance) of the hypertrophied wall, these benefits come at the expense of higher than normal diastolic ventricular pressures, which are transmitted to the left atrium and pulmonary vasculature (Fig. 9.8).

The pattern of hypertrophy that develops depends on whether the ventricle is subjected to chronic volume or pressure overload. Chronic chamber dilation owing to *volume* overload (e.g., chronic mitral or aortic regurgitation) results in the synthesis of new sarcomeres in *series* with the old. The radius of the ventricular chamber therefore enlarges, does so in proportion to the increase in wall thickness, and is termed *eccentric* hypertrophy. Chronic *pressure* overload (e.g., due to hypertension or aortic stenosis) results in the synthesis of sarcomeres in *parallel* with the old, termed *concentric* hypertrophy. In this situation, the wall thickness increases without proportional chamber dilatation, so that wall stress may be substantially reduced.

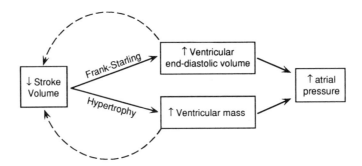

Figure 9.8. Compensatory mechanisms in heart failure. Both the Frank-Starling mechanism (which is invoked by the rise in ventricular end-diastolic volume) and myocardial hypertrophy (in response to pressure or volume overload) serve to maintain forward stroke volume (dashed lines). However, the chronic rise in EDV by the former, and increased ventricular stiffness by the latter, cause an increase in atrial pressure, which may result in manifestations of "backward" failure (e.g., pulmonary congestion in the case of left-sided heart failure).

Neurohormonal Activation

Neurohormonal stimulation is an important compensatory mechanism in heart failure that involves: 1) the adrenergic nervous system, 2) the renin-angiotensin system, and 3) increased production of antidiuretic hormone (ADH), all in response to decreased cardiac output (Fig. 9.9). In part, these mechanisms serve to increase systemic vascular resistance, thereby attenuating any fall in blood pressure, even in the setting of a reduced cardiac output. That is, since blood pressure (BP) is equal to the product of cardiac output (CO) and total peripheral resistance (TPR):

$$BP = CO \times TPR$$

a rise in TPR induced by these compensatory mechanisms can nearly balance the fall in CO, and in the early stages of heart failure maintain a fairly normal blood pressure. In addition, neurohormonal activation results in salt and water retention, which in turn increases intravascular volume and left ventricular preload, so as to maximize stroke volume via the Frank-Starling mechanism.

While the acute effects of neurohormonal stimulation are "compensatory" and beneficial, chronic activation of these mechanisms often ultimately proves deleterious to the failing heart, as discussed below.

Adrenergic Nervous System

The fall in cardiac output in heart failure is sensed as decreased perfusion pressure by baroreceptors in the carotid sinus and aortic arch. These receptors decrease their rate of firing in proportion to the fall in blood pressure, and the signal is transmitted by the 9th and 10th cranial nerves to the cardiovascular control center in medulla. As a result, sympathetic outflow to the heart and peripheral circulation is increased, and parasympathetic tone is diminished. Three immediate consequences arise (Fig. 9.9): 1) an increase in heart rate, 2) an increase in ventricular contractility, and 3) vasoconstriction due to stimulation of α-receptors on the systemic veins and arteries. The increased heart rate and ventricular contractility directly augment cardiac output. Vasoconstriction of the venous and arterial circulations is also *initially* beneficial. Venous constriction results in augmented blood return to the heart, which increases preload and raises stroke volume through the Frank-Starling mechanism, if the ventricle is operating on the ascending portion of its ventricular performance curve (Fig. 9.3). Arteriolar constriction increases the peripheral vascular resistance and therefore helps to maintain blood pressure (recall that BP = CO × TPR). The regional distribution of α-receptors is such that during sympathetic stimulation, blood flow is redistributed to

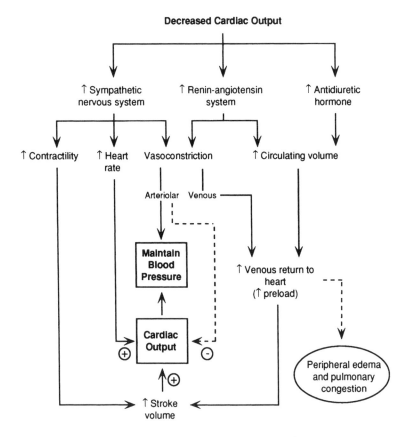

Figure 9.9.   Compensatory neurohormonal stimulation develops in response to the reduced forward cardiac output and blood pressure of heart failure. Increased activity of the sympathetic nervous system, renin-angiotensin system, and antidiuretic hormone serve to support the cardiac output and blood pressure (boxes). However, adverse consequences of these activations (dashed lines) include an increase in afterload from excessive vasoconstriction (which may impede the cardiac output) and excess fluid retention, which contributes to peripheral edema and pulmonary congestion.

vital organs (e.g., heart and brain) at the expense of the skin, splanchnic viscera, and kidneys.

The Renin-Angiotensin System

This system is also activated in patients with heart failure (Fig. 9.9). In this condition, the main stimuli for renin secretion from the juxtaglomerular cells of the kidney include: 1) decreased renal artery perfusion pressure secondary to low cardiac output, 2) decreased salt delivery to the macula densa due to alterations in intrarenal hemodynamics in heart failure, and 3) direct stimulation of juxtaglomerular β_2-receptors by the activated adrenergic nervous system.

Renin acts on circulating angiotensinogen to form angiotensin I, which is then rapidly cleaved by angiotensin converting enzyme (ACE) to form angiotensin II (AII), a potent vasoconstrictor (see Chapter 13). The increased levels of AII raise total peripheral resistance and thereby help maintain systemic blood pressure. In addition, AII acts to increase intravascular volume by two mechanisms: 1) at the hypothalamus, it stimulates thirst and therefore water intake, and 2) it acts at the adrenal cortex to increase aldosterone secretion. The latter hormone promotes sodium reabsorption from the distal convoluted tubule of the kidney into the circulation (see Chapter 17). The rise in intravascular volume increases left ventricular preload and thereby augments cardiac output via the Frank-Starling mechanism in patients on the ascending portion of the ventricular performance curve (Fig. 9.3).

Antidiuretic Hormone

Secretion of this hormone by the posterior pituitary is also increased in many patients with heart failure, presumably mediated through left atrial and arterial baroreceptors, and by increased levels of AII. ADH contributes to increased intravascular volume because it promotes water retention in the distal nephron (see Chapter 17). The increased intravascular volume serves to augment left ventricular preload and cardiac output.

Although these three neurohormonal activations are initially beneficial in heart failure, ultimately, they prove harmful. For example, the increased circulating volume and augmented venous return to the heart may worsen the engorgement of the lung vasculature, exacerbating congestive pulmonary symptoms. Furthermore, the elevated arteriolar resistance increases the afterload against which the failing left ventricle contracts, and may further impair stroke volume and reduce cardiac output (Fig. 9.9). An increased heart rate increases metabolic demand and can therefore reduce the performance of the failing heart. Finally, the continuous sympathetic nervous system activation results in the down-regulation of cardiac β-adrenergic receptors and up-regulation of inhibitory G-proteins, contributing to a decrease in the myocardium's sensitivity to circulating catecholamines and *reduced* inotropic response. Because the adverse consequences of neurohormonal activation often outweigh their benefits, much of the pharmacologic therapy of heart failure is designed to moderate these neurohormonal "compensatory" mechanisms.

Conversely, *atrial natriuretic peptide* is a counter-regulatory hormone secreted by the atria in response to increased intracardiac pressures. Its actions are largely opposite to those of the other hormone systems activated in heart failure, resulting in excretion of sodium and water, vasodilation, inhibition of renin secretion, and antagonism of the effects of AII on vasopressin and aldosterone secretion. Although plasma levels of this apparently beneficial peptide are elevated in heart failure, its effects may be blunted by end-organ, particularly renal, hyporesponsiveness.

CELLULAR DYSFUNCTION

The myocardium in heart failure is abnormal at the ultrastructural and molecular levels. Mechanical wall stress and neurohormonal activation, the same stimuli that induce myocyte hypertrophy, are believed to activate changes in the genetic expression of contractile proteins, ion channels, catalytic enzymes, surface receptors, and secondary messengers in the myocyte. Recent experimental evidence has demonstrated such changes at the subcellular level that affect intracellular calcium handling by the sarcoplasmic reticulum, decrease the responsiveness of the myofilaments to calcium, impair excitation-contraction coupling, and alter cellular energy production. It is believed that the most important cellular factors contributing to dysfunction in heart failure are: 1) a reduced cellular ability to maintain calcium homeostasis, and/or 2) changes in the production, availability, and utilization of high-energy phosphates. However, the actual subcellular alterations that result in heart failure have not yet been elucidated, and this remains one of the most active areas of cardiovascular research.

PRECIPITATING FACTORS

Many patients with chronic heart failure remain asymptomatic for extended periods either because the impairment is mild or because cardiac dysfunction is balanced by the compensatory mechanisms described above. Often the clinical manifestations of heart failure occur only in the presence of precipitating factors that increase the cardiac workload and tip the balanced state into one of decompensation. Common precipitating factors are listed in Table 9.3. Conditions of increased metabolic demand such as fever or infection may not be matched by a sufficient increase in output by the failing heart, so that symptoms of cardiac insufficiency are precipitated. Tachyarrhythmias precipitate heart failure by decreasing diastolic ventricular filling time (and hence reduce cardiac output) and by increasing myocardial oxygen demand. Excessively low heart rates (bradyarrhythmias) directly cause a drop in cardiac output (remember cardiac output = heart rate × stroke volume) and may thereby precipitate failure. An increase in salt ingestion, renal failure, or failure to take prescribed diuretics may result in an increase in circulating volume, thus promoting systemic and pulmonary venous engorgement and congestive symptoms. Uncontrolled hypertension depresses systolic contractile function because of excessive afterload confronting the LV. A large pulmonary embolism results in both hypoxemia (and therefore decreased myocardial oxygen supply) and a substantial increase in right ventricular afterload. Superimposed ischemic insults (i.e., myocardial ischemia or infarction), ethanol ingestion, or negative in-

otropic medications (e.g., β-blockers and certain calcium channel blockers), can all depress myocardial contractility and precipitate symptoms in the otherwise compensated congestive heart failure patient.

CLINICAL MANIFESTATIONS

The clinical manifestations of heart failure may include impaired forward cardiac output and/or elevated venous pressures, and relate to which of the ventricles has failed (Table 9.4). A patient may present with the chronic progressive symptoms of heart failure described here, or in certain cases with sudden decompensation of left-sided heart function, known as acute pulmonary edema (described below).

Symptoms

The most prominent symptom of chronic left ventricular failure is dyspnea (breathlessness) on exertion. Controversy regarding the cause of this symptom has centered on whether it is primarily a manifestation of pulmonary venous congestion or decreased forward cardiac output. When the pulmonary venous pressure exceeds 20 mmHg, there is transudation of fluid into the pulmonary interstitium and congestion of the lung parenchyma. The resulting reduction in pulmonary compliance contributes to an increase in the work of breathing as the patient must generate a greater negative intrathoracic pressure in order to move the same volume of air. Moreover, the excess fluid in the intersitium compresses the walls of the bronchioles and alveoli, increasing the resistance to airflow and requiring greater effort of respiration. In addition, increased interstitial lung volumes stimulate juxtacapillary receptors (J receptors) that mediate rapid shallow breathing. However, the heart failure patient can suffer from dyspnea even in the absence of pulmonary congestion, because reduced forward blood flow to the overworked respiratory muscles and accumulation of lactic acid may also contribute to that sen-

TABLE 9.3. Factors That May Precipitate Symptoms in Compensated Heart Failure

Increased metabolic demands
  Fever
  Infection
  Anemia
  Tachycardia
  Hyperthyroidism
  Pregnancy
Increased circulating volume (increased preload)
  Excessive sodium content in diet
  Excessive fluid administration
  Renal failure
Conditions that increase afterload
  Uncontrolled hypertension
  Pulmonary embolism (increased right ventricular afterload)
Conditions that impair contractility
  Negative inotropic medications (e.g., β-blockers)
  Myocardial ischemia or infarction
  Ethanol ingestion
Failure to take prescribed heart failure medications
Excessively slow heart rate

TABLE 9.4. Most Common Symptoms and Physical Findings in Heart Failure

Symptoms	Physical Findings
Left-sided	
Dyspnea	Diaphoresis (sweating)
Orthopnea	Tachycardia, tachypnea
Paroxysmal nocturnal dyspnea	Pulmonary rales
Fatigue	Loud P_2
	S_3 gallop ($\pm$ S_4)
Right-sided	
Peripheral edema	Jugular venous distention
Right upper quadrant discomfort	Hepatomegaly
(due to hepatic enlargement)	Peripheral edema

sation. Heart failure may initially cause dyspnea only on exertion, but more severe dysfunction results in symptoms at rest, as well.

Other manifestations of low forward output in heart failure may include a dulled mental status because of a fall in cerebral perfusion and reduced urine output during the day because of decreased renal perfusion. The latter often gives way to increased urinary frequency at night (nocturia) when, while supine, blood flow is redistributed to the kidney, promoting renal perfusion and diuresis. Reduced skeletal muscle perfusion may result in fatigue and weakness.

Other congestive manifestations of heart failure include orthopnea, paroxysmal nocturnal dyspnea (PND), and nocturnal cough. Orthopnea is the sensation of labored breathing while lying flat, and is relieved by sitting upright. It results from the redistribution of intravascular blood from the gravity-dependent portions of the body (abdomen and lower extremities) toward the lungs after lying down. The degree of orthopnea is generally assessed by the number of pillows on which the patient sleeps to avoid breathlessness. Sometimes, orthopnea is so marked that the patient may try to sleep upright in a chair.

PND is severe breathlessness that awakens the patient from sleep 2 to 3 hours after retiring to bed. This frightening symptom results from the gradual reabsorption into the circulation of lower extremity interstitial edema after lying down, with subsequent expansion of intravascular volume and increased venous return to the heart and lungs. A nocturnal cough is another symptom of pulmonary congestion and is produced by a similar mechanism as orthopnea. Hemoptysis (coughing bright red blood) may result from rupture of engorged bronchial veins.

In right-sided heart failure, the elevated systemic venous pressures can result in right upper quadrant abdominal discomfort because the liver becomes engorged, and its capsule is stretched. Similarly, anorexia (decreased appetite) and nausea may result from edema within the GI tract. Peripheral edema, especially in the ankles and feet, also reflects increased hydrostatic venous pressures. Because of the effects of gravity, it tends to worsen while the patient is upright during the day and is often improved by the morning after lying supine at night. Even before peripheral edema develops, the patient may note an unexpected weight gain due to the accumulation of interstitial fluid.

The symptoms of heart failure are often graded according to the New York Heart Association classification (Table 9.5).

Physical Signs

The physical signs of heart failure depend on the severity and chronicity of the condition, and can be divided into those due to left or right cardiac dysfunction (Table 9.4). Those individuals with only mild impairment may appear well. In general, however, the patient with chronic, severe heart failure may demonstrate ca-

TABLE 9.5. New York Heart Association Classification of Heart Failure

Class I:	No limitation of physical activity
Class II:	Slight limitation of activity. Dyspnea and fatigue with moderate physical activity (e.g., walking up stairs quickly)
Class III:	Marked limitation of activity. Dyspnea with minimal activity (e.g., slowly walking up stairs).
Class IV:	Severe limitation of activity. Symptoms are present even at rest.

chexia (a frail, wasted appearance) due in part to poor appetite and to the increased metabolic demands of the increased effort of breathing. In decompensated left-sided heart failure, the patient may appear dusky (decreased cardiac output) and diaphoretic (sweating due to increased sympathetic nervous activity), and the extremities are cool because of peripheral arterial vasoconstriction. Tachypnea (rapid breathing) is common. The pattern of Cheyne-Stokes respiration may also be present in advanced heart failure, characterized by periods of hyperventilation separated by intervals of apnea (absent breathing). This pattern is related to the prolonged circulation time between the lungs and respiratory center of the brain in heart failure that interferes with the feedback mechanism of systemic oxygenation. Sinus tachycardia (due to increased sympathetic nervous system activity) is also common. Pulsus alternans (alternating strong and weak contractions detected in the peripheral pulse) may be present as a sign of advanced ventricular dysfunction.

In left-sided heart failure, the ausculatory finding of pulmonary rales is created by the "popping open" of small airways that had been closed off by edema fluid prior to inspiration. This finding is initially apparent at the lung bases, where hydrostatic forces are greatest, but more severe pulmonary congestion is associated with additional rales higher in the lung fields. Compression of conduction airways by pulmonary congestion may also produce coarse rhonchi and wheezing; the latter finding is termed "cardiac asthma."

Depending on the cause of heart failure, palpation of the heart may show that the left ventricular impulse is not focal, but diffuse (in dilated cardiomyopathy), sustained (in pressure overload states such as aortic stenosis or hypertension), or lifting in quality (in volume overload states such as mitral regurgitation). Because elevated left heart filling pressures result in an increase in pulmonary vascular pressures, the pulmonic component of the second heart sound is often loud, as the pulmonic valve is forcefully closed. An early diastolic sound (S_3) is frequently heard in adults with heart failure, and is due to abnormal filling of the dilated chamber (see Chapter 2). A late diastolic sound (S_4) results from forceful atrial contraction into a stiffened ventricle and is common in states of decreased left ventricular compliance (diastolic dysfunction). The murmur of mitral regurgitation is sometimes auscultated in left-sided heart failure if the valve annulus is stretched and the papillary muscles are spread widely apart from one another because of left ventricular dilatation, thus preventing full closure of the mitral leaflets in systole.

In the presence of right-sided heart failure, additional physical findings are present. Cardiac examination may reveal a palpable parasternal right ventricular "heave," representing right ventricular enlargement, or a right-sided S_3 or S_4 gallop. The murmur of tricuspid regurgitation may be auscultated, and is due to right ventricular enlargement, analogous to the mitral regurgitation that develops from left ventricular dilatation. The elevated systemic venous pressure produced by right heart failure is manifested by distention of the jugular veins, as well as hepatic enlargement with abdominal right upper quadrant tenderness. Edema accumulates in the dependent portions of the body, beginning in the ankles and feet of ambulatory patients, and in the presacral regions of bedridden individuals.

Pleural effusions may develop in either left- or right-sided heart failure, because the pleural veins drain into both the systemic and pulmonary venous beds. The presence of pleural effusions is suggested on physical examination by dullness to percussion over the posterior lung bases.

Laboratory Tests

Normally the mean left atrial (LA) pressure is ≤ 10 mmHg. When the left atrial pressure exceeds approximately 15 mmHg, the chest radiograph shows upper zone vascular redistribution, such that the vessels supplying the upper lung lobes are larger than those supplying the lower lobes (see Fig. 3.5). This is explained as follows: When a patient is in the upright position, blood flow is normally greater to the lung bases than to the apices because of the effect of gravity. Redistribution of flow occurs when interstitial and perivascular edema develop, because such edema is most prominent at the lung bases, where the hydrostatic pressure is the highest, and compresses the blood vessels in that region, whereas flow into the upper lung zones is less affected. When the LA pressure surpasses 20 mmHg, interstitial edema is usually manifested as indistinctness of the vessels and the presence of Kerley B lines (short linear markings at the periphery of the lower lung fields) indicative of interlobular edema. If the LA pressure exceeds 25 to 30 mmHg, alveolar pulmonary edema may develop, with opacification of the air spaces. The relationship between LA pressure and the chest radiograph findings is modified in patients with chronic heart failure because of enhanced lymphatic drainage, such that higher pressures can be accommodated with fewer radiologic signs.

Depending on the cause of heart failure, the chest radiograph may show cardiomegaly, defined as a cardiothoracic ratio of greater than 0.5 on the posteroanterior film (see Chapter 3). A high right atrial pressure also causes enlargement of the azygous vein, a finding visualized by chest radiography. Pleural effusions may be present in either right- or left-sided heart failure, but are most common when bilateral failure is present.

The cause of heart failure in an individual is often evident from the history, such as a patient who has sustained a large myocardial infarction, or by physical examination, as in an individual with the murmur of mitral stenosis. In other cases, the cause is not clear on the basis of clinical evaluation. In most cases, the critical step in the differential diagnosis of heart failure is to determine whether systolic ventricular function is normal or depressed (Fig. 9.6). Ventricular function can be assessed by a number of noninvasive tests, including echocardiography and radionuclide ventriculography (these techniques are described in Chapter 3). In a minority of cases, cardiac catheterization is necessary to determine the cause of heart failure, including valvular and ischemic etiologies.

PROGNOSIS

The prognosis of heart failure is dismal in the absence of a correctable underlying cause: Only 50% of patients remain alive 5 years after the diagnosis of heart failure is made. Patients with severe symptoms (i.e., New York Heart Association Class III or IV) fare the least well, having a 1-year survival rate of only 40%. The greatest mortality is due to refractory heart failure, but a large number of patients die suddenly, presumably because of ventricular arrhythmias. Recent studies have demonstrated that survival may be prolonged in heart failure patients by including certain vasodilator drugs in their treatment regimens, as discussed below.

TREATMENT

The treatment of chronic congestive heart failure depends on the etiology of the disorder. Here we concentrate on the treatment of systolic left ventricular dysfunction, the most common cause. There are four main goals of therapy:

1. Identification and correction of the underlying condition causing heart failure. In some individuals, this may require surgical repair or replacement of dys-

functional cardiac valves, coronary artery bypass graft surgery, aggressive treatment of severe hypertension, or cessation of alcohol consumption.

2. Elimination of the acute precipitating cause of symptoms in patients with heart failure who were previously in a compensated state. This may include, for example, treatment of acute infections or arrhythmias.

3. Treatment of the acute symptoms of congestive heart failure:

   a) Treatment of pulmonary and systemic vascular congestion. This is most readily accomplished by means of dietary sodium restriction and pharmacologic therapy. The most direct means of ridding excess sodium and water from the circulation is by the use of diuretics. In addition, inotropic drugs and certain vasodilators are used to reduce vascular congestion by augmenting forward cardiac output, thereby increasing renal perfusion and effecting diuresis (see below).

   b) Increase forward cardiac output and perfusion of vital organs. The agents most useful in this regard include inotropic drugs, which increase the force of myocardial contraction, and vasodilators, through the mechanisms described below.

4. Improvement in long-term survival. There is now convincing evidence that longevity is enhanced by certain vasodilator drug regimens, as described below.

Diuretics

The mechanism of action and pharmacology of diuretic drugs are summarized in Chapter 17. By promoting the elimination of sodium and water via the kidney, diuretics reduce intravascular volume and thus venous return to the heart. Therefore, the preload of the left ventricle is decreased, and its diastolic pressure falls out of the range that promotes pulmonary congestion (Fig. 9.10, point b). The judicious use of di-

uretics does not significantly reduce cardiac output in the congestive heart failure patient, because the heart is operating on the "flat" portion of a depressed Frank-Starling curve. The intent is to reduce the end-diastolic pressure (and therefore hydrostatic forces contributing to pulmonary congestion) without a significant fall in stroke volume. However, overly vigorous diuresis *can* lower the left ventricular filling pressures into the steep portion of the ventricular performance curve, resulting in an undesired fall in cardiac output (Fig. 9.10, point b'). Thus, diuretics are used only if there is evidence of pulmonary congestion (rales) or peripheral interstitial fluid accumulation (peripheral edema).

Diuretics that act primarily at the renal loop of Henle are the most potent in congestive heart failure (furosemide, bumetanide, ethacrynic acid). Thiazides are also useful, but are less potent in the setting of decreased renal perfusion, which is often present in this condition. The general side effects of diuretics are described in Chapter 17. The most important adverse side effects with respect to heart failure include overdiuresis resulting in a fall in cardiac output, and electrolyte disturbances, particularly hypokalemia and hypomagnesemia, which may contribute to dangerous arrhythmias. When diuretics are used in patients with pure diastolic left ventricular dysfunction to relieve congestive symptoms, one must be especially careful to avoid overdiuresis, as these patients *require* elevated diastolic filling pressures in order to adequately fill their stiffened left ventricles (Fig. 9.7B). One must therefore often accept some degree of elevated filling pressures in patients with diastolic ventricular dysfunction.

Inotropic Drugs

The inotropic drugs include digitalis glycosides, β-adrenergic agonists, and phosphodiesterase inhibitors, which are described in Chapter 17. By increasing the availability of intracellular calcium, each of these groups of drugs increases the force of ventricular contraction and therefore shifts

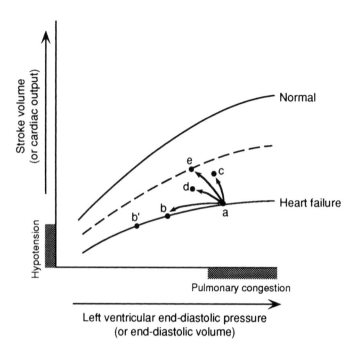

Figure 9.10. Examples of the effect of heart failure treatment on the left ventricular (LV) Frank-Starling curve. Point a represents the failing heart on a curve that is shifted downward compared with normal: The stroke volume is reduced (bordering on hypotension), and the end-diastolic pressure (LVEDP) is increased, resulting in symptoms of pulmonary congestion. Therapy with a diuretic or pure venous vasodilator (point b on the same Frank-Starling curve) reduces LV pressure without much change in stroke volume (SV). However, excessive diuresis or venous vasodilatation may result in an undesired fall in SV with hypotension (point b'). Inotropic drug therapy (point c) and arteriolar (or "balanced") vasodilator therapy (point d) augment SV, and because of improved LV emptying during contraction, the LVEDP becomes less. Point e represents the potential added benefit of combining an inotrope and vasodilator together. The dashed line shows one example of how the Frank-Starling curve shifts upward during inotropic/vasodilator therapy, but does not achieve the level of a normal ventricle.

the Frank-Starling curve in an upward direction (Fig. 9.10). As a result, stroke volume and cardiac output are augmented at any given ventricular end-diastolic volume (preload). Therefore, these agents are useful in the treatment of systolic ventricular dysfunction, but not in patients with pure diastolic failure.

The β-*adrenergic agonists*, especially dobutamine and dopamine, are administered intravenously for temporary hemodynamic support in acutely ill, hospitalized patients. Their long-term use is limited by the lack of an oral form of administration, and by the rapid development of drug tolerance. The latter refers to the progressive decline in effectiveness during continued administration of the drug, possibly due to downregulation of myocardial adrenergic receptors. The role of *phosphodiesterase inhibitors*,

much like that of the β-adrenergic agonists, is limited to the treatment of congestive heart failure in acutely ill patients via intravenous administration. Despite the initial promise of effective oral phosphodiesterase inhibitors, studies thus far have not demonstrated improved survival among patients so treated.

A commonly used form of inotropic therapy is *digitalis* (discussed in Chapter 17), which can be administered intravenously or orally. Digitalis preparations enhance contractility, reduce cardiac enlargement, improve symptoms, and augment cardiac output in patients with heart failure. Digitalis also increases the sensitivity of the baroreceptors, so that the compensatory sympathetic drive in heart failure is blunted, a desired effect that reduces left ventricular afterload. Digitalis has an added benefit in patients with congestive heart failure and concurrent atrial fibrillation in that it helps control the rate of ventricular contractions in such patients. Although digitalis can improve symptomatology in heart failure patients, this therapy does not improve long-term survival. Digitalis is not useful in the treatment of diastolic left ventricular dysfunction, because it does not improve the relaxation properties of the ventricle.

β-Blockers

Historically, β-blockers have been relatively contraindicated in patients with systolic dysfunction, as their negative inotropic effect would be expected to worsen symptomatology. However, recent studies have shown that in some patients with dilated cardiomyopathy, β-blocker therapy can paradoxically *improve* cardiac output and reduce hemodynamic deterioration. The explanation for this observation remains unclear, but may relate to the reduction in heart rate, the blunting of chronic sympathetic activation, or the anti-ischemic properties of β-blocker therapy. The use of β-blockers in the treatment of heart failure remains largely investigational at this time.

Vasodilators

The most important group of drugs to be introduced for the treatment of congestive heart failure are the vasodilators, particularly, the class of vasodilators known as angiotensin converting enzyme (ACE) inhibitors. As described above, neurohormonal compensatory mechanisms in heart failure often lead to harmful excessive vasoconstriction and volume retention. Vasodilator drugs help to reverse these adverse consequences. In addition, multiple studies have shown that certain vasodilator regimens significantly extend survival in patients with heart failure. The pharmacology of these drugs is described in Chapter 17.

Venous vasodilators (e.g., nitrates) in-

crease venous capacitance, decrease venous return to the heart, and therefore, reduce left ventricular preload. As a result, left ventricular diastolic pressures fall. This is reflected as a decline in the pulmonary capillary hydrostatic pressure, similar to the hemodynamic effects of diuretic therapy. As a result, pulmonary congestion improves, and as long as the heart failure patient is on the relatively "flat" part of the depressed Frank-Starling curve (Fig. 9.10), the cardiac output does not fall despite the reduction in ventricular filling pressure. However, venous vasodilatation in a patient who is operating on the steeper part of the curve may result in an undesired fall in stroke volume, cardiac output, and blood pressure, with reduced perfusion of the peripheral tissues.

Pure *arteriolar vasodilators* (e.g., hydralazine) reduce systemic vascular resistance, and therefore LV afterload, which in turn permits increased ventricular muscle fiber shortening during systole (Fig. 9.5B). This results in an augmented stroke volume and is represented on the Frank-Starling diagram as a shift in an upward and leftward direction (Fig. 9.10). While one might conclude that an arterial vasodilator would necessarily reduce blood pressure, an undesired effect in patients with heart failure who may already be hypotensive, this generally does not occur. As resistance is reduced by arteriolar vasodilatation, a concurrent *rise* in cardiac output usually occurs, such that blood pressure remains constant or decreases only mildly.

Some groups of drugs result in vasodilatation of both the venous and arteriolar circuits ("balanced" vasodilators). Of these, the most important are the *angiotensin converting enzyme inhibitors* (*ACEI*). These function as vasodilators by inhibiting the formation of the vasoconstrictor AII, the production of which is otherwise stimulated in heart failure. In addition, because aldosterone levels fall in response to ACEI therapy, sodium elimination is facilitated, resulting in a reduction of intravascular volume, and therefore, improvement of systemic and pulmonary vascular congestion. Additionally, ACEI have been proved to be beneficial following acute myocardial infarction (see Chapter 7), especially in individuals with reduced systolic contractile function.

In addition to ACE inhibitors' beneficial hemodynamic effects, recent large clinical trials have convincingly shown that ACEI therapy extends survival in patients with chronic heart failure. As a result, ACE inhibitors are now the standard first-line chronic therapy for patients with LV systolic dysfunction. Chronic therapy using the combination of the venous dilator isosorbide dinitrate and the arteriolar dilator hydralazine has also been shown to improve survival in patients with moderate symptoms of heart failure. However, when administration of the ACE inhibitor enalapril was compared with the hydralazine-isorbide dinitrate (H-ISDN) combination, the ACE inhibitor was shown to produce the greater improvement in survival. The H-ISDN is generally substituted only if a patient cannot tolerate ACEI therapy.

In summary, routine therapy of congestive heart failure associated with left ventricular systolic dysfunction may include vasodilators (especially ACEI), diuretics, and the digitalis glycosides. The general sequence of initiation of therapy is to start with an ACEI and to add a diuretic if pulmonary or systemic congestive symptoms are present. If a patient is unable to tolerate the ACEI, then hydralazine plus isosorbide dinitrate may be substituted. If symptoms persist or forward output remains inadequate on this regimen, then digitalis is added.

Other therapies commonly administered to patients with systolic dysfunction include: 1) anticoagulation to prevent thromboembolism in patients with markedly impaired left ventricular systolic function (a controversional therapy, as clear benefit has not yet been demonstrated by clinical trials), and 2) treatment of atrial and ventricular arrhythmias that frequently accompany chronic heart failure (see Chapter 12). Patients with severe left ventricular dysfunction that is refractory to maximal medical management may be candidates for cardiac transplantation.

Treatment of Diastolic Dysfunction

Correctable causes of impaired diastolic function should be considered and addressed. For example, pericardiectomy would be undertaken for constrictive pericarditis (see Chapter 14), or therapy would be directed at coronary artery disease if transient ischemia is the mechanism of diastolic dysfunction. There is no role for inotropic drugs in the treatment of pure diastolic dysfunction. Diuretics may reduce pulmonary congestion and peripheral edema, but must be used cautiously to avoid decreased cardiac output or hypotension, as the stiffened left ventricle relies on higher filling pressures than normal in order to maintain its output. Calcium channel blockers are occasionally beneficial in diastolic dysfunction due to hypertension or hypertrophic cardiomyopathy (see Chapter 10), but have not been shown to be helpful in diastolic dysfunction caused by other disorders.

ACUTE PULMONARY EDEMA

A severe, acute form of left-sided heart failure is cardiogenic pulmonary edema, in which elevated capillary hydrostatic pressure causes rapid accumulation of fluid within the interstitium and alveolar spaces of the lung. This condition is frequently accompanied by hypoxemia because of shunting of pulmonary blood flow through regions of hypoventilated alveoli. Pulmonary edema may appear suddenly in a previously asymptomatic individual in, for example, the setting of an acute myocardial infarction, or in patients with chronic compensated congestive heart failure following a precipitating event (Table 9.3). Pulmonary edema is a horrifying experience for the patient, resulting in severe dyspnea and marked anxiety while struggling to breathe.

On examination, the patient is tachycardic and demonstrates cold, clammy skin due to peripheral vasoconstriction in response to the increased sympathetic outflow. Tachypnea and coughing of "frothy" sputum represent transudation of fluid into the alveoli. Rales are present initially at the bases and then throughout the lung fields, sometimes accompanied by wheezing because of edema fluid within the conductance airways.

In the presence of normal plasma oncotic pressure, pulmonary edema generally develops when the pulmonary capillary wedge pressure, which reflects LV diastolic pressure, exceeds 25 mmHg (or greater than 30 mmHg in those with a chronically elevated PCW).

Pulmonary edema is a life-threatening emergency that requires immediate improvement of systemic oxygenation and elimination of the underlying cause. The patient should be seated upright to permit pooling of blood within the systemic veins of the lower body, so as to reduce venous return to the heart. Supplemental oxygen is provided by face mask. Morphine sulphate is administered intravenously to reduce anxiety and as a venous dilator to facilitate pooling of blood peripherally. A rapidly acting diuretic, such as intravenous furosemide, is administered in an attempt to further reduce left ventricular preload and pulmonary capillary hydrostatic pressure. Other means of reducing preload include administration of nitrates (often intravenously), or in extreme cases, venous phlebotomy. Inotropic drugs can also be administered intravenously to augment forward cardiac output. During resolution of the pulmonary congestion and hypoxemia, attention is directed at identifying and treating the underlying cause.

SUMMARY

1. Heart failure is present when cardiac output fails to meet the metabolic demands of the body, or meets those demands only if the cardiac filling pressures are abnormally high. Heart failure most often results from impaired left ventricular systolic function, but may also arise from ventricular diastolic dysfunction and other cardiac abnormalities that interfere with ventricular filling or emptying.

2. Compensatory mechanisms in heart failure that help maintain cardiac output and blood pressure include: 1) augmented stroke volume via the Frank-Starling mechanism, 2) ventricular hypertrophy, and 3) activation of neurohormonal systems.

3. Symptoms of heart failure may be exacerbated by precipitating factors that increase metabolic demand, increase circulating volume, increase afterload, or decrease contractility (summarized in Table 9.3).

4. Successful treatment of heart failure requires identification of the underlying cause of the condition and elimination of precipitating factors. Medical treatment of heart failure includes the judicious application of vasodilators (particularly ACE inhibitors), diuretics, and inotropic drugs.

ADDITIONAL READING

Braunwald E, Ross J Jr, Sonnenblick EH. Mechanisms of Contraction of the Normal and Failing Heart. 2nd ed. Boston: Little, Brown & Co., 1976.

Colucci WS, Braunwald E. Pathophysiology of heart failure. In: Braunwald E, ed. Heart Disease: A Textbook of Cardiovascular Medicine. 5th ed. Philadelphia: WB Saunders, 1997:394–420.

Cohn JN. The management of chronic heart failure. N Engl J Med 1996;335:490–498.

The CONSENSUS Trial Study Group. Effects of enalapril on mortality in severe congestive heart failure: Results of the cooperative north scandinavian enalapril survival study (CONSENSUS). N Engl J Med 1987;316:1429–1435.

Dzau VJ. Autocrine and paracrine mechanisms in the pathophysiology of heart failure. Am J Cardiol 1992;70:4C–11C.

Figueredo VM, Camacho SA. Basic mechanisms of myocardial dysfunction: cellular pathophysiology of heart failure. Curr Opin Cardiol 1994;9:272–279.

Gaasch WH. Diagnosis and treatment of heart failure based on left ventricular systolic or diastolic dysfunction. JAMA 1994;271:1276–1280.

Garg R, Yusef S. Overview of randomized trials of angiotensin-converting enzyme inhibitors on mortality and morbidity in patients with heart failure. JAMA 1995;273:1450–1456.

Gottlieb SS. β-Blockers for heart failure: where are we now? Curr Opin Cardiol 1994;9:295–300.

Katz AM. Physiology of the Heart. 2nd ed. New York: Raven Press, 1992.

Kelly RA, Smith TW. Pharmacologic treatment of heart failure. In: Goodman and Gilman's Pharmacological Basis of Therapeutics. 9th ed. New York: McGraw Hill, 1996:809–838.

Lenihan DJ, Gerson MC, Hoit BD, et al. Mechanisms,

diagnosis and treatment of diastolic heart failure. Am. Heart J 1995;130:153–166.

Pfeffer MA, Braunwald E, et. al. Effect of captopril on mortality and morbidity in patients with left ventricular dysfunction after myocardial infarction: results of the survival and ventricular enlargement trial. N Engl J Med 1992;327:678–684.

The SOLVD Investigators. Effect of enalapril on survival in patients with reduced left ventricular ejection fraction and congestive heart failure. N Engl J Med 1991;325:293–302.

The SOLVD Investigators. Effect of enalapril on mortality and the development of heart failure in asymptomatic patients with reduced left ventricular ejection fractions. N Engl J Med 1992;327:685–691.

Williams JF, Bristow MR, Fowler MB, et al. Guidelines for the evaluation and management of heart failure: Report of the American College of Cardiology/American Heart Association Task Force on Practice Guidelines. Circulation 1995;92:2764–2784.

Acknowledgments   The previous edition of this chapter was written by Arthur Coday, Jr., MD, Vikram Janakiraman, MD, and Michael A. Fifer, MD.

The Cardiomyopathies

David Grayzel, G. William Dec, and Leonard S. Lilly

The cardiomyopathies are a group of heart disorders in which the major structural abnormality is limited to the myocardium. These conditions often result in symptoms of heart failure, and while the underlying cause of myocardial dysfunction can sometimes be identified, the etiology frequently remains unknown. Excluded from the definition of this group of diseases is heart muscle impairment due to other known cardiac conditions, such as hypertension, valvular, or coronary artery disease.

Cardiomyopathies can be classified into three types by the anatomic appearance and abnormal physiology of the left ventricle (Fig. 10.1). **Dilated** cardiomyopathy is characterized by ventricular enlargement with impaired *systolic* contractile function; **hypertrophic** cardiomyopathy by an abnormally thickened ventricle with abnormal *diastolic* relaxation; and **restrictive** cardiomyopathy by an abnormally stiffened myocardium (because of fibrosis or an infiltrative process) such that diastolic relaxation is impaired, but systolic contractile function is usually preserved.

DILATED CARDIOMYOPATHY (DCM)

Etiology

Cardiac enlargement in DCM is due to ventricular dilatation, with only minor hypertrophy. Myocyte damage leading to this condition results from a wide spectrum of toxic, metabolic, and infectious causes (Table 10.1). Although the majority of cases are "idiopathic," in that the cause is undetermined, examples of conditions that *are* commonly recognized causes of DCM are viral myocarditis and alcohol toxicity. A familial form of DCM has also been identified.

Acute viral myocarditis generally afflicts young, previously healthy individuals, and is most often the result of Coxsackie group B or echovirus infection. It is usually a self-limited condition with full recovery, but for unclear reasons, some patients progress to DCM. It is hypothesized that myocardial destruction and fibrosis result from immune-mediated injury triggered by viral constituents. Nonetheless, immunosuppressive drugs have not been shown to improve the prognosis of this condition. Transvenous right ventricular biopsy during acute myocarditis may demonstrate active inflammation, and Coxsackie B RNA sequences have been demonstrated in some infected individuals.

Alcoholic cardiomyopathy develops in a small number of individuals who imbibe alcoholic beverages chronically. Although the pathophysiology is unknown, ethanol is thought to impair cellular function by inhibiting mitochondrial oxidative phosphorylation and fatty acid oxidation. Its clinical presentation and histologic features are similar to other dilated cardiomyopathies,

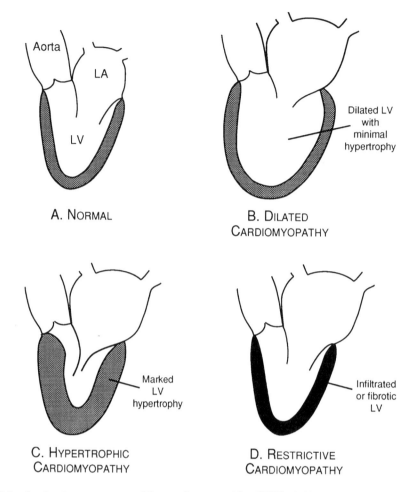

Figure 10.1. Anatomic appearance of the cardiomyopathies (CMP). A. Normal heart demonstrating left ventricle (LV) and left atrium (LA). **B.** Dilated CMP is characterized by ventricular dilatation with only mild hypertrophy. **C.** Hypertrophic CMP demonstrates marked ventricular hypertrophy, often predominantly involving the intraventricular septum. **D.** Restrictive CMP is due to infiltration or fibrosis of the ventricles, usually without enlargement of the cavities. Note that LA enlargement is common to all three types of CMP.

but it is important to identify because it is one of the few potentially *reversible* causes, in that cessation of alcohol consumption can result in dramatic improvement of ventricular function.

Pathology

Marked enlargement of all four cardiac chambers is typical of DCM (Fig. 10.2), although sometimes the disease is limited to only the left or right side of the heart. The thickness of the ventricular walls may be increased, but chamber dilatation is out of proportion to any hypertrophy. Microscopically, there is evidence of myocyte degeneration with irregular hypertrophy and atrophy

of myofibers. Interstitial and perivascular fibrosis is often extensive.

Pathophysiology

The hallmark of dilated cardiomyopathy is ventricular dilatation with decreased contractile function (Fig. 10.3). Most often in DCM, both ventricles are impaired, but sometimes dysfunction is limited to the LV, and even less commonly to the RV.

As ventricular stroke volume and cardiac output decline because of impaired myocyte contractility, two compensatory effects are called into action: 1) the Frank-Starling mechanism, in which the elevated ventricular diastolic volume increases the

TABLE 10.1. Examples of Dilated Cardiomyopathies

Idiopathic
Inflammatory
  Infectious (especially viral)
  Noninfectious
    Connective tissue diseases
    Peripartum cardiomyopathy
    Sarcoidosis
Toxic
  Chronic alcohol ingestion
  Chemotherapeutic agents (e.g., adriamycin)
Metabolic
  Hypothyroidism
  Chronic hypocalcemia or hypophosphatemia
Neuromuscular
  Muscular or myotonic dystrophy

stretch of the myofibers, thereby increasing their subsequent stroke work, and 2) neurohormonal activation, initially mediated by activation of the sympathetic nervous system (see Chapter 9). The latter contributes to an increase in heart rate and contractility, which help to buffer the fall in cardiac output. These compensations may render the patient asymptomatic during the early stages of ventricular dysfunction, but as progressive myocyte degeneration and volume overload ensue, clinical symptoms of heart failure develop.

With persistent reduction of cardiac output, the decline in renal blood flow prompts the kidneys to elaborate increased amounts of renin. This activation of the renin-angiotensin system results in an increase in peripheral vascular resistance (mediated through angiotensin II) and intravascular volume (because of increased aldosterone). As described in Chapter 9, these effects are also initially helpful in buffering the fall in cardiac output.

Ultimately however, the "compensatory" effects of neurohormonal activation prove detrimental. Arteriolar vasoconstriction and increased systemic resistance render it more difficult for the LV to eject blood in the forward direction, and the rise in intravascular volume further burdens the ventricles, resulting in pulmonary and systemic congestion.

Furthermore, as the cardiomyopathic process causes the ventricles to enlarge over time, the mitral and tricuspid valves fail to coapt properly in systole, and valvular regurgitation ensues. Such regurgitation has two detrimental consequences: 1) volume and pressure loads are placed on the atria, causing them to dilate, often leading to atrial fibrillation, and 2) regurgitation of blood into the left atrium further decreases forward stroke volume into the aorta and systemic circulation.

Clinical Findings

The clinical manifestations of DCM are typically those of congestive heart failure. The most common symptoms of low forward cardiac output include fatigue, lightheadedness, and exertional dyspnea, asso-

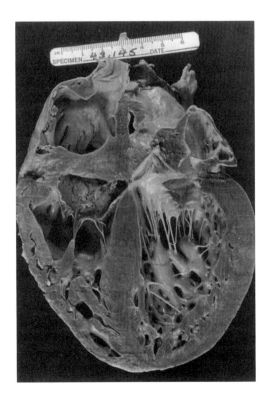

Figure 10.2. Postmortem heart specimen from a patient who died with dilated cardiomyopathy. The ventricles are dilated without proportional increase in wall thickness.

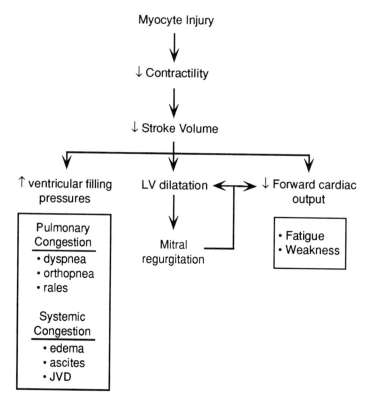

Figure 10.3. Pathophysiology of dilated cardiomyopathy. The reduced ventricular stroke volume results in decreased forward cardiac output and increased ventricular filling pressures. The listed clinical manifestations follow. JVD, jugular venous distension.

ciated with decreased tissue perfusion. Pulmonary congestion results in dyspnea, orthopnea, paroxysmal nocturnal dyspnea, whereas systemic venous congestion is responsible for peripheral edema. Because these symptoms may develop insidiously, the patient may complain only of recent weight gain (because of interstitial edema) and shortness of breath upon exertion.

Physical Examination

Signs of decreased cardiac output are often present and include cool extremities (due to peripheral vasoconstriction), low arterial pressure, and tachycardia. Pulmonary venous congestion is responsible for pulmonary rales, and basilar chest dullness may be present because of pleural effusions. Cardiac examination shows an enlarged heart with leftward displacement of the dif-

fuse, poorly contractile chamber. On auscultation, an S_3 is common as a sign of poor systolic function. The murmur of mitral valve regurgitation is common, in association with marked left ventricular dilatation. If right ventricular heart failure has developed, signs of systemic venous congestion include jugular vein distension, hepatomegaly, ascites, and peripheral edema. Right ventricular enlargement and contractile dysfunction is often accompanied by the murmur of tricuspid valve regurgitation.

Diagnostic Studies

The *chest radiograph* shows an enlarged cardiac silhouette. If heart failure has developed, then pulmonary vascular redistribution, interstitial and alveolar edema, and pleural effusions are evident (see Fig. 3.5).

The *EKG* usually demonstrates atrial and

ventricular enlargement. Patchy fibrosis of the myofibers results in a wide array of arrhythmias (most importantly atrial fibrillation and ventricular tachycardia). Conduction defects (left or right bundle branch block) occur in the majority of cases. Diffuse repolarization (ST and T wave) abnormalities are common. In addition, regions of dense myocardial fibrosis may produce localized Q waves, resembling the pattern of myocardial infarction.

Echocardiography is valuable in the diagnosis of this condition. It demonstrates four-chamber cardiac enlargement with little hypertrophy, and usually global reduction of systolic contractile function. Mitral and/or tricuspid regurgitation is frequently detected. At some hospitals, noninvasive *radionuclide ventriculography* (also termed blood pool imaging, as described in Chapter 3) is used in addition to, or in place of, echocardiography to assess cardiac enlargement and to quantify the ventricular ejection fractions.

Cardiac catheterization is often performed to determine whether coronary artery disease is contributing to the impaired ventricular function. This procedure is most useful diagnostically in patients who describe episodes of angina pectoris or have evidence of previous myocardial infarction on the electrocardiogram. Typically, hemodynamic measurements show elevation of right- and left-sided diastolic pressures (due to incomplete chamber emptying) and diminished cardiac output. While in the catheterization laboratory, a transvenous biopsy of the right ventricle is sometimes performed in an attempt to clarify the etiology of the cardiomyopathy. There is only a limited role for such a biopsy, however, because it is rarely diagnostic in patients with DCM, and only infrequently alters therapeutic decisions.

Treatment

The goal of therapy in DCM is to improve the quality of life by relieving symptoms, to prevent devastating complications associated with this disorder, and to improve long-term survival. Therefore, the therapeutic approach addresses: 1) treatment of the underlying cause, if identified, 2) prevention of progressive ventricular dilatation, 3) relief of pulmonary and systemic congestion, 4) augmentation of low cardiac output, 5) prevention of life-threatening arrhythmias, 6) prevention of thrombo-emboli, and 7) consideration of cardiac transplantation.

Approaches to the relief of vascular congestion and improvement in forward cardiac output are the same as standard approaches to heart failure described in Chapter 9. Initial therapy of congestion includes salt restriction and diuretics. The most important advance in the past two decades has been the introduction of vasodilator therapy: Improvement in hemodynamic measurements, quality of life, and survival has been shown with the chronic oral use of angiotensin converting-enzyme inhibitors, and to a lesser extent with the combination of hydralazine (an arteriolar vasodilator) plus isosorbide dinitrate (a venous vasodilator). In addition, recent studies have shown that ACE inhibitor therapy can even benefit *asymptomatic* individuals with left ventricular dysfunction by slowing the progression to the symptomatic stages of heart failure. Thus, ACE inhibitors are first-line therapy for patients with dilated cardiomyopathy, while the combination of hydralazine plus isosorbide dinitrate is used when ACE inhibitors are not tolerated. In some patients with dilated cardiomyopathy, digitalis glycosides may be used to improve symptoms, but they have not been shown to reduce long-term mortality in this condition.

Atrial and ventricular arrhythmias are common in advanced DCM, and approximately 40% of deaths in this condition are due to ventricular tachycardia and fibrillation. It is important to maintain serum electrolytes (notably potassium and magnesium) within their normal ranges, especially during diuretic therapy, so as to not further promote serious arrhythmias. Unfortunately, studies to date have *not* shown that antiarrhythmic drugs prevent death related to ventricular arrhythmias in DCM;

in fact, when used in patients with poor LV function, many antiarrhythmic drugs may *worsen* the rhythm disturbance (see Chapter 17). At present, only the implantation of a permanent automatic defibrillator has been shown to reduce arrhythmic deaths in patients with DCM and severe ventricular rhythm disorders.

Stasis of blood flow within the poorly contractile ventricles promotes thrombus formation. Right ventricular thrombus may lead to pulmonary emboli, whereas thrombo-emboli of left ventricular origin may lodge in any systemic artery, resulting in, for example, devastating cerebral, myocardial, or renal infarctions. Chronic oral anticoagulation therapy (i.e., warfarin) is therefore commonly administered to DCM patients who have severe depression of ventricular function (e.g., LV ejection fraction < 30%). It should be noted however, that prospective studies to evaluate the effectiveness (and risks) of long-term anticoagulation therapy in patients with DCM have not been performed.

As described in Chapter 9, β-blockers have been shown, paradoxically, to improve symptoms and exercise capacity in some patients with DCM. The reasons for the effectiveness of β-blockers in this setting is not known, but excessive sympathetic discharge and chronically elevated catecholamine levels in DCM patients may have deleterious effects on the myocardium. A reduced density of β_1 adrenergic receptors has been documented in DCM, most likely because of long-term sympathetic overstimulation. Therefore, beta-blockers may be efficacious by blunting the effects of increased sympathetic nervous system activation and allowing "upregulation" of myocardial β-receptors. At present, the use of β-blockers in this syndrome remains largely investigational.

Finally, in suitable patients with severe symptoms of congestive heart failure, cardiac transplantation offers a substantially better 5-year prognosis than the standard therapy for DCM described above. The current 5- and 10-year survival rates after transplantation are 74% and 55%, respectively. However, the scarcity of donor hearts greatly limits the availability of this technique. Because of this limitation, fewer than 2500 transplants are performed per year, compared with approximately 20,000 patients who could potentially benefit from the procedure.

Prognosis

Despite advances in therapy, the prognosis for patients with DCM who do not undergo cardiac transplantation is poor and depends on the magnitude of ventricular dysfunction. For example, the average 5-year survival rate without transplantation is less than 50%. Methods to reduce progressive LV dysfunction by early intervention in asymptomatic or minimally symptomatic patients, and the prevention of sudden cardiac death remain major research goals in the treatment of this disorder.

HYPERTROPHIC CARDIOMYOPATHY

Hypertrophic cardiomyopathy (HCM) receives occasional notoriety in the lay press, because it is the most common cardiac abnormality found in young athletes who die suddenly during vigorous physical exertion. This condition is characterized by left ventricular hypertrophy that is not due to chronic pressure overload (i.e., *not* the result of systemic hypertension or aortic stenosis). Other terms frequently used to describe this disease are hypertrophic obstructive cardiomyopathy (HOCM), or idiopathic hypertrophic subaortic stenosis (IHSS). In this condition, systolic LV contractile function is vigorous, but the thickened muscle is stiff, resulting in impaired ventricular relaxation and high diastolic pressures.

Etiology

HCM may occur either as a familial or a sporadic form. Inheritance of the familial type appears to follow an autosomal dominant pattern with variable penetrance. Such transmission has recently been shown to be genetically heterogeneous and mutations in at least five different genes have been associated with this condition. Proteins encoded by three of these genes have been identified: β-myosin heavy chain (β-MHC), cardiac troponin T, and α-tropomyosin. Alterations at the loci that encode these sarcomeric proteins are thought to account for approximately 70% of all familial cases.

The pathophysiology and natural history of familial hypertrophic cardiomyopathy (FHC) are quite variable and appear related to particular mutations within the disease-causing gene, rather than the actual gene involved. For example, disease progression in families with mutations in the β-MHC gene can be clinically indistinguishable from that in families with mutations in the troponin T gene. Conversely, two unrelated families with unlike mutations in the β-MHC gene may have vastly different degrees of cardiac hypertrophy and mortality rates.

Life expectancy data for families with FHC have been extensively compiled, and it is from that data that specific genetic mutations have been shown to portend a worse prognosis. In particular, β-MHC mutations that alter the charge of the coded amino acid confer a higher mortality rate than mutations that do not alter the charge.

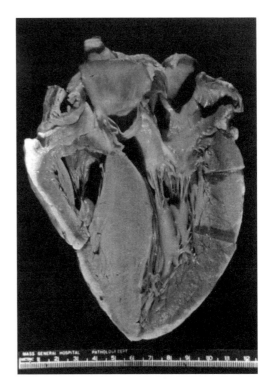

Figure 10.4. Postmortem heart specimen from a patient with hypertrophic cardiomyopathy. Marked left ventricular hypertrophy is seen, especially of the interventricular septum.

array may be in part responsible for the abnormal diastolic stiffness and the arrhythmias that are so common in this disorder.

Pathology

Although hypertrophy in HCM may involve any portion of the ventricles, asymmetric hypertrophy of the ventricular septum (Fig. 10.4) is most common (approximately 90% of cases). Less often, the hypertrophy involves the ventricular walls symmetrically, or is localized to the apex or midregions of the LV.

Unlike ventricular hypertrophy due to hypertension, in which the myocytes enlarge uniformly and remain orderly, the histology of HCM is unusual: The myocardial fibers are in a pattern of extensive disarray (Fig. 10.5). Short, wide, hypertrophied fibers are oriented in chaotic directions and surrounded by loose connective tissue. This dis-

Pathophysiology

The predominant feature of HCM is marked ventricular hypertrophy that reduces the compliance and relaxation (*diastolic* function) of the chamber, such that normal filling becomes impaired (Fig. 10.6). Patients who have asymmetric hypertrophy of the upper interventricular septum may display additional findings due to transient obstruction of left ventricular outflow during *systole*. In that case, the mechanism of systolic obstruction is thought to involve abnormal motion of the anterior mitral valve leaflet toward the LV outflow tract where the thickened septum protrudes (Fig. 10.7). This process is explained as follows: 1) during ventricular contraction,

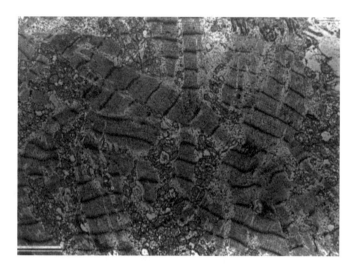

Figure 10.5.   Electron microscopy of the myocardium from a patient with hypertrophic cardiomyopathy. Note the disarray of the myofibers.

ejection of blood past the upper septum is more rapid than usual, as it must flow through an outflow tract that is narrowed by the thickened septum; 2) this rapid flow creates Venturi forces that abnormally draw the anterior mitral leaflet toward the septum during contraction; 3) the anterior mitral leaflet approaches and transiently abuts the hypertrophied septum, causing brief obstruction of blood flow into the aorta.

It is useful to consider the pathophysiology of HCM based on whether transient systolic obstruction is present:

HCM Without Outflow Tract Obstruction

Although systolic contraction of the left ventricle is usually vigorous in HCM, the hypertrophied walls result in increased stiffness and impaired diastolic relaxation of the chamber. The reduced ventricular compliance alters the normal pressure-volume relationship, such that the passive diastolic filling curve shifts upward (Fig. 9.7B). The associated rise in diastolic LV pressure is transmitted backward, leading to elevated left atrial, pulmonary venous, and pulmonary capillary pressures. Dyspnea, especially during exertion, is thus a common symptom in this disorder.

HCM With Outflow Obstruction

In patients with outflow obstruction, elevated left atrial and pulmonary capillary wedge pressures are due both to decreased ventricular compliance and to the outflow obstruction during contraction. During systolic obstruction, a pressure gradient develops between the body of the LV and the outflow tract distal to the obstruction (Fig. 10.7). The elevated ventricular systolic pressure increases wall stress and myocardial oxygen consumption, possibly resulting in anginal chest discomfort (Fig. 10.6). In addition, because obstruction is due to abnormal motion of the anterior mitral leaflet toward the septum (and therefore *away* from the posterior mitral leaflet), the mitral valve does not close properly during systole, and mitral regurgitation may result. This further elevates left atrial and pulmonary venous pressures, and may worsen symptoms of dyspnea.

The systolic pressure gradient observed in obstructive HCM is "dynamic" in that its magnitude varies during contraction, and depends at any given time on the distance between the anterior leaflet of the mitral valve and the hypertrophied septum. Situations that *decrease* LV cavity size (e.g., reduced venous return because of intravascu-

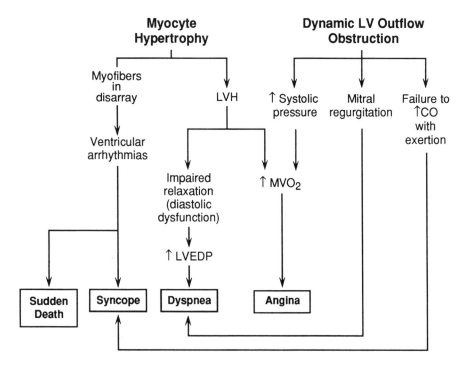

Figure 10.6. Pathophysiology of hypertrophic cardiomyopathy. The bizarre and hypertrophied myocytes may result in ventricular arrhythmias (which can cause syncope or sudden death) and impaired diastolic left ventricular (LV) relaxation (which causes elevated LV filling pressures and dyspnea). If dynamic left ventricular outflow obstruction is present, mitral regurgitation often accompanies it (which contributes to dyspnea) and the impaired ability to raise cardiac output with exertion can lead to exertional syncope. The thickened LV wall and systolic outflow tract obstruction both contribute to increased myocardial oxygen consumption (MVO_2) and can precipitate angina. LVH, LV hypertrophy; LVEDP, LV end-diastolic pressure; CO, cardiac output.

lar volume depletion) bring the mitral leaflet and septum into closer proximity and *promote* obstruction. Conversely, conditions that *enlarge* the LV (e.g., augmented intravascular volume) increase the distance between the anterior mitral leaflet and septum and *reduce* the obstruction. Positive inotropic drugs (which augment the force of contraction) also force the mitral leaflet and septum into closer proximity and contribute to obstruction, whereas negative inotropic drugs (e.g., β-blockers, verapamil) have the opposite effect.

Although dynamic systolic outflow tract obstruction creates impressive murmurs and receives great attention, the symptoms of obstructive HCM appear to be primarily due to the increased LV stiffness and diastolic dysfunction that is also present in the nonobstructive form.

Clinical Findings

The symptoms of HCM vary widely, from the asymptomatic individual to those with marked physical limitations. The average age of presentation is in the mid-20s.

The most frequent symptom is *dyspnea* due to elevated diastolic LV (and therefore pulmonary capillary) pressures. This symptom is further provoked by the high systolic LV pressure and mitral regurgitation seen in individuals with the outflow tract obstructive form.

Angina is often described by patients with HCM, even in the absence of obstructive coronary artery disease. Myocardial ischemia may be contributed to by: 1) the high oxygen demand of the increased muscle mass, and 2) the presence of thickened and narrowed small branches of the coro-

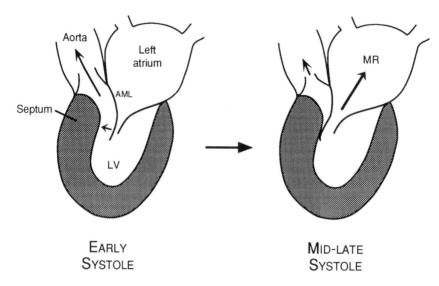

EARLY   MID-LATE
SYSTOLE   SYSTOLE

Figure 10.7.   Pathophysiology of aortic outflow obtruction and mitral regurgitation in hypertrophic cardiomyopathy (HCM). Left panel. The LV outflow tract is abnormally narrowed between the hypertrophied interventricular septum and the anterior leaflet of the mitral valve (AML). The rapid ejection velocity along the narrowed tract in early systole draws the AML toward the septum (small arrow). **Right panel.** As the mitral valve abnormally moves anteriorly and contacts the septum, outflow into the aorta is transiently obstructed. Since the mitral leaflets do not coapt normally in systole, mitral regurgitation (MR) also results.

nary arteries within the hypertrophied ventricular wall (i.e., decreased vasodilator reserve, hence reduced myocardial oxygen supply). If outflow tract obstruction is present, the high systolic ventricular pressure also increases myocardial oxygen demand, because of the increased wall stress.

Syncope in HCM may result from cardiac arrhythmias that develop because of the structurally abnormal myofibers (see below). In patients with outflow tract obstruction, syncope may be further provoked by exertion, when the pressure gradient is made worse by the increased force of contraction, thereby causing a transient fall in cardiac output. Orthostatic lightheadedness is also common in patients with outflow tract obstruction. This occurs because venous return to the heart is reduced upon standing by the gravitational pooling of blood in the lower extremities, the LV thereby decreases in size, and outflow tract obstruction intensifies, transiently reducing cardiac output and cerebral perfusion.

Unfortunately, the first manifestation of HCM may be *sudden death* due to ventricu-

lar fibrillation, particularly among young adults during strenuous physical exertion.

Physical Examination

Patients with mild forms of HCM are often asymptomatic, and the physical examination may be entirely normal. However, a common finding is the presence of a fourth heart sound (S_4). It is generated by left atrial contraction into the stiffened LV (see Chapter 2). The forceful atrial contraction may also result in a palpable presystolic impulse over the cardiac apex (known as a "double" apical impulse).

In patients with systolic outflow obstruction, other findings are common: The carotid pulse rises briskly in early systole, but then quickly declines, as obstruction to cardiac outflow appears. The characteristic murmur of LV outflow obstruction is rough and crescendo-decrescendo in shape, heard best at the left lower sternal border (due to turbulent flow through the narrowed outflow tract). However, as the stethoscope is moved toward the apex, the murmur may take on a more blowing, pansystolic quality (because of the mitral regurgitation component). Although the murmur may be soft at rest, bedside maneuvers that alter preload and afterload can dramatically increase its intensity (Table 10.2) and help differentiate this murmur from other conditions, such as aortic stenosis.

Diagnostic Studies

The *EKG* typically shows left ventricular hypertrophy. Prominent Q waves are common in the inferior and lateral leads, and are thought to represent the forces of initial depolarization by the hypertrophied ventricular septum. Atrial and ventricular arrhythmias are frequent, and potentially dangerous: Atrial fibrillation is not well-tolerated, because cardiac output may decline as much as 25% when the stiffened left ventricle loses the contribution of its "atrial kick." Ventricular arrhythmias are particularly ominous because they may herald ventricular fibrillation and death, even in previously asymptomatic patients.

Echocardiography is most helpful in the evaluation of HCM. The left ventricle is hypertrophied, and asymmetric wall thickness can be readily identified. Signs of left ventricular outflow obstruction may be demonstrated, and include abnormal anterior motion of the mitral valve as it is drawn toward the hypertrophied septum during systole, and partial closure of the aortic valve in midsystole as flow across it is transiently obstructed. Doppler recordings during echocardiography accurately measure the outflow gradient and quantify any associated mitral regurgitation. Children and adolescents with apparently mild HCM should undergo serial echocardiographic assessment over time, as the degree of hypertrophy may increase during puberty and early adulthood.

Cardiac catheterization is reserved for situations in which the diagnosis is uncertain or if cardiac surgery is planned. The major feature is the presence of a pressure gradient within the outflow portion of the left ventricle, either at rest or during maneuvers that transiently reduce LV size and promote outflow tract obstruction. Myocardial biopsy at the time of catheterization is not necessary, since histologic findings do not predict disease severity or long-term prognosis.

Although genetic testing for HCM is not currently feasible on a wide-scale basis, future genotyping may provide a noninvasive technique for definitive diagnosis and risk stratification among families with this condition.

Treatment

β-blockers are standard therapy of HCM because they: 1) reduce myocardial oxygen demand by slowing the heart rate and the force of contraction (and therefore diminish angina and dyspnea), 2) lessen the LV outflow gradient during exercise by reducing the force of contraction (allowing the chamber size to increase, thus separating the anterior leaflet of the mitral valve from the ventricular septum), and 3) decrease the frequency of ventricular ectopic beats. Despite the latter antiarrhythmic effect, β-blockers have not been shown to prevent sudden arrhythmic death in this condition.

Calcium channel antagonists appear to reduce ventricular stiffness and are sometimes useful in improving exercise capacity in patients who fail to respond to β-blockers. *Antiarrhythmic drugs* are used to reduce symptomatic rhythm disturbances, but no regimen has been conclusively shown to reduce sudden death in this syndrome; amiodarone (see Chapter 17) appears to be the most promising. Strenuous exercise and competitive athletics should be avoided in patients with HCM because of the propen-

---

TABLE 10.2. Effect of Maneuvers on Murmurs of Aortic Stenosis (AS) and Hypertrophic Cardiomyopathy (HCM)

	Valsalva	Squatting	Standing
Preload	↓	↑	↓
Afterload	↓	↑	↓
HCM murmur	↑	↓	↑
AS murmur	↓	↑ (usually)	↓

sity of sudden death during such activity. For those individuals who demonstrate potentially lethal arrythmias (e.g., ventricular tachycardia), an implanted cardiac defibrillator may be recommended.

Infective endocarditis can develop in patients with obstructive HCM because of turbulent blood flow through the narrowed LV outflow tract and the associated mitral regurgitation; *antibiotic prophylaxis* (see Chapter 8) is therefore indicated during surgical procedures that result in bacteremia, to prevent endocardial infection.

Surgical therapy (*myomectomy*) is considered for patients who do not respond to pharmacologic therapy. This procedure involves excision of portions of the hypertrophied muscle mass and usually results in improved symptomatology.

Some studies have shown clinical improvement when patients with obstructive HCM are treated with a dual-chamber permanent pacemaker, the electrodes of which are placed in the right atrium and right ventricle. The LV outflow gradient may become reduced by this procedure, possibly by altering the normal sequence of ventricular contraction, such that septal-mitral valve apposition becomes less prominent. This technique seems to be useful for only a small percentage of patients.

Genetic counseling should be provided to all patients with HCM. As this is an autosomal dominant disease, children of affected individuals have a 50% chance of inheriting the abnormal gene. In addition, first-degree relatives of patients with HCM should be screened for the condition by echocardiography. Even if affected individuals are asymptomatic, they are at increased risk of complications, including sudden death, and must be closely monitored.

Prognosis

The incidence of sudden cardiac death in HCM is 2%–4% per year in adults and 4%–6% in children and adolescents. Factors associated with the worst prognosis include an early age of diagnosis, a familial form of HCM with known sudden cardiac death in first-degree relatives, a history of syncope, myocardial ischemia, and the presence of ventricular arrhythmias.

RESTRICTIVE CARDIOMYOPATHY

The restrictive cardiomyopathies are less common than DCM and HCM. They are characterized by abnormally rigid (but not necessarily thickened) ventricles with impaired diastolic filling but usually normal systolic function. This condition results from either: 1) fibrosis or scarring of the endomyocardium, or 2) infiltration of the myocardium by an abnormal substance, such as amyloid (Table 10.3).

Pathophysiology

Reduced compliance of the ventricles due to fibrosis or infiltration results in an upward shift of the passive ventricular filling curve (Fig. 9.7B) such that intraventricular pressure is abnormally high throughout diastole. There are two major consequences: 1) elevated systemic and pulmonary venous pressures, with signs of right- and left-sided vascular congestion, and 2) reduced ventricular cavity size with decreased stroke volume and cardiac output.

TABLE 10.3. Examples of Restrictive Cardiomyopathy

Myocardial	Endomyocardial
Noninfiltrative	Endomyocardial fibrosis
Idiopathic	Hypereosinophilic syndrome
Scleroderma	Metastatic tumors
Infiltrative	Radiation therapy
Amyloidosis	
Sarcoidosis	
Storage diseases	
Hemochromatosis	
Glycogen storage	
diseases	

Clinical Findings

It follows from the underlying pathophysiology that signs of left- and right-sided heart failure are expected (Fig. 10.8). Decreased cardiac output is manifested by fatigue and decreased exercise tolerance. Systemic congestion (often more prominent than pulmonary congestion in this syndrome) leads to jugular venous distension, peripheral edema, and ascites with a large, tender liver.

Diagnostic Studies

As described in Chapter 14, the restrictive cardiomyopathies share nearly identical symptoms, physical signs, and hemodynamic profiles with constrictive pericarditis. However, it is important to distinguish between these two entities, because constrictive pericarditis is a treatable condition, whereas the restrictive cardiomyopathies generally are not.

The most useful diagnostic tools to differentiate restrictive cardiomyopathy from constrictive pericarditis are transvenous endomyocardial biopsy, computed tomography (CT), and magnetic resonance imaging (MRI). For example, in restrictive cardiomyopathy, a transvenous endomyocardial biopsy may demonstrate the presence of infiltrative matter such as amyloid, iron deposits (hemochromatosis), or metastatic tumors. Conversely, CT or MRI scans are useful to identify the thickened

pericardium of constrictive pericarditis, a finding that is not expected in restrictive cardiomyopathy.

Treatment

Restrictive cardiomyopathy typically has a very poor prognosis, except when treatment can be targeted at an underlying cause. For example, phlebotomy and iron chelation therapy may be helpful in the early form of hemochromatosis (iron storage disease). Symptomatic therapy includes salt restriction and cautious use of diuretics to improve symptoms of systemic and pulmonary congestion. Unlike the dilated cardiomyopathies, digitalis and vasodilators are not helpful, because systolic function is usually preserved. Some restrictive cardiomyopathies are prone to intraventricular thrombus formation, in which case chronic oral anticoagulant therapy is warranted.

SUMMARY

1. The cardiomyopathies are diseases of heart muscle that are classified by their pathophysiologic presentation into dilated, hypertrophic, or restrictive types (Table 10.4).
2. The dilated cardiomyopathies are characterized by ventricular dilatation with impaired systolic function. Progressive left ventricular enlargement often leads to symptomatic heart failure, ventricular

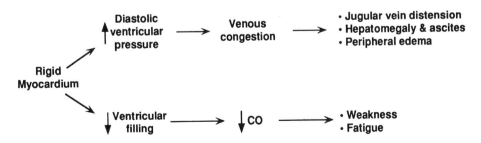

Figure 10.8. Pathophysiology of restrictive cardiomyopathy. The rigid myocardium results in elevated ventricular diastolic pressures and decreased ventricular filling. The resultant symptoms can be predicted from these abnormalities.

TABLE 10.4. Summary of the Cardiomyopathies

	Dilated cardiomyopathy	Hypertrophic cardiomyopathy	Restrictive cardiomyopathy
Ventricular morphology	Dilated LV with little hypertrophy	Marked hypertrophy, often asymmetric	Fibrotic or infiltrated myocardium
Symptoms	Fatigue, weakness, dyspnea, orthopnea, PND (symptoms of congestive heart failure)	Dyspnea, angina, syncope	Dyspnea, fatigue
Physical exam	Pulmonary rales, S3; If RV failure present: JVD, hepatomegaly, peripheral edema	S4; If outflow obstruction present: systolic murmur loudest at left sternal border, accompanied by mitral regurgitation	Signs of RV failure: JVD, hepatomegaly, peripheral edema
Pathophysiology	Impaired systolic contraction	Impaired diastolic relaxation; LV systolic function vigorous, often with dynamic obstruction	"Stiff" LV with impaired diastolic relaxation but normal systolic function
Cardiac size on chest radiograph	Dilated	Normal or dilated	Usually normal
Echocardiogram	Dilated, poorly contractile LV	LV hypertrophy, often more pronounced in septum; systolic anterior movement of MV with mitral regurgitation	Usually normal systolic contraction; "speckled" appearance in infiltrative disorders

LV, left ventricle; MV, mitral valve; PND, paroxysmal nocturnal dyspnea; JVD, jugular venous distension

arrhythmias, or embolic complications. Angiotensin converting-enzyme inhibitor therapy improves the long-term prognosis.

3. Hypertrophic cardiomyopathy is characterized by a markedly thickened left ventricle and impaired diastolic relaxation. Dynamic LV outflow tract obstruction during systole may be present. The most common symptoms are dyspnea and exertional angina. Ventricular arrhythmias may lead to sudden cardiac death.

4. The restrictive cardiomyopathies are uncommon and are characterized by impairment of diastolic ventricular relaxation due to an infiltrated or fibrotic myocardium. Symptoms of heart failure are typical.

ADDITIONAL READING

Costanzo NW, Augustine S, Bourge R, et al. Selection and treatment of candidates for heart transplantation. A statement for health professionals from the Committee on Heart Failure and Cardiac Transplantation of the Council of Clinical Cardiology, American Heart Association. Circulation 1995;92: 3593–3612.

Dec GW, Fuster VF. Idiopathic dilated cardiomyopathy. N Eng J Med 1994;331:1564–1575.

Hess M. Molecular pathology of dilated cardiomyopathies. Curr Probl Cardiol 1996;1:102–144.

Kushwaha SS, Fallon JT, Fuster V. Medical progress: restrictive cardiomyopathy. N Engl J Med 1997;336: 267–276.

Lenihan DJ, Gerson M, Holt BD, et al. Mechanisms, diagnosis, and treatment of diastolic heart failure. Am Heart J 1995;130:153–166.

Marian AJ, Roberts R. Recent advances in the molecular genetics of hypertrophic cardiomyopathy. Circulation 1995;92:1336–1347.

Richardson P, McKenna W, Bristow M, et al. Report of the 1995 World Health Organization/International Society and Federation of Cardiology Task Force on the Definition and Classification of Cardiomyopathies. Circulation 1996;93:841–842.

Wigle ED, Rakowski H, Kimball BP, et al. Hypertrophic cardiomyopathy. Clinical spectrum and treatment. Circulation 1995;92:1680–1692.

Acknowledgments The previous edition of this chapter was written by Kay Fang, MD, G.William Dec, MD, and Leonard S. Lilly, MD.

Mechanisms of Cardiac Arrhythmias

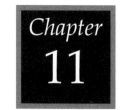

Chapter
11

Marc S. Sabatine, Elliott M. Antman, Leonard I. Ganz, Gary R. Strichartz, and Leonard S. Lilly

Normal Impulse Formation
  Ionic Basis of Automaticity
  Native and Latent Pacemakers
  Overdrive Suppression
  Electrotonic Interactions
Altered Impulse Formation
  Alterations in Sinus Node Automaticity
  Escape Rhythms
  Enhanced Automaticity of Latent Pacemakers

Abnormal Automaticity
Triggered Activity
Altered Impulse Conduction
  Conduction Block
  Reentry
Approach to Antiarrhythmic Treatment
  Bradyarrhythmias
  Tachyarrhythmias

Normal cardiac function relies on the flow of electrical impulses through the heart in an exquisitely coordinated fashion. Abnormalities of the electrical rhythm are known as *arrhythmias* (also termed *dysrhythmias*), and are among the most common clinical problems encountered. Their presentations range from benign palpitations to severe symptoms of low cardiac output and death, so that a thorough understanding of these disorders, their diagnosis, and their treatment is important to the daily practice of medicine.

This chapter describes the mechanisms by which arrhythmias develop, followed by a general description of their treatment. The next chapter summarizes specific rhythm disorders and how to recognize them.

Disorders of heart rhythm result from alterations of **impulse formation,** of **impulse conduction,** or both. We first address how alterations of impulse formation and conduction occur and under what circumstances they cause arrhythmias. Figure 11.1 provides an organizational schema for this discussion.

NORMAL IMPULSE FORMATION

As presented in Chapter 1, electrical impulse formation in the heart arises from the intrinsic automaticity of specialized cardiac cells. **Automaticity** refers to a cell's ability to depolarize itself to a threshold voltage in a rhythmic fashion, such that *spontaneous* action potentials are generated. Although atrial and ventricular myocytes do not have this property under normal conditions, the cells of the specialized conducting system do possess natural automaticity, and are therefore termed **pacemaker cells.** The specialized conducting system includes the SA node, the AV nodal region, and the ventricular conducting system. The latter is composed of the bundle of His, the bundle branches, and the Purkinje fibers. In *pathologic situations,* myocardial cells outside the conducting system may also acquire the property of automaticity.

Ionic Basis of Automaticity

Cells with natural automaticity do not have a static resting potential. Rather, they

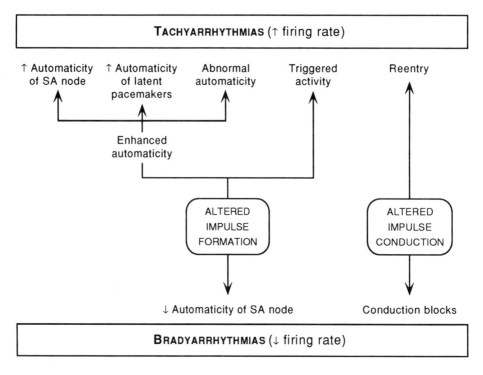

Figure 11.1. Arrhythmias result from alterations in impulse formation and/or impulse conduction. Tachyarrhythmias are characterized by an increased firing rate of action potentials, whereas bradyarrhythmias are associated with a decreased firing rate.

display a gradually upsloping phase 4 of the action potential (Fig. 11.2), which represents spontaneous diastolic depolarization. An important ionic flow largely responsible for this phase 4 depolarization is known as the **pacemaker current (I_f).** This current, carried mainly by sodium ions, passes through specific membrane channels that open during cellular repolarization, when the membrane voltage becomes more negative than approximately -50 mV (these channels are *different* from the fast sodium channels responsible for rapid phase 0 depolarization in nonpacemaker cells). The slow inward flow of Na$^+$, driven by its concentration gradient and the negative intracellular charge, forces the membrane potential to depolarize toward the threshold voltage.

In the pacemaker cells of the sinoatrial node, alterations in two other ionic currents also contribute to phase 4 depolarization: 1) a slow inward calcium current, the channels of which become activated at voltages near

the end of phase 4, and 2) a progressive decline of an *outward* potassium current. The latter current is responsible for cellular repolarization during phase 3 of the action potential, and it progressively diminishes during phase 4. The combination of the inward I_f, inward Ca^{++}, and reduced outward K$^+$ currents acts to gradually depolarize the SA nodal cells to the threshold potential.

When the pacemaker cell potential reaches the threshold value, the upstroke of the action potential is generated. In distinction to the phase 0 upstroke of nonpacemaker cells, that of the pacemaker cell is much less rapid (Fig. 11.2; compare with Fig. 1.13). This is so because the fast sodium channels in pacemaker cells are chronically inactivated by the persistently less negative voltages, compared with atrial and ventricular myocytes (i.e., pacemaker cell voltages never approach the maximum negative membrane potential of -90 mV seen in myocardial cells). Thus, the action potential

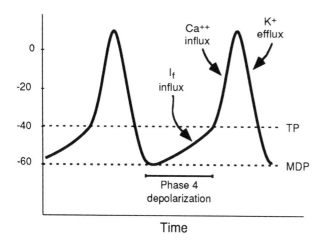

Figure 11.2. The action potential (AP) of a pacemaker cell. Note the slow phase 4 depolarization, largely caused by the I_f (pacemaker) current, which drives the cell to threshold potential (approximately -40mV). The upstroke of the AP is due to the slow inward current of Ca^{++} ions. Inactivation of the calcium channels and K^+ efflux through potassium channels are responsible for repolarization. MDP, maximum diastolic potential; TP, threshold potential.

upstroke relies solely on calcium ion inflow, through the relatively slower opening Ca^{++} channels.

The repolarization phase of pacemaker cells depends on inactivation of the calcium channels, as well as K^+ efflux from the cell through specific voltage-gated potassium channels.

Native and Latent Pacemakers

The different populations of automatic cells in the specialized conduction pathway have distinct intrinsic rates of firing. These rates are determined by three variables that influence how fast the membrane potential reaches threshold: 1) the rate (i.e., the slope) of phase 4 spontaneous depolarization, 2) the maximum negative diastolic potential, and 3) the threshold potential. A more negative maximum diastolic potential, or a less negative threshold potential, slows the rate of impulse initiation because it takes longer to reach that threshold value (Fig. 11.3). Conversely, the greater the I_f, the steeper the slope of phase 4, and the faster the cell depolarizes. The rate of I_f depends on the number and kinetics of the individual pacemaker channels through which this current flows. Therefore, the cell population with the greatest number and most active pacemaker channels possesses the highest intrinsic firing rate.

Since all of the healthy myocardial cells are electrically connected by gap junctions, an action potential generated in one part of the myocardium will ultimately spread to all other regions. When an impulse arrives at a cell that has not yet depolarized, that cell will fire regardless of how close its intrinsic I_f has brought it to threshold. Thus, it should be clear that the pacemaker cells with the fastest rate of depolarization set the heart rate. In the normal heart, the dominant pacemaker is the *sinoatrial node,* which usually initiates impulses at a rate of 60–100 beats per minute (bpm). Because this sinus node firing rate is faster than that of the other tissues that possess automaticity, the SA node impulses preempt the spontaneous firing of other potential pacemaker sites.

Since the SA node normally sets the heart rate, it is known as the **native pacemaker**. Other cells within the specialized conduction system harbor the potential to act as pacemakers when called upon to do so, and are therefore called **latent pacemakers** (also termed **ectopic pacemakers**). In contrast to the SA node, the AV node and the bundle of His have an intrinsic firing rate of approximately 50 to 60 bpm and cells of the Purkinje system about 30 to 40 bpm. These latent pacemakers may initiate impulses and take over the pacemaking function at their intrinsic firing rates if the faster pacemakers (i.e., cells of the SA node) fail, or if conduction abnormalities block the normal wave of depolarization from reaching the latent pacemaker sites.

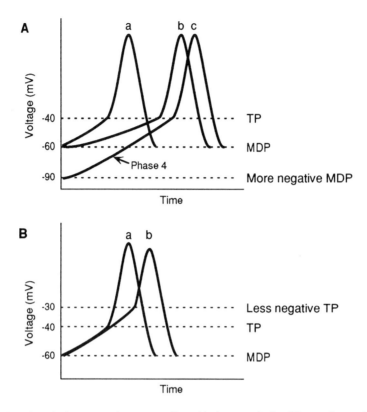

Figure 11.3. **A.** Alterations in the pacemaker current (I_f) and in the magnitude of the maximum diastolic potential (MDP) alter the cell firing rate. (a), The normal action potential (AP) of a pacemaker cell. (b), Reduced I_f renders the slope of phase 4 less steep; thus the time required to reach threshold potential (TP) is increased. (c), The MDP is more negative; therefore the time required to reach TP is increased. **B.** Alterations in TP alter the firing rate of the cell. Compared with the normal TP (a), the TP in (b) is less negative; thus the duration of time to achieve threshold is increased, and the firing rate decreases.

Overdrive Suppression

Not only does the cell population with the fastest intrinsic beat preempt all other automatic cells from spontaneously firing, it also directly *suppresses* the automaticity of other conduction pathway cells. This phenomenon is called overdrive suppression. Cells maintain their trans-sarcolemmal ion distributions because of the continuously active Na^+/K^+-ATPase pump that extrudes three Na^+ ions out of the cell in exchange for two K^+ ions transported in (Fig. 11.4). Because its net transport effect is one positive charge in the outward direction, the Na^+/K^+ pump creates a *hyperpolarizing* current (i.e., it tends to make the inside of the cell *more negative*). As such, it constantly antagonizes the spontaneous depolariza-

tion that otherwise occurs in automatic (pacemaker) cells. However, pacemaker cells firing at their own intrinsic beat have an I_f current sufficiently large to overcome this hyperpolarizing influence (Fig. 11.4).

When a cell is forced to fire faster than its intrinsic pacemaker rate, the balance between hyperpolarizing and depolarizing currents is altered. The more frequently the cell is depolarized, the greater the quantity of Na^+ ions that enter the cell per unit time. As a result, the Na^+/K^+ pump becomes more active, so as to restore the normal transmembrane Na^+ gradient. This increased pump activity provides a larger hyperpolarizing current that more substantially counters the depolarizing current, I_f. As the balance in these cells shifts toward hyperpolarization (i.e., the maximum nega-

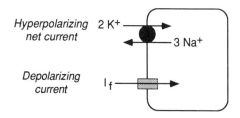

Figure 11.4. Competition between the depolarizing pacemaker current (I_f) and the Na$^+$/K$^+$ pump, which produces a hyperpolarizing current: It transports three positive charges outside the cell for every two it pumps in. The hyperpolarizing current acts to suppress automaticity, and contributes to overdrive suppression in cells that are stimulated more rapidly than their intrinsic firing rate.

tive potential becomes more negative), additional time is required for spontaneous phase 4 depolarization to reach the threshold voltage (Fig. 11.3A), and therefore, the cell *spontaneously* initiates action potentials at a slower rate. In this fashion, overdrive suppression decreases a cell's automaticity when that cell is forced to fire faster than its intrinsic firing rate. Thus, not only do faster pacemaker cells preempt others downstream, they also inhibit the automaticity of those cells through overdrive suppression.

Electrotonic Interactions

In addition to the effect of overdrive suppression on latent pacemakers, evidence exists that *anatomic connections* between pacemaker and nonpacemaker cells are important in the suppression of latent pacemaker foci. Myocardial cells that are not part of the specialized conducting system repolarize to a resting potential of -90 mV, whereas pacemaker cells repolarize to a maximum diastolic potential of about -60 mV. When these two cell types are adjacent to one another, *electrical coupling* occurs through their intercalated disks. This coupling results in a hyperpolarizing current flowing away from the automatic cell tending to equilibrate the electrical potentials (Fig. 11.5). The hyperpolarizing current competes with I_f, thereby reducing the cell's automaticity. This mechanism may be particularly important in suppressing auto-

maticity in the AV node (via connections between atrial myocytes and AV nodal cells) and in the distal Purkinje fibers (which are anatomically adjacent to nonautomatic ventricular myocardial cells). Decoupling of this mechanism (e.g., by ischemic damage) may remove the inhibitory influence, and therefore lead to enhanced automaticity and an ectopic rhythm generated by the latent pacemaker tissue.

ALTERED IMPULSE FORMATION

Arrhythmias may arise from altered impulse formation at the SA node or from other sites, such as the specialized conduction pathways or from abnormal regions of cardiac muscle. The two main abnormalities of impulse initiation that lead to arrhythmias are: 1) **altered automaticity** (of the sinus node, of latent pacemakers within the specialized conduction pathway, or development of abnormal automaticity by atrial or ventricular myocytes) and 2) **triggered activity**.

Alterations in Sinus Node Automaticity

The rate of impulse initiation by the sinus node, as well as by the latent pacemakers of the specialized conducting system, is regulated primarily by neurohumoral factors, as described in this section.

Increased Sinus Node Automaticity

The most important modulator of normal sinus node automaticity is the autonomic nervous system. Sympathetic stimulation, or an increased concentration of circulating catecholamines, acting through β_1-adrenergic receptors, increases the probability of the pacemaker channels being open, as illustrated in Figure 11.6. Therefore, a pacemaker channel at a membrane potential within its excitable range is more likely to be open after sympathetic stimulation than before. This results in an increased

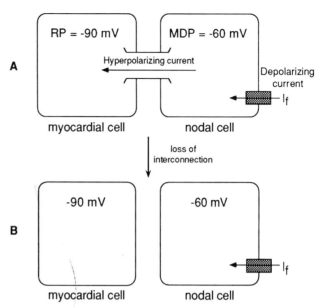

Figure 11.5. Electrotonic interaction between pacemaker (e.g., AV nodal) and nonpacemaker (myocardial) cells. Nodal cells have a maximum negative potential (MDP) of approximately −60 mV, whereas myocardial cells have a resting potential (RP) of approximately −90 mV. When these cell populations neighbor one another, they may be connected electrically by intercalated discs (**A**). In this situation, a positive electrical current flows from the nodal cell toward the myocardial cell, tending to hyperpolarize the former and depolarize the latter. This action opposes I_f of the nodal pacemaker cell and therefore, suppresses cellular automaticity. **B.** If a disease state causes the loss of the intercellular connection, then the nodal cell is no longer hyperpolarized by the neighboring cell, and thus depolarizes to threshold more readily.

number of available channels through which I_f can flow. The subsequent increase in the magnitude of I_f leads to a steeper slope of phase 4 depolarization. This causes the SA node to reach threshold and fire earlier than in the absence of sympathetic stimulation, and the heart rate increases.

In addition, sympathetic stimulation shifts the action potential threshold to more negative voltages, by increasing the probability that voltage-sensitive Ca^{++} channels are open (recall that it is calcium that carries the current of phase 0 depolarization in pacemaker cells). Therefore, automaticity is increased by adrenergic stimulation in two ways: by causing the action potential threshold to become more negative, and by increasing I_f.

Examples of this physiologic effect occur during exercise or emotional stress, whereby increased sympathetic stimulation appropriately increases the heart rate.

Decreased Sinus Node Automaticity

A decrease in SA node automaticity is mediated primarily by the parasympathetic nervous system, which antagonizes the sympathetic influence. While the sympathetic nervous system exerts a dominant ef-

fect on the heart rate during times of stress, the parasympathetic nervous system is the major mediator of heart rate at rest.

Cholinergic (i.e., parasympathetic) stimulation via the vagus nerve acts at the SA node to reduce the probability of the pacemaker channels being open (Fig. 11.6). Thus, I_f and the slope of phase 4 depolarization are reduced, and the intrinsic firing rate of the cell is slowed. In addition, the probability of the Ca^+ channels being open is decreased, thus the action potential threshold moves closer to zero (i.e., further away from the resting potential). Furthermore, cholinergic stimulation increases the probability of certain K^+ channels being open at rest. Because positively charged K^+ ions exit through these channels, the cell becomes hyperpolarized, and the maximum diastolic potential becomes more negative. The net effect of reduced I_f, more negative maximum diastolic potential, and a less negative threshold level, is a slowing of the intrinsic firing rate (i.e., decreased automaticity), and therefore a reduced heart rate.

It follows that the use of pharmacologic agents that modify the effects of the autonomic nervous system will also affect the firing rate of the SA node. For example, beta-blocking drugs antagonize the beta-adrenergic sympathetic effect, and there-

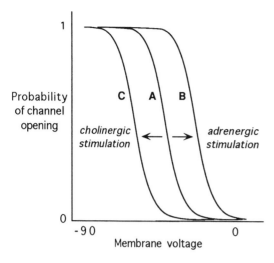

Figure 11.6.   The channels through which the pacemaker current (I_f) flows are voltage-gated, opening at more negative membrane potentials. At any given voltage, there exists a probability between 0 and 1 that a specific channel will be open. Compared with normal baseline behavior (curve A), sympathetic stimulation (curve B) shifts this probability to a higher value for any given level of membrane voltage, thus increasing the number of open channels and the rate at which the cell will fire. Curve C shows that parasympathetic stimulation has the opposite effect, decreasing the probability of a channel being open, and therefore inhibiting depolarization.

fore *decrease* the rate of phase 4 depolarization of the SA node, and slow the heart rate. Conversely, atropine, an anticholinergic drug has the opposite effect: by blocking the parasympathetic response, the rate of phase 4 depolarization *increases*, and the heart rate accelerates.

Escape Rhythms

If the sinus node becomes suppressed and fires less frequently than normal, the site of impulse formation usually shifts to a latent pacemaker within the specialized conduction pathway. When a latent pacemaker initiates an impulse because the SA node rate has slowed, it is called an **escape beat**. Persistent impairment of the SA node will allow a continued series of escape beats, termed an **escape rhythm**. Escape rhythms represent protective mechanisms

that prevent the heart rate from becoming too slow when SA node firing is impaired.

As discussed in the previous section, suppression of the sinus node may occur because of parasympathetic influences. Different regions of the heart vary in their sensitivity to parasympathetic (vagal) stimulation and its neurotransmitter acetylcholine (ACh). The SA node and the AV node are most sensitive to vagal influences, followed by atrial tissue. The ventricular conducting system is the least sensitive. Therefore, moderate vagal stimulation slows the sinus rate, and allows the pacemaker to shift to another atrial site. However, very strong vagal stimulation suppresses the SA node and atrial tissue, can cause conduction block at the AV node, and may therefore result in the emergence of a ventricular escape pacemaker.

Enhanced Automaticity of Latent Pacemakers

Another means by which a latent pacemaker can assume control of impulse formation is if it develops an intrinsic rate of depolarization *faster* than that of the sinus node. Termed an **ectopic beat,** the impulse is *premature* in terms of the normal rhythm, whereas an escape beat occurs *late*, terminating a pause caused by slowing of the sinus rhythm. When similar ectopic beats occur in series, it is called an **ectopic rhythm**.

Ectopic beats may arise in several circumstances. For example, high *catecholamine* concentrations can enhance the automaticity of latent pacemakers, and if the resulting rate of depolarization exceeds that of the sinus node, then an ectopic rhythm will develop. Ectopic beats are also commonly induced during periods of hypoxemia, ischemia, electrolyte disturbances, and because of certain drug toxicities (such as digitalis, as described in Chapter 17).

Abnormal Automaticity

Cardiac tissue injury may lead to pathologic changes in impulse formation whereby myocardial cells *outside* the specialized conduction system acquire automaticity and spontaneously depolarize. Although such activity may appear similar to impulses originating from latent pacemakers within the specialized conduction pathways, these ectopic beats arise from cells that do not usually possess automaticity. If the rate of depolarization of such cells exceeds that of the sinus node, they transiently take over the pacemaker function and become the source of an abnormal ectopic rhythm.

Because these myocardial cells have few or no activated pacemaker channels, they do not normally carry I_f. How injury allows these cells to spontaneously depolarize has not been fully elucidated. However, when cells become injured, their membranes become "leaky." As such, they are unable to maintain the concentration gradients of ions, and the resting potential becomes less negative (i.e., the cell becomes partially depolarized). When a cell's membrane potential is reduced to a value less negative than -60 mV, gradual phase 4 depolarization can be demonstrated even among nonpacemaker cells. This slow spontaneous depolarization is probably related to a slow calcium current, as well as by closure of a subset of K^+ channels that normally help repolarize the cell.

Triggered Activity

Under certain conditions, a normal action potential can abnormally "trigger" additional depolarizations that can lead to extra heart beats or rapid arrhythmias. This process may occur when the first action potential leads to oscillations of the membrane voltage known as *afterdepolarizations*. As illustrated in Figures 11.7 and 11.8 afterdepolarizations are of two types. *Early* afterdepolarizations occur during the repolarization phase of the inciting beat. *Delayed* afterdepolarizations occur shortly after repolarization has been completed. In either case, abnormal action potentials are triggered if the afterdepolarization reaches a threshold voltage. Ectopic beats due to afterdepolarizations differ from those related

to enhanced automaticity because the latter do not depend on a preceding triggering stimulus.

Early afterdepolarizations represent sudden changes of the membrane potential in the positive direction during repolarization (Fig 11.7). They can occur either during the plateau of the action potential (phase 2) or during rapid repolarization (phase 3). Early afterdepolarizations are more likely to develop in conditions that prolong the action potential duration (and therefore the electrocardiographic QT interval), as may occur during therapy with certain drugs (as described in Chapter 17).

The ionic current responsible for an early afterdepolarization depends on the membrane voltage at which the triggered event occurs. If the early afterdepolarization occurs during phase 2 (the plateau) of the action potential, when most of the Na^+ channels are in an inactivated state, the upstroke of the triggered beat relies on an inward Ca^{++} current. If, however, the early afterdepolarization occurs during phase 3 (when the membrane voltage is more negative), there is partial recovery of the fast Na^+ channels, which are then available to contribute to the current.

An early afterdepolarization-triggered action potential can be self-perpetuating and lead to a series of depolarizations (Fig. 11.7). Long sequences of early afterdepolarizations appear to be the mechanism responsible for the arrhythmia known as "torsades de pointes" discussed in the next chapter.

When **delayed afterdepolarizations** occur, they appear shortly after repolarization is complete (Fig. 11.8). They most commonly develop in states of *high intracellular calcium*, as may be present with digitalis intoxication (see Chapter 17), or during marked catecholamine stimulation. Through an incompletely understood mechanism, intracellular Ca^{++} accumulation causes the activation of certain Na^+ channels, and the resulting inward sodium current generates the delayed afterdepolarization.

As with early afterdepolarizations, if the amplitude of the delayed afterdepolarization reaches a threshold voltage, an action

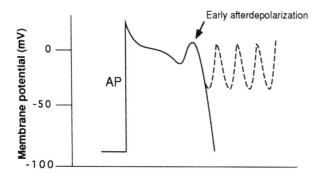

Figure 11.7. Triggered activity: An early afterdepolarization (arrow) occurs before the triggering action potential (AP) has fully repolarized. Repetitive afterdepolarizations (dashed curve) may produce a rapid sequence of triggered action potentials, and hence a tachyarrhythmia.

potential will be initiated. Such an action potential can also be self-perpetuating and lead to a series of depolarizations (i.e., a tachyarrhythmia). For example, many arrhythmias associated with digitalis toxicity are thought to be the result of delayed afterdepolarizations (described in Chapter 17).

ALTERED IMPULSE CONDUCTION

Alterations in impulse conduction may also lead to arrhythmias. The mechanisms primarily responsible for aberrant impulse conduction are: 1) conduction blocks, and 2) reentry. Conduction blocks generally lead to slow heart rates (bradyarrhythmias) and reentry to fast rhythms (tachyarrhythmias).

Conduction Block

A propagating impulse is blocked when it encounters a region of the heart that is electrically unexcitable. Conduction block can be either transient or permanent, and may be unidirectional (i.e., conduction proceeds when the involved region is stimulated from one direction, but not when stimulated from the opposite direction) or bidirectional (conduction is blocked in both directions). A variety of conditions may cause conduction block, including ischemia, fibrosis, and trauma. Conduction block may also be precipitated temporarily by certain drugs. Most commonly, conduction block occurs because a propagating impulse encounters cardiac cells that are either still refractory (from a previous depolarization) or tissue that is intrinsically unable to conduct because of fibrosis or scarring.

A blocked impulse within the specialized conducting system prevents normal propagation from the sinus node to more distal sites and thus removes the normal overdrive suppression that keeps latent pacemakers in check. Thus, conduction block anywhere along the specialized con-

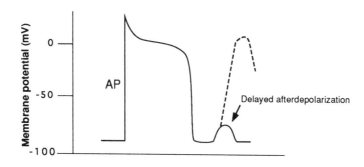

Figure 11.8. Triggered activity: A delayed afterdepolarization (arrow) arises after the triggering action potential (AP) has fully repolarized. If the delayed afterdepolarization reaches the threshold voltage, a propagated action potential is fired (dashed curve).

duction pathway usually results in escape beats or escape rhythms, as more distal sites within the conduction pathway assume the cardiac pacemaker function.

Conduction blocks between the atria and ventricles (termed AV blocks) are particularly common, and the major types of AV block are presented in the next chapter.

Reentry

A common mechanism by which altered stimulus conduction leads to tachyarrhythmias is termed **reentry**. A reentrant rhythm is caused by a self-sustaining electrical circuit that repeatedly depolarizes a region of cardiac tissue.

During normal cardiac conduction, each electrical impulse that originates in the SA node travels in an orderly fashion through the rest of the heart, and then the impulse dies out. Each region of the conduction system and myocardium depolarizes exactly once with each impulse, because cellular refractoriness prevents reactivation of tissue that was just stimulated. In contrast, Figure 11.9 illustrates the conditions by which reentry may occur. The figure depicts electrical activity as it flows through a branch point anywhere within the conduction pathways of the heart. Panel A shows propogation of a normal action potential. At point "x," the impulse reaches two parallel pathways (α and β) and travels down each into the more distal conduction tissue. Since the α and β pathways have identical conduction velocities and refractory periods, a portion of each wave front will collide in the distal conduction tissue and extinguish each other.

Panel B shows what happens if conduction is blocked in one limb of the pathway. In this example, the action potential is blocked when it encounters the β pathway from above, and therefore propagates only down the α tract into the distal tissue. As the impulse continues within the distal tissue, it will encounter the distal end of the β pathway (at point "y"). If the tissue in the distal β tract is also unable to conduct, then the impulse will simply continue to propagate

into the more distal tissue, and reentry will not occur. However, if the impulse at point "y" *is* able to propagate retrogradely (backward) into pathway β, one of the necessary conditions for reentry will be met.

When an action potential is able to pass retrogradely in a conduction pathway, whereas it had been prevented from doing so in the forward direction, **unidirectional block** is said to be present. Unidirectional block may occur in states of cellular dysfunction, in tissues with pathologic differences in the refractory periods of neighboring cells, and in contiguous fibers with functionally different electrophysiologic properties.

As shown in Figure 11.9, Panel C, if the impulse is able to propagate retrogradely up the β pathway, it will again arrive at point x. If at that time the α pathway has not yet repolarized from the previous action potential that had just occurred moments earlier, then that limb will be refractory to repeat stimulation, and the returning impulse will die out at that point.

However, in panel D, consider what happens if the velocity of retrograde conduction in the diseased β path is not normal, but *slower than normal*. In that case, sufficient time may have elapsed for the α pathway to repolarize before the returning impulse reaches point x from the β limb. Then, the impulse is free to stimulate the α pathway once again, and the cycle repeats itself. This circular action can continue indefinitely, and each pass of the impulse through the loop excites cells of the distal conduction tissue, which propagates to the rest of the myocardium, resulting in various tachyarrhythmias.

The slowed conduction demonstrated in panel D is usually, but not always, a requirement for the development of a reentrant circuit. That is, in order for reentry to occur, the propogating impulse must continuously encounter excitable tissue. Thus, the time it takes for the impulse to travel around the reentrant loop must be greater than the refractory period of the tissue to be restimulated (pathway α in this example). If the loop conduction time is shorter, the impulse will encounter refractory tissue and

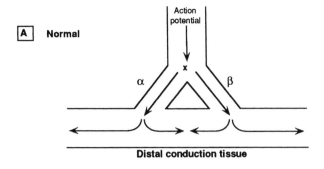

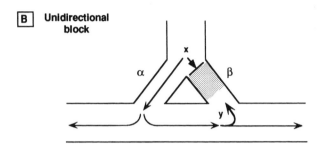

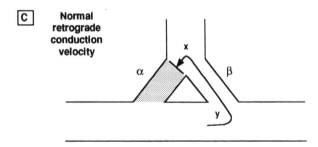

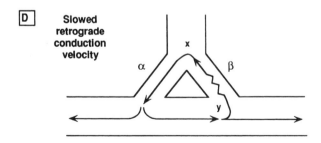

Figure 11.9.   Mechanism of reentry. A. Normal conduction. When an action potential (AP) reaches a division in the conduction pathway (point x), the impulse travels down both fibers α and β to excite distal conduction tissue. **B.** Unidirectional block. Forward passage of the impulse is blocked in the β pathway, but proceeds normally down the α pathway. When the impulse reaches point y, if retrograde conduction of the β pathway is intact, the AP can enter β from below, and conduct in a retrograde fashion. **C.** When point x is reached, if the α pathway has not had sufficient time to repolarize, then the impulse dies out. **D.** However, if conduction through the retrograde pathway is abnormally slow (jagged line), it reaches point x after the α pathway has completed repolarization. Thus the impulse is free to excite pathway α again, and a reentrant loop is formed.

die out. Since normal conduction velocity is approximately 50 cm/sec, and the average effective refractory period is about 200 msec, the circuit would need to be at least 10 cm long in order for reentry to occur. Most clinical occurences of reentry occur within much smaller regions of tissue. Therefore, slowing of the conduction velocity within the reentrant loop, as described in this example, is usually necessary in order to sustain the aberrant rhythm.

In practice, a region of cardiac tissue may

develop reentry if two main conditions are met: 1) unidirectional block, and 2) slowed conduction through the loop of tissue. These conditions may exist if neighboring cells display different conduction velocities and refractory periods. This may occur, for example, in the AV node of an otherwise normal heart (see next chapter), in the presence of an anatomic **bypass tract** (see below), or within diseased cardiac tissue. Ischemic myocardium, for example, provides a nidus for reentry because such tissue is a mosaic of nonexcitable and partially excitable zones.

Bypass Tracts

In the normal heart, the impulse generated by the SA node propagates through atrial tissue to the AV node, where there is a short delay before continuing on to the ventricular conducting system. In some individuals, this is not the only available conduction tract from the atria to the ventricles. Rather, there is an additional "accessory" pathway that bypasses the AV node (hence the term "bypass tract"). The most common accessory pathway is called the bundle of Kent, which consists of a normal band of myocardium (similar electrically to atrial tissue) that is abnormally positioned such that it connects atrial to ventricular myocardium, as shown in Figure 11.10. Because accessory tract tissue conducts impulses rapidly, the conduction delay that normally occurs at the AV node does not take place, stimulation of the ventricles occurs earlier than normal, and therefore the PR interval of the EKG is *shortened* (usually to less than 0.12 seconds (i.e., <3 small boxes)). Furthermore, ventricular depolarization in such individuals represents the combination of conduction via the accessory tract and that over the normal conducting system. This results in a *wider than normal* QRS complex on the EKG, with an *earlier than normal* upstroke, known as the "delta wave" (Fig. 11.10).

In the presence of a bypass tract, a large anatomic loop may be created, with the abnormal tract serving as one limb and the normal conduction pathway through the AV node as the other. Because the conduction velocity and refractory period of the bypass tract are usually different from those

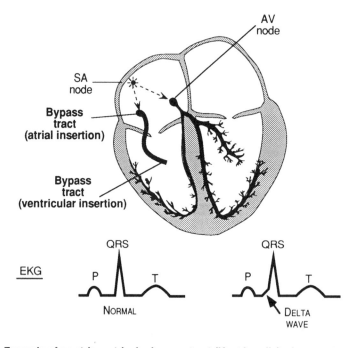

Figure 11.10.   Example of an atrioventricular bypass tract (Kent bundle), shown schematically, which can conduct impulses from the atrium directly to the ventricles, bypassing the AV node. The EKG demonstrates a shortened PR interval and "delta" wave, due to early excitation of the ventricles through the bypass tract.

of the normal conduction pathway, an appropriately timed stimulus may set the stage for reentrant rhythms, as described in the next chapter.

The mechanisms of altered impulse formation and conduction are the basis of all common arrhythmias, which can be divided into two groups: abnormally slow rhythms (bradyarrhythmias) and those that are abnormally fast (tachyarrhythmias). Table 11.1 lists the underlying mechanisms, with examples of their commonly associated arrhythmias (discussed in the next chapter).

APPROACH TO ANTIARRHYTHMIC TREATMENT

The treatment of arrhythmias is aimed at correcting the basic mechanisms of altered impulse formation and conduction. This section summarizes the common modalities of antiarrhythmic therapy, and the next chapter describes how these are used to treat specific rhythm disorders.

Bradyarrhythmias

Treatment of slow heart rhythms includes pharmacologic therapy and electronic pacemakers.

Pharmacologic Therapy

Pharmacologic therapies modify the autonomic input to the heart:

1. Anticholinergic drugs: Vagal stimulation reduces the heart rate and decreases conduction through the AV node through the release of acetylcholine onto muscarinic receptors. Anticholinergic drugs, such as atropine, block the vagal effect, and thus increase the heart rate and enhance AV nodal conduction.
2. β_1-receptor agonists mimic the effect of endogenous catecholamines, which increase heart rate and speed AV nodal conduction. An example of this class is isoproterenol.

Atropine and isoproterenol are administered intravenously. Though useful in treat-

---

TABLE 11.1. Mechanisms of Arrhythmia Development

Abnormality	Mechanism	Examples (described in next chapter)
Bradyarrhythmias		
Altered impulse formation		
• Decreased automaticity	Decreased phase 4 depolarization (e.g., cholinergic stimulation)	Sinus bradycardia
Altered impulse conduction		
• Conduction blocks	Ischemic, anatomic, or drug-induced impaired conduction	1°, 2°, 3° AV blocks
Tachyarrythmias		
Altered impulse formation		
• Enhanced automaticity		
Sinus node	Increased phase 4 depolarization (e.g. sympathetic stimulation)	Sinus tachycardia
Ectopic focus	Acquires phase 4 depolarization	Ectopic atrial tachycardia
• Triggered activity		
Early afterdepolarization	Prolonged action potential duration	Torsades de pointes
Delayed afterdepolarization	Intracellular calcium overload (e.g., digitalis toxicity)	APBs, VPBs, digitalis-induced SVTs
Altered impulse conduction		
• Reentry	Unidirectional block plus slowed conduction	Paroxysmal SVTs, atrial flutter and fibrillation, ventricular tachycardia and fibrillation

APB, atrial premature beat; VPB, ventricular premature beat; SVT, supraventricular tachycardia

ing certain slow heart rhythm disorders acutely, these agents cannot be administered over the long term for persistent bradyarrhythmias.

Electronic Pacemakers

Electronic pacemakers are devices that apply repeated electrical stimulation to the heart, thereby assuming control of an otherwise slow cardiac rhythm. Pacemakers may be installed on a temporary or a permanent basis. Temporary units are used to stabilize patients who are awaiting implantation of a permanent pacemaker, or to treat transient bradyarrhythmias. For example, a bradyarrhythmia brought on by drug toxicity requires pacing only until the drug effect resolves.

There are two types of temporary pacemakers. The first uses **transthoracic** stimulation. That is, through wire electrodes, a current is applied *externally* to the patient's chest, which indirectly stimulates the heart. As you might imagine, this technique can be quite uncomfortable, as it also stimulates contraction of the thoracic muscles. Nonetheless, in an emergency, this form of pacing can be applied rapidly. The other option for temporary pacing is a **transvenous** device, in which an electrode-tipped catheter is passed into the heart through a peripheral vein, and connected to an external power source. This type of pacemaker is effective for several days; but after 48 to 72 hours the risk of infection and thrombosis increases.

Permanent pacemakers are more sophisticated than the temporary variety. Different configurations can sense and capture the electrical activity of the atria and/or ventricles. The electrodes are generally passed transvenously into the right-sided cardiac chambers. The power source, not much larger than a silver dollar, is implanted under the skin, and typically lasts 5–15 years. Modern permanent pacemakers are programmable, in that their modes of action can be altered noninvasively via transcutaneous radio signals that are received by onboard circuits in the implanted generator.

Tachyarrhythmias

The treatment of tachyarrhythmias is directed at the specific mechanism responsible for the abnormal rhythm. Pharmacologic agents and cardioversion/defibrillation are the most commonly used therapies, but innovative electrical devices and transvenous catheter-based techniques are revolutionizing the chronic treatment of these disorders.

Pharmacologic Therapy

Pharmacologic management of tachyarrhythmias attacks the abnormal mechanisms responsible for their formation: abnormal automaticity, reentrant circuits, or triggered activity. Many antiarrhythmic drugs are available, the pharmacology and actions of which are addressed in Chapter 17. The choice of drug relies on an understanding of the cause of the specific arrhythmia. From the mechanisms presented in this chapter, the following strategies emerge:

To eliminate rhythms due to *increased automaticity*, desired drug effects include the following:

1. To reduce the slope of phase 4 spontaneous depolarization of the automatic cells
2. To make the diastolic potential more negative
3. To make the threshold potential less negative

By altering the diastolic and/or threshold potentials, or slowing the rate of spontaneous diastolic depolarization, the firing rate of ectopic pacemakers can be inhibited.

To interrupt *reentrant circuits*, desired antiarrhythmic effects include the following:

1. Decrease cellular conduction velocity, such that impulse propagation within the slowly conducting limb of the circuit becomes even slower and eventually dies out, aborting the reentrant rhythm
2. Increase the refractory period within the reentrant circuit so that a propagating

impulse finds tissue within the loop un-excitable, and the impulse dies out

To eliminate *triggered activity,* desired antiarrhythmic drug effects include the following:

1. Shorten the action potential duration (to prevent early afterdepolarizations)
2. Correct conditions of calcium overload (to prevent delayed afterdepolarizations)

For each of the tachyarrhythmia mechanisms, the treatment goals can be achieved by antiarrhythmic drugs that modulate the action potential through interactions with ion channels, surface receptors, and transport pumps. Please look through the antiarrhythmic drug section of Chapter 17 at this time, to familiarize yourself with the general mechanisms of action, and names of the antiarrhythmic drugs.

Vagal Maneuvers

A useful bedside technique that is frequently employed to arrest certain reentrant tachyarrhythmias is **carotid sinus massage**. Located at the bifurcation of the internal and external carotid arteries on either side of the neck, the carotid sinuses respond to stimulation (such as rubbing one of them firmly in a circular fashion for 3–5 secs) by enhancing CNS parasympathetic outflow and inhibiting sympathetic activity. The result is a decrease in the sinus node rate of discharge, as well as slowing of AV nodal conduction. The latter may interrupt rhythms in which the AV node is a part of a reentrant circuit. Vagal discharge can also be stimulated by instructing the patient to perform the Valsalva maneuver (straining against a closed glottis), or by dunking the face in a tub of ice water (the "diving reflex").

Antitachycardia Pacemakers

Reentrant supraventricular tachyarrhythmias can in some cases be terminated by rapid stimulation of the atria by a temporary artificial pacemaker. The idea is to electrically capture and depolarize a portion of a reentrant circuit, thus rendering it refractory to further immediate depolarization. Consequently, when a reentrant impulse returns to the zone already stimulated by the pacemaker, it encounters unexcitable tissue. The impulse cannot propagate further, breaking the reentrant circuit.

Electrical Cardioversion

Cardioversion and defibrillation are similar techniques used in the treatment of some tachycardias, in which an electrical current is momentarily discharged across the chest in order to simultaneously depolarize the bulk of the myocardial tissue. This allows the sinus node (the site of fastest spontaneous discharge) to regain pacemaker control. Tachyarrhythmias that are due to reentry will likely terminate by this procedure, whereas those associated with enhanced automaticity may not be stopped, if the responsible ectopic focus continues to discharge at a rate faster than the SA node.

Cardioversion is performed by briefly sedating the patient, then placing two electrode paddles against the chest on either side of the heart. The electrical discharge is electronically *synchronized* to fire at the time of a QRS complex (i.e., when ventricular depolarization occurs). This prevents the possibility of discharge during the relative refractory period of the ventricle, which could induce ventricular fibrillation.

Defibrillation is performed in emergency situations for ventricular fibrillation (described in the next chapter). Unlike cardioversion, in this technique the electrical discharge is *not synchronized* to the QRS complex, because the latter is not discernible. An increasingly common procedure for the treatment of recurrent ventricular fibrillation, in selected patients, is to implant a small defibrillator into the body (known as an implantable cardioverter-defibrillator, or ICD), which automatically detects ventricular tachycardia or fibrillation and fires an electrical discharge to abort the

rhythm. Modern versions of this sophisticated device are also capable of performing
antitachycardic pacing functions, that may
revert ventricular tachycardia without producing a painful electric shock.

Ablative Therapy

For patients with recurrent supraventricular or ventricular arrhythmias, it is possible, through **electrophysiologic mapping**
techniques, to localize the region of myocardium or conduction tissue responsible
for the disturbance. It is then often possible
to ablate crucial elements of reentrant circuits, as well as foci of ectopic arrhythmias,
via transvenous catheter techniques. Such
procedures have revolutionized the management of patients with many types of
supraventricular tachycardias, as they offer
a permanent therapeutic solution that
spares individuals the need for chronic antiarrhythmic drugs.

SUMMARY

1. Arrhythmias result from disorders of impulse formation, impulse conduction, or
both.
2. Bradyarrhythmias develop because of
decreased impulse formation (e.g., sinus
bradycardia), or decreased impulse
conduction (e.g., AV nodal conduction
blocks).
3. Tachyarrhythmias result from: 1) increased automaticity (of the SA node, latent pacemakers, or abnormal myocardial sites), 2) triggered activity, or 3)
reentrant pathways.
4. Bradyarrhythmias are usually treated by
drugs that accelerate the rate of sinus
node discharge and enhance AV nodal
conduction (atropine, isoproterenol) or
electronic pacemakers.
5. Tachyarrhythmias respond to pharmacologic therapy directed at the mechanism
of arrhythmia formation. For refractory
tachyarrhythmias, or in emergency situations, electrical cardioversion/defibrilla-
tion is employed. Catheter-based ablative
techniques are becoming a popular
method for long-term control of certain
tachyarrhythmias.

The next chapter summarizes the recognition and treatment of the most common
arrhythmias. Additional reading suggestions are listed at the end of that chapter.
Chapter 17 describes currently available antiarrhythmic drugs.

*Acknowledgments.   The previous edition of this
chapter was written by Wendy Armstrong, MD,
Nicholas Boulis, MD, Elliott M. Antman, MD, and
Leonard S. Lilly, MD.*

Diagnosis of Cardiac Arrhythmias

Chapter 12

Marc S. Sabatine, Elliott M. Antman,
Leonard I. Ganz, and Leonard S. Lilly

Bradyarrhythmias
  SA Node
  Escape Rhythms
  Atrioventricular Node

Tachyarrhythmias
  Supraventricular Arrhythmias
  Ventricular Arrhythmias
  Differentiation of Wide Complex Tachycardias

The previous chapter presented the mechanisms by which abnormal heart rhythms develop. The purpose of this chapter is to describe how to recognize and treat specific common arrhythmias. Table 12.1 categorizes the rhythm disorders considered in this chapter.

There are five basic questions to consider when confronted with a patient with an abnormal heart rhythm, as detailed in the sections that follow:

1. Definition: What is the arrhythmia?
2. Pathogenesis: What is the basic mechanism that causes it?
3. Cause: What underlying conditions provoke it?
4. Clinical Presentation: What symptoms and signs accompany the arrhythmia?
5. Treatment: What to do about it?

BRADYARRHYTHMIAS

Bradyarrhythmias are abnormal rhythms in which the heart rate is < 60 bpm. They arise from disorders of impulse formation or impaired impulse conduction (conduction pathway blocks).

SA Node

Sinus Bradycardia

Sinus bradycardia (Fig. 12.1) is simply a slowing of the normal heart rhythm as a re-

sult of decreased firing of the SA node, to a rate below 60 bpm. Trained athletes and normal elderly individuals at rest may have perfectly benign sinus bradycardia. Therefore, it is incumbent on the physician to decide whether bradycardia in a particular patient is appropriate or pathologic. This decision can be made on the basis of a patient's age, underlying heart disease, and whether the heart rate increases appropriately in response to exercise.

Sinus bradycardia can result from either abnormally high vagal tone or decreased intrinsic automaticity of the SA node. It can occur physiologically (e.g., well-trained athletes, elderly individuals), pharmacologically (e.g., therapy with β-blockers, verapamil or diltiazem), or pathologically (e.g., hypothermia or hypothyroidism).

Sinus bradycardia is usually asymptomatic, but a pronounced reduction of the heart rate can lead to fatigue and syncope. Treatment is necessary only if the patient is symptomatic. If so, acute therapy with intravenous anticholinergic drugs (e.g., atropine) or β-adrenergic agents (e.g., isoproterenol) may speed the rate transiently. Permanent pacemakers are implanted for chronic symptomatic bradycardia.

Sick Sinus Syndrome

When SA node function is disturbed, its rate of impulse formation may become markedly variable and a condition known

TABLE 12.1. Common Arrhythmias

Location	Bradyarrhythmias	Tachyarrhythmias
SA node	Sinus bradycardia Sick sinus syndrome	Sinus tachycardia
Atria		Atrial premature beats Atrial flutter Atrial fibrillation Paroxysmal supraventricular tachycardias (reentrant and nonreentrant) Multifocal atrial tachycardia
AV node	Conduction blocks (1°, 2°, 3°) Junctional escape rhythm	Paroxysmal reentrant tachycardias (AV or AV nodal)
Ventricles	Ventricular escape rhythm	Ventricular premature beats Ventricular tachycardia Torsades de pointes Ventricular fibrillation

as sick sinus syndrome (SSS) develops (Fig. 12.2). In this situation, paroxysmal dizziness, confusion, or syncope results from intermittent reduction of cardiac output related to periods of excessive bradycardia and/or tachycardia.

A common form of SSS is called the *bradycardia-tachycardia syndrome,* generally seen in elderly individuals, in which periods of sinus node slowing transiently follow atrial tachyarrhythmias such as atrial flutter or fibrillation. Treatment generally requires the combination of antiarrhythmic drug therapy to suppress the tachyarrhythmias, and a permanent pacemaker to prevent symptomatic bradyarrhythmias.

Escape Rhythms

Suppression of SA node activity or blockade within the conduction pathway can lead to escape rhythms by more distal latent pacemakers. **Junctional escape beats** (Fig.

12.3) arise at the junction of the AV node and the bundle of His. They are characterized by a normal, narrow QRS complex that occurs at a rate of 40–60 bpm. The QRS complexes are not preceded by normal P waves because the impulse originates below the atria. However, *retrograde P waves* may sometimes be observed because of stimulation of the atria from the more distal portion of the conducting system. Retrograde P waves typically *follow* the QRS complex and are *inverted* (negative deflection on the EKG) in limb leads II, III, and aV$_F$ indicative of activation of the atria from below.

Ventricular escape beats are characterized by even slower rates (30–40 bpm) and a widened QRS complex, because such impulses are conducted outside of the normal, rapidly propagating Purkinje fibers.

Junctional and ventricular escape rhythms serve as protective mechanisms that maintain a heart rate during periods of decreased sinus node firing or atrioventricular conduction blocks. The major clinical finding is a slow pulse rate, sometimes with

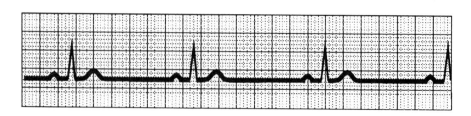

Figure 12.1. Sinus bradycardia. The P wave and QRS complexes are normal, but the rate is < 60 bpm.

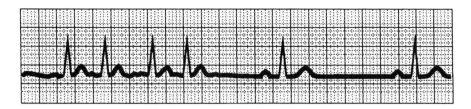

Figure 12.2.   Sick sinus syndrome. A brief irregular tachycardia is followed by slow sinus node discharge.

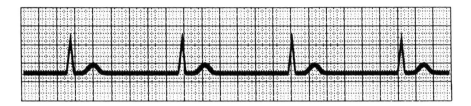

Figure 12.3.   Junctional escape rhythm. Normal-width QRS complexes at a slow, constant rate are not preceded by P waves.

symptoms of low cardiac output, such as lightheadedness or syncope. Treatment of symptomatic individuals includes intravenous atropine acutely and, if persistent, an electronic pacemaker.

Atrioventricular Node

There are three "degrees" (types) of **conduction block** that can occur between the atria and ventricles.

First-Degree AV Block

First-degree AV block (1° AV block), shown in Figure 12.4, indicates prolongation of the normal delay between atrial and ventricular depolarization, such that the P-R interval is > 0.2 sec (> 5 small boxes on the standard EKG recording). This abnormality is caused either by a transient influence or by structural defects of the conduction pathway, usually at the AV node. *Reversible* causes include heightened vagal tone, transient AV nodal ischemia, and the effects of digitalis glycosides, β-blockers, and Ca^{++} channel antagonists. *Structural* causes of 1° AV block include myocardial infarction and chronic degenerative diseases of the conduction system. Generally, 1° AV block is a

benign, asymptomatic condition that does not require treatment.

Second-Degree AV Block

Second-degree AV block is characterized by *intermittent* failure of AV conduction, such that not every P wave is followed by a QRS complex. It can take one of two forms: in **Mobitz Type I** block (also termed **Wenckebach** block) shown in Figure 12.5, the conduction defect becomes progressively more pronounced with each beat until an impulse is completely blocked, such that ventricular stimulation does not follow a P wave for a single beat. The EKG shows a progressive increase in the P-R interval from one beat to the next until a single QRS complex is absent, and then the cycle starts anew. The AV node (rather than the bundle of His) is almost always the site of this form of block. It is usually benign and may be seen in children, trained athletes, and individuals with increased vagal tone. It may also develop during an acute inferior wall MI, because of vagal stimulation, but is usually transient. Treatment is typically not necessary, but in symptomatic cases, this rhythm responds to atropine.

Mobitz Type II block is a more ominous form of second-degree AV block. In this

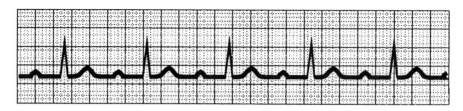

Figure 12.4. First-degree AV block. The PR interval is prolonged.

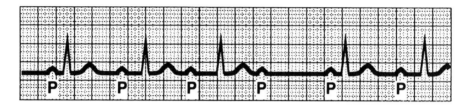

Figure 12.5. Second-degree AV block: Möbitz I (Wenckebach). The P-wave rate is constant, but the PR interval progressively lengthens, until a QRS is completely blocked (after 4th P wave).

case, AV conduction intermittently ceases unexpectedly, without the warning of progressive PR prolongation in previous beats (Fig. 12.6). The block may persist for two or more beats (i.e., two sequential P waves not followed by QRS complexes), in which case it is known as **high-grade** AV block (Fig. 12.7). Although Type II second-degree block may originate in the AV node, it usually indicates disease more distally in the His-Purkinje system. As a result, the QRS complexes may be abnormally wide, simulating right or left bundle branch block. This type of block may arise from extensive infarction or chronic degeneration of the conduction pathway. Because the underlying disease associated with Type II block tends to be severe, the rhythm may progress to third-degree block without warning. Treatment of Type II block with a pacemaker is

therefore necessary, even in asymptomatic patients.

Third-Degree AV Block

Third-degree AV block (Fig. 12.8) occurs when there is complete failure of conduction between the atria and ventricles. In adults, the most common causes of complete block are acute MI, drug toxicity (especially digitalis), and chronic degeneration of the conduction pathway. Third-degree AV block divides the heart into two unconnected zones: There is no relationship between the P waves and QRS complexes, as the atria depolarize in response to SA node activity, while an escape rhythm drives the ventricles independently, at an intrinsic rate of 30 to 55 bpm. As a result of the slow

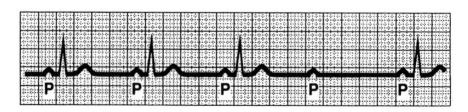

Figure 12.6. Second-degree AV block: Möbitz II. A QRS complex is blocked (after the 4th P wave), without gradual lenghthening of the preceeding PR intervals.

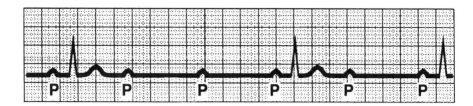

Figure 12.7. High-grade AV block: Sequential QRS complexes are blocked (after the 2nd and 3rd P waves).

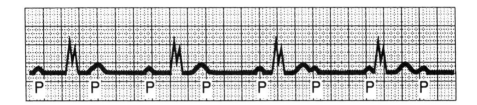

Figure 12.8. Third-degree AV block. The P wave and QRS rhythms are independent of one another. The QRS complexes are widened as they originate within the distal ventricular conduction system, not at the bundle of His. The second and fourth P waves are superimposed on normal T waves.

rate, lightheadedness or syncope may occur. Permanent pacemaker therapy is almost always necessary.

The term **atrioventricular dissociation (AV dissociation)** refers to any situation in which the atria and ventricles are activated and beat independently, without any direct relationship between P waves and QRS complexes. Third-degree AV block is one example of AV dissociation.

TACHYARRHYTHMIAS

Whenever the heart rate is > 100 bpm for three beats or more, a tachyarrhythmia is said to be present. Recall from the previous chapter that tachyarrhythmias result from mechanisms that cause an increased firing rate. Increased firing may be due to: 1) enhanced cellular automaticity, 2) triggered activity, or 3) reentry. Tachyarrhythmias are categorized into those that arise *above* (supraventricular) and those that arise *within* the ventricles, and can usually be differentiated by the width of the QRS complex, the morphology and rate of the P waves, the relationship between the P waves and the QRS complexes, and the re-

sponse of the rhythm to vagal maneuvers such as carotid sinus massage (Fig. 12.9).

Supraventricular Arrhythmias

Sinus Tachycardia

Sinus tachycardia (ST) is characterized by an SA node discharge rate of 100 to 180 bpm, and normal P waves and QRS complexes (Fig. 12.10). This rhythm most often arises from increased sympathetic stimulation of the SA node, with resultant enhanced automaticity. For example, sinus tachycardia is a normal physiologic response to exercise. However, sympathetic stimulation may also result from pathologic conditions, including fever, hyperthyroidism, and hypoxemia. Because the increased rate is usually a response to stimuli external to the heart, the treatment of sinus tachycardia is directed at the underlying cause.

Atrial Premature Beats

Atrial premature beats (APBs) are common in healthy, as well as diseased hearts

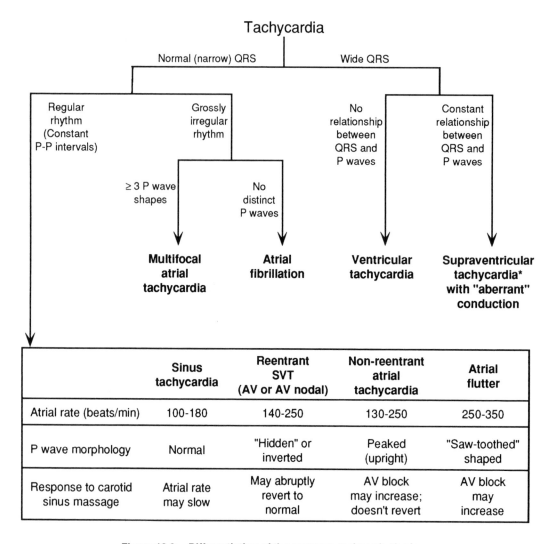

Figure 12.9.   Differentiation of the common tachyarrhythmias.

(Fig. 12.11), and they are caused by the same conditions that result in sinus tachycardia. They are usually asymptomatic, but occasionally a sensation of palpitation accompanies them. An APB appears as an earlier-than-expected P wave with an *abnormal shape* (the impulse doesn't arise from the SA node, such that conduction through the atria is abnormal), followed by a normal QRS, as ventricular conduction is not impaired. Note that if the abnormal focus fires very quickly after the previous beat, the impulse may encounter an AV node still refractory to excitation, and ventricular depolarization does not occur. This would appear as a premature P wave with abnormal morphology *not* followed by a QRS complex (termed a "blocked" APB). Similarly, if the ectopic focus fires just a bit later in diastole, it may encounter portions of the His-Purkinje system still in their refractory periods, and the impulse is then conducted through those territories and to the ventricles in a slower than normal rate, resulting in a QRS that is aberrantly widened.

Treatment is required only if APBs are symptomatic. Because caffeine ingestion, alcohol, and adrenergic stimulation (e.g., emotional stress) all predispose to APB formation, it is important to reduce these exposures. β-blockers (class II antiarrhyth-

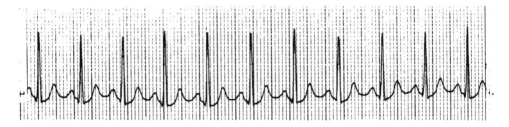

Figure 12.10. Sinus tachycardia. The P wave and QRS complexes are normal, but the rate is > 100 bpm.

mics) are the preferred pharmacologic treatment, if needed.

Atrial Flutter

Atrial flutter is characterized by rapid, coarse "sawtooth" appearing atrial activity, at a rate of 250 to 350 bpm (Fig. 12.12). Many of these fast impulses reach the AV node during its refractory period, so that the ventricular rate is generally lower, and often in an even fraction of the atrial rate. Thus, if the atrial rate is 300 bpm, and 2:1 block occurs at the AV node (i.e., each alternate atrial impulse finds the AV node refractory), then the ventricular rate would be 150 bpm. Because vagal maneuvers (e.g., carotid sinus massage) decrease AV nodal conduction, that technique is often useful for temporarily slowing the ventricular rate, allowing better visualization of the underlying atrial activity. Reentry within the right atrium appears to be the mechanism that underlies most instances of atrial flutter.

Atrial flutter generally occurs in individuals with preexisting heart disease. It may be paroxysmal and transient, or persistent, lasting for weeks or longer. Frequently, it degenerates into atrial fibrillation. Atrial flutter may paradoxically become more dangerous if the atrial rate *slows* somewhat, either spontaneously or due to pharmacologic intervention, to a rate that allows the AV node more time to recover between impulses. In that situation, the AV node may begin to conduct in a 1:1 fashion, producing very rapid ventricular rates. For example, consider a patient with atrial flutter at an atrial rate of 280 bpm with 2:1 conduction block at the AV node. The ventricular rate in this circumstance would be 140 bpm. If the atrial rate slows to 220 bpm, then the AV node may be able to recover sufficiently between depolarizations to conduct in a 1:1 fashion—that is, the ventricular rate *accelerates* to 220 bpm. In individuals with limited cardiac reserve, this acceleration may result in a profound reduction of cardiac output and hypotension.

There are several approaches to the treatment of atrial flutter:

1. The most expiditious therapy is electrical cardioversion, which is undertaken directly for highly symptomatic patients. This technique is also used to revert chronic refractory atrial flutter that has not responded to other approaches.
2. Rapid atrial stimulation by a temporary

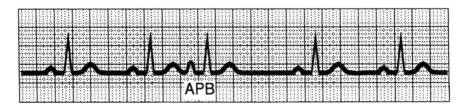

Figure 12.11. Atrial premature beat (APB). The P wave occurs earlier than expected, and its shape is abnormal.

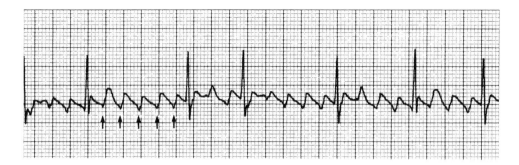

Figure 12.12. Atrial flutter is typified by rapid "saw-toothed" atrial activity (arrows).

artificial pacemaker is sometimes used to capture the atrial rhythm (see Chapter 11) and break the reentrant circuit. This procedure can be undertaken, for example, in patients who develop atrial flutter soon after open heart surgery, using temporary pacing wires that are implanted routinely at the time of operation.

3. For patients without the immediate need for cardioversion, pharmacologic therapy is begun: First, the ventricular rate is slowed by drugs that increase AV block (beta-blockers, calcium channel blockers (i.e., verapamil, diltiazem), or digoxin). Once the rate is effectively slowed, attempts are made to convert back to sinus rhythm using drugs from specific antiarrhythmic classes (IA, IC or III, described in Chapter 17). Should such drugs fail to convert the rhythm, elective electrical cardioversion is ultimately undertaken. Once sinus rhythm has been restored, antiarrhythmic drugs (class IA, IC or III) are then administered on a chronic basis to prevent recurrences.

4. In some patients with recurrent atrial flutter, it is possible to localize, and ab-

late (via transvenous catheter techniques), the responsible reentrant loop within the right atrium, thereby preventing additional episodes.

Atrial Fibrillation

Atrial fibrillation (AF) is a chaotic rhythm that results in an atrial rate of 350 to 600 discharges/min, so that discrete atrial P waves are not discernible on the EKG (Fig. 12.13). Like atrial flutter, the high rate of impulse bombardment frequently encounters refractory tissue at the AV node, so that only some of the depolarizations are conveyed to the ventricles, in a very irregular fashion; the average ventricular rate in untreated AF is about 160 bpm. Because discrete P waves are not visible on the EKG, the baseline shows low amplitude undulations punctuated by QRS complexes and T waves.

The mechanism of atrial fibrillation appears to involve multiple micro-reentrant circuits within the atria, and it is common to observe the rhythm repetitively shift be-

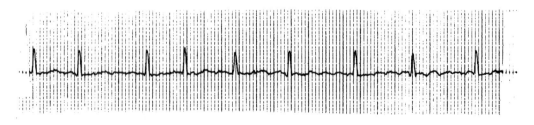

Figure 12.13. Atrial fibrillation is characterized by chaotic atrial activity without organized P waves, and irregularity of the ventricular (QRS) rate.

tween fibrillation and atrial flutter. AF may occur in an otherwise normal individual, but is most often precipitated either by right or left atrial enlargement (e.g., from mitral stenosis or regurgitation). AF is also common in patients with hypertension, coronary artery disease, thyrotoxicosis, or pulmonary embolism.

AF is potentially dangerous for two reasons: 1) rapid ventricular rates may compromise cardiac output, resulting in hypotension and pulmonary congestion, particularly in individuals with hypertrophied or "stiff" left ventricles in whom normal organized atrial contraction contributes significantly to left ventricular filling, and 2) the absence of organized atrial contraction results in blood stasis in the atria, leading to possible thrombus formation. Individuals who remain in chronic AF are therefore at increased risk of thromboemboli, including stroke, and should receive long-term anticoagulation therapy.

Antiarrhythmic drug treatment of chronic AF is similar to that of atrial flutter. β-blockers or Ca^{++} channel antagonists (diltiazem, verapamil) are administered to promote block at the AV node, to reduce the ventricular rate. Digitalis preparations are less effective and do not act as quickly. For patients who remain symptomatic despite adequate rate control of AF, conversion back to sinus rhythm is attempted (after several weeks of anticoagulant therapy), by drugs of the class IA, IC or III antiarrhythmic groups (see Chapter 17). If chemical conversion does not succeed, electrical cardioversion can be undertaken. Once successfully converted to sinus rhythm, antiar-

rhythmic drugs are often continued in order to prevent recurrences.

Because of potentially serious, sometimes lethal, side effects of antiarrhythmic drugs (as described in Chapter 17), it is common to avoid their use in patients with chronic AF who are rendered asymptomatic with rate control agents, and instead to continue the rate control drug and anticoagulation therapy (i.e., warfarin) indefinitely.

Paroxysmal Supraventricular Tachycardias (PSVTs)

Paroxysmal supraventricular tachycardias (Fig. 12.14) are manifest by: 1) sudden onset and termination, 2) atrial rates of 140 to 250 bpm, 3) and narrow (normal) QRS complexes (unless "aberrant conduction" is present, as described below). The mechanism of PSVT is most often reentry, while enhanced automaticity and triggered activity are less often the cause.

Reentrant tachycardias. Reentry is the cause of PSVT more than 90% of the time, with the reentrant circuit involving the AV node, the SA node, or atrial muscle. A special form of reentrant PSVT loops through an accessory bypass tract, as discussed below.

AV nodal reentrant tachycardia (AVNRT) is a common form of PSVT. In most patients with AVNRT, the AV node is composed of two functionally distinct pathways, designated the slow (or "α") pathway and the fast (or "β") pathway (Fig. 12.15). The fast pathway has a rapid conduction velocity but a

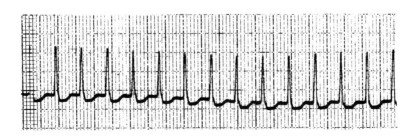

Figure 12.14. Paroxysmal supraventricular tachycardia (originating at the AV nodal junction). Retrograde P waves in this example occur simultaneously with, and are "hidden" in, the QRS complexes.

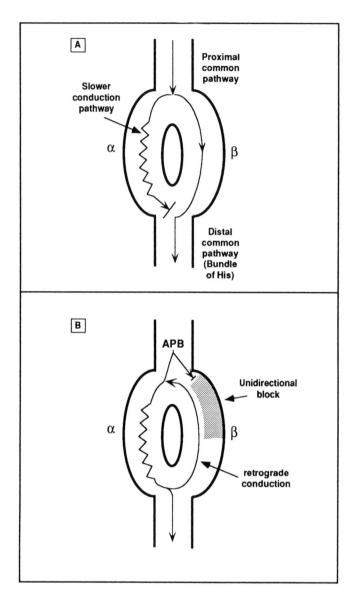

Figure 12.15. Common mechanism of AV nodal reentry. A. In patients with AV nodal reentry, two functionally distinct tracts exist within the AV node (termed α and β). The α pathway conducts slowly and has a short refractory period, whereas the β pathway conducts more rapidly but has a long refractory period. Impulses from above conduct down both pathways; because the β impulse reaches the distal common pathway first, it continues to the bundle of His. Conversely, the α pathway impulse arrives later and encounters refractory tissue. **B.** A premature beat (APB) arrives at the entrance of the two pathways; the β pathway is still refractory, but the α pathway has repolarized and is able to conduct. When the impulse reaches the distal portion of the β pathway after traveling down the α fiber, β has repolarized and is able to conduct the impulse in a retrograde direction (unidirectional block). A reentrant loop is initiated.

relatively long refractory period. The slow pathway has a less rapid conduction velocity but a shorter refractory period. Thus, although the β pathway conducts quickly, it takes longer to recover between impulses than the α pathway. This difference in elec-trical characteristics of the two pathways is one of the fundamental requirements for reenty to occur in AVNRT.

Normally, a stimulus arriving at the AV node travels down both pathways, but the impulse traveling down the faster β pathway reaches the bundle of His first. By the time the impulse traversing the slower α limb reaches the distal part of that pathway, it encounters refractory tissue, and is extinguished. Thus under normal conditions, only the β pathway impulse makes its way to the bundle of His and ventricles.

However, following an atrial premature beat (APB), the situation may be different. The fast pathway, because of its long refractory period, may be temporarily unexcitable, and cannot conduct the premature impulse. The slow pathway, on the other hand, has already repolarized (remember, it has a shorter refractory period). The APB is able to travel down the slow pathway and, by the time it reaches the bundle of His, the fast pathway *has* had time to repolarize and is no longer refractory (i.e., the fast pathway exhibits unidirectional block while the slow pathway demonstrates slowed conduction—the conditions for reentry). Thus the impulse not only continues to travel distally through the bundle of His into the ventricles, but also returns *retrogradely* up the now excitable fast β pathway. Upon reaching the top of the β pathway, the impulse is free to reenter the slow α pathway, and a sustained "endless loop" reentrant rhythm within the AV node occurs.

On the EKG, P waves may not be apparent in AVNRT, because any retrograde atrial depolarization typically occurs simultaneously with ventricular depolarization. Therefore, the P wave is "hidden" in the QRS complex. When P waves *are* visualized, they are superimposed on the terminal portion of the QRS complex and are inverted (upside down) in limb leads II, III, and aV_F because of the caudocranial direction of activation.

AV nodal reentrant tachyarrhythmias show no predisposition to specific age groups, but are better tolerated among the young, who may simply sense rapid palpitations during an episode. In elderly patients, or those with underlying heart disease, more severe symptoms may result, such as syncope, angina, or pulmonary edema.

Many treatment options exist. Vagal maneuvers, such as carotid sinus massage, may abruptly terminate the arrhythmia by increasing parasympathetic input to the AV node, slowing and eventually blocking AV conduction, thereby breaking the reentrant circuit. The most rapidly effective pharmacologic therapy is intravenous adenosine (see Chapter 17). Other drug options include intravenous calcium channel antagonists (especially verapamil and diltiazem) or β-blockers, each of which slows conduction and blocks the reentrant circuit in the AV node. Digitalis also slows conduction through the AV node, but is less useful in treating an acute episode of PSVT because of its slow onset of action.

Long-term suppression of AVNRT can often be achieved by oral β-blocker, Ca^{++} channel blocker, digoxin, or specific antiarrhythmic (e.g., class IA or IC) drugs. If pharmacologic therapy fails, or if there are frequent recurrences, the patient can be referred for transcatheter ablation of the reentrant circuit, a highly successful procedure.

Atrioventricular reentrant tachycardias (AVRTs) are similar to AV nodal reentrant tachycardias except that in the former, one limb of the reentrant loop is an accessory pathway rather than a second pathway within the AV node itself. Such rhythms are discussed in greater detail below.

Nonreentrant supraventricular tachycardias are due to either increased automaticity or triggered activity. These are much less common than reentrant PSVTs, and because they often originate from an ectopic atrial focus, the P wave is upright, precedes the QRS, and is of abnormal shape. A major cause of nonreentrant atrial tachycardias is digitalis toxicity. Treatment in this case involves withdrawal of digitalis and correction of hypokalemia, if present (see Chapter 17). Unlike reentrant SVTs, vagal maneuvers usually have no effect on atrial discharges from the ectopic pacemaker focus.

Multifocal Atrial Tachycardia

Multifocal atrial tachycardia (MAT) is due to enhanced automaticity within the atria, resulting in abnormal discharges from several ectopic foci (Fig. 12.16). This arrhythmia most often occurs in the setting of severe pulmonary disease and hypoxemia. The EKG shows an irregular rhythm with multiple (at least three) P wave morphologies, and the average atrial rate is > 100 bpm. Because individuals with this rhythm are usually critically ill from the underlying disease, the mortality is high, and treatment is aimed at resolving the causative disorder. The Ca^{++} channel blocker verapamil is often effective in slowing the ventricular rate as a temporizing measure.

Preexcitation Syndrome (Wolff-Parkinson-White Syndrome)

The characteristic EKG pattern of Wolff-Parkinson-White syndrome (WPW) results from an abnormal connection between atria and ventricles through an accessory bypass tract (Figure 12.17). Although different types of bypass tracts have been identified, the bundle of Kent (see Fig. 11.10) is the most common and can usually conduct in both the anterograde and retrograde directions. In an individual with WPW, atrial impulses can pass to the ventricles through both the AV node *and* the accessory pathway. Because the latter pathway bypasses the AV node, the ventricles are stimulated *earlier* than by the normal impulse traversing the AV node. As a result, the EKG (Fig. 12.17) shows three characteristic abnormalities: 1) the PR interval is shortened (since there is no delay prior to initial ventricular stimulation); 2) a slurred, rather than sharp upstroke of the QRS (termed the "delta wave") is apparent; and 3) the QRS complex is abnormally widened, because of fusion of the impulses arriving at the ventricles by the two separate routes.

Accessory pathways do not always result in EKG findings of ventricular preexcitation, since 25% of such pathways are capable of only *retrograde* conduction. In this case, the accessory pathway is called a *concealed* bypass tract, as its presence is not apparent during sinus rhythm on the EKG (there is no delta wave). However, since the abnormal pathway *is* capable of retrograde conduction, it can form a limb of a reentrant circuit, and contribute to tachyarrhythmia development.

Individuals with the preexcitation syndrome may be asymptomatic. However, serious arrhythmias can occur, as the bypass tract, in conjunction with normal conduction across the AV node, constitute a reentrant loop. The resulting PSVTs are similar to the AV nodal reentrant rhythms described above, but the ventricular rates may be much faster, because conduction through the bypass tract is usually rapid.

The most common form of PSVT in patients with the WPW syndrome is *orthodromic* atrioventricular reentrant tachycardia (AVRT), in which the impulses travel *antegradely* down the AV node, His bundle, and bundle branches into the ventricular myocardium, then *retrogradely* up the accessory tract and back to the atrium (Fig 12.18B). Since the ventricles are depolarized during each cycle via the normal conduction system (through the AV node and bundle of His), there is no delta wave during the tachycardia and the width of the QRS is nor-

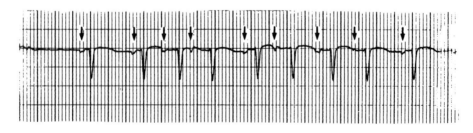

Figure 12.16. Multifocal atrial tachycardia. Each QRS is preceded by a P wave (arrows) of varying morphology. (Courtesy of Dr. Eric Isselbacher, Massachusetts General Hospital, Boston, Massachusetts.)

mal. Retrograde P waves are usually visible soon after each QRS complex (as the atria are stimulated from below via retrograde conduction through the bypass tract).

In a minority of patients with AVRT in-volving an accessory pathway (< 10% of patients), the reentrant arrhythmia travels in the opposite direction. Impulses conduct *antegradely* down the accessory pathway and *retrogradely* up the AV node (Fig

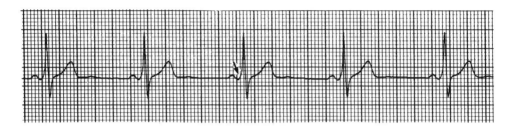

Figure 12.17. Wolff-Parkinson-White syndrome. The delta wave (arrow) indicates preexcitation of the ventricles (Courtesy of Dr. Eric Isselbacher, Massachusetts General Hospital, Boston, Massachusetts.)

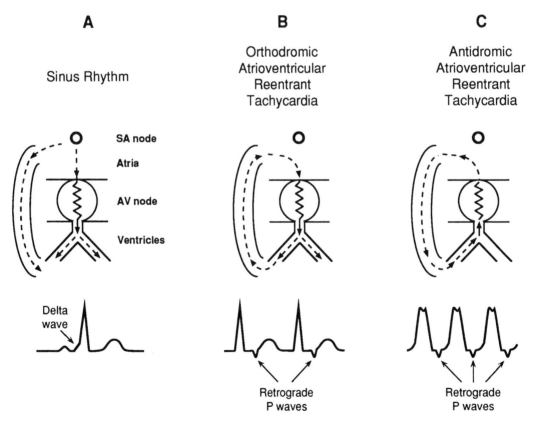

Figure 12.18. Wolff-Parkinson-White syndrome. A. During normal sinus rhythm, the shortened PR interval, delta wave, and widened QRS complex indicate fusion of ventricular activation via the AV node and accessory pathway. **B.** An APB can trigger an orthodromic atrioventricular reentrant tachycardia, in which impulses are conducted antegradely down the AV node and retrogradely up the accessory pathway. Retrograde P waves are visible immediately after the QRS complex. There is no delta wave because antegrade ventricular stimulation passes exclusively through the AV node. **C.** Antidromic atrioventricular reentrant tachycardia, in which impulses are conducted antegradely down the accessory tract and retrogradely up the AV node. The QRS complex is wide and bizarre because the ventricles are stimulated by abnormal conduction through the accessory pathway.

12.18C). Termed *antidromic* AVRT, its EKG pattern is characterized by a *widened* QRS complex, because the ventricles are activated entirely from anterograde conduction over the accessory pathway (thus representing an exaggerated form of the delta wave).

Pharmacologic management of arrhythmias in patients with the preexcitation syndrome requires greater caution than in the case of AVNRT. For example, digitalis and Ca^{++} channel blockers can, in some patients with WPW, shorten the refractory period of the accessory pathway, thus *speeding* conduction, and the heart rate, during tachycardias. As a result, Na^+ channel blockers (specifically, class IA and IC antiarrhythmics), which slow conduction and prolong the refractory period of accessory pathways, are among the preferred treatments. Permanent resolution of bypass tract- mediated tachycardias may be accomplished by transvenous catheter ablation of the accessory pathway.

Ventricular Arrhythmias

The common ventricular arrhythmias are: 1) ventricular premature beats, 2) ventricular tachycardia, and 3) ventricular fibrillation. Ventricular arrhythmias are usually more dangerous than supraventricular rhythm disorders.

Ventricular Premature Beats (VPBs)

Similar to atrial premature beats, ventricular premature beats are common, even among healthy individuals, and are often asymptomatic and benign (Fig. 12.19). They arise, for example, when an ectopic ventricular focus triggers an action potential. On the EKG, a VPB appears as a *widened* QRS complex, because the impulse travels from its ectopic site through the ventricles via slow cell-to-cell connections rather than through the normal rapid conduction system pathway. Furthermore, the ectopic beat is not related to a preceding P wave.

VPBs take on added significance in patients with structural heart disease. For example, they are common following an acute MI. When VPBs occur frequently in that setting (more than 10/hour), or appear in **couplets** (two in a row) or **triplets** (three in a row), they are markers of increased mortality. VPBs can also occur in a grouped pattern in which a fixed number of normal beats are followed by a VPB, then the series repeats. When every alternate beat is a VPB, the rhythm is termed **bigeminy**. When two normal beats precede every VPB it is **trigeminy;** then there's quadrigeminy, and so on.

In asymptomatic healthy individuals, treatment for VPBs is not necessary. Individuals who are symptomatic are often effectively treated with β-blockers (class II antiarrhythmic drugs).

Ventricular Tachycardia

Ventricular tachycardia (VT) is a series of three or more VPBs in a row (Fig. 12.20). VT is divided arbitrarily into two categories. If it persists for more than 30 seconds or requires termination because of severe symp-

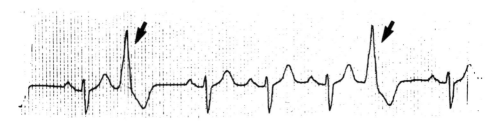

Figure 12.19. Ventricular premature beats (arrows).

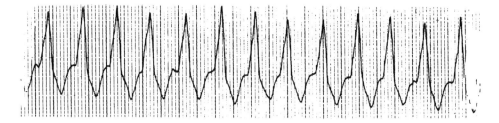

Figure 12.20. Ventricular tachycardia.

toms, it is called **sustained VT,** otherwise it is termed **nonsustained VT**. Both forms are usually associated with structural heart disease, but occasionally occur in otherwise healthy individuals.

Clinically, the symptoms of VT vary depending on the duration of the tachycardia, the rate, and the underlying condition of the heart. When VT provokes symptoms, the major manifestations are hypotension and loss of consciousness due to low cardiac output.

In VT, the QRS complexes are abnormally broad and occur at a rate of 100 to 200 bpm. The QRS complexes may all be of the same shape (monomorphic) or as continually changing forms (polymorphic), indicating that the abnormal depolarizations arise from several ventricular foci. Other arrhythmias may mimic VT, such as atrial tachycardias with bundle branch block patterns, and differentiation relies heavily on observing the relationship between the P waves and QRS complexes (there is no consistent relationship between them in VT). The basic electrophysiologic mechanism of VT varies among patients. Although both enhanced automaticity and reentry have been implicated, current evidence suggests

that reentry is the cause in the majority of patients.

Symptomatic or sustained episodes of VT are dangerous because they can deteriorate into ventricular fibrillation, which is fatal if not quickly corrected. Acute treatment usually consists of electrical cardioversion, followed by antiarrhythmic drugs (described in Chapter 17) for chronic suppression. Under some circumstances, a permanent internal defibrillator is implanted. At present, appropriate therapy for asymptomatic or nonsustained VT is less clear, because antiarrhythmic drugs have not been shown to improve long-term prognosis, and they may actually worsen the outcome because of adverse (pro-arrhythmic) side effects.

Torsades De Pointes

Torsades de pointes ("twisting of the points") is a form of ventricular tachycardia, typified by varying amplitudes of the QRS, as if the complexes are "twisting" about the baseline (Fig. 12.21). It can be produced by afterdepolarizations (triggered activity) in diseased tissues, particularly in

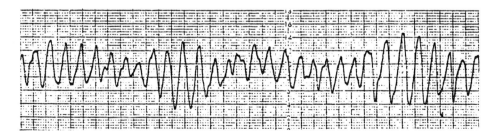

Figure 12.21. **Torsades de pointes.** The widened QRS complexes demonstrate sinusoidal patterns.

patients who have a *prolonged QT interval*. The latter may occur with some drugs (such as with certain *anti*-arrhythmics, including up to 2% of patients taking quinidine), electrolyte disturbances (especially hypokalemia or hypomagnesemia), and congenital prolongation of the QT interval.

Torsades de pointes is usually symptomatic, but often self-limited. Its danger results from syncope during the rhythm, or its degeneration into ventricular fibrillation. When it is drug- or electrolyte-induced, correcting that underlying cause abolishes the arrhythmia. Intravenous magnesium is also sometimes of benefit in stabilizing the rhythm. Other strategies aimed at shortening the QT, thereby preventing recurrences of this rhythm, include the use of intravenous isoproterenol or overdrive artificial pacing. Conversely, when this rhythm appears in patients with congenital prolongation of the QT interval, beta-blocking drugs are the treatment of choice, because sympathetic stimulation aggravates the arrhythmia in that case.

Ventricular Fibrillation

Ventricular fibrillation (VF) is the most life-threatening arrhythmia (Fig. 12.22). It results in disordered rapid stimulation of the ventricles, preventing them from contracting in a coordinated fashion. The result is a severe drop in cardiac output and death if not quickly reversed. This rhythm most often occurs in individuals with severe heart disease, and is the major cause of death in acute MI.

VF is thought to result from multiple small wavelets of reentry. On the EKG, it is characterized by a chaotic irregular appearance with complexes of varying amplitude and morphology, without discrete QRS waveforms.

Untreated, VF rapidly leads to death; the only effective therapy is electrical defibrillation. As soon as the heart has been converted to a safe rhythm, the underlying cause of the arrhythmia must be corrected (e.g., electrolyte imbalances, hypoxemia, or acidosis). Intravenous antiarrhythmic drug therapy is administered to prevent recurrences while the inciting cause is investigated.

Differentiation of Wide Complex Tachycardias

Ventricular tachycardia can usually be distinguished from supraventricular tachycardias by the width of the QRS complex: It is routinely wide in the former, and narrow (i.e., normal) in the latter, as illustrated in Figure 12.9. However, under certain circumstances, arrhythmias that arise from sites above the ventricles *can* result in wide QRS complexes. This may occur either because: 1) the patient has an underlying conduction abnormality (usually a bundle branch block), such that the QRS is abnormally wide even when in normal sinus rhythm, or 2) repetitive rapid stimulation of the ventricles from a supraventricular tachycardia finds portions of the ventricular conduction system refractory, because of insufficient time to recover from the previous depolarization. As a result, the impulse propagating through the ventricles is partially blocked, such that the QRS becomes

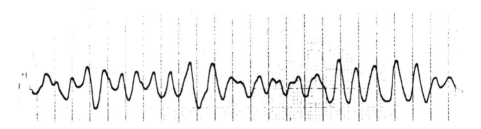

Figure 12.22. Ventricular fibrillation

TABLE 12.2. Differentiation of Wide Complex Tachycardias

Supports SVT with "aberrant" conduction	Supports ventricular tachycardia

• QRS morphology same as when in sinus rhythm
• Rhythm responds to vagal maneuvers (see Fig. 12.9)
	• No relationship between P wave and QRS complexes
	• Concordance of QRS complexes in the chest leads (V_1-V_6)
	• Extremely wide QRS:
	    > 0.14 sec if RBBB pattern
	    > 0.16 sec if LBBB pattern
	• Unusual mean QRS axis:
	    Left axis deviation with RBBB pattern
	    More negative than$-90°$ with LBBB pattern

SVT, all supraventricular tachycardias

distorted and widened (termed "aberrant" conduction).

Certain features help to distinguish wide QRS complexes of ventricular tachycardia from those of supraventricular rhythms with aberrant conduction. For example, a *supraventricular* tachyarrhythmia is more likely if the morphology of the QRS at the rapid rate is similar to that on the patient's EKG tracing obtained while in sinus rhythm (i.e., the complex is widened because of a persistent underlying bundle branch block). A supraventricular tachycardia with aberrancy is also more likely if vagal maneuvers (such as carotid sinus massage) effect the rhythm, as indicated in Figure 12.9.

Conversely, *ventricular* tachycardia is more likely the cause of a wide complex tachycardia if any of the following crieria are met: 1) there is no relationship between the rhythm of the QRS complexes and any observed P waves (atrioventricular "dissociation"); 2) the QRS complexes in each of the chest leads (V_1 through V_6) are oriented in the same direction (i.e., they are all either positive or negative ("concordance" of the precordial QRS complexes)); 3) the QRS complexes are extremely wide (> 0.14 sec [> 3.5 small boxes] when there is a right bundle branch block (BBB) configuration or > 0.16 sec [> 4 small boxes] if a left BBB configuration is present); 4) the mean QRS axis is highly abnormal (e.g., if *left* axis deviation is present when the QRS morphology is that of right BBB, or there is *extreme* left axis deviation (more negative than $-90°$) when the morphology is that of left BBB. These dif-

ferentiating features are summarized in Table 12.2.

SUMMARY

Disorders of impulse formation and conduction result in bradyarrhythmias and tachyarrhythmias, the most common of which are presented in this chapter. Through careful analysis of the EKG, it is usually possible to distinguish between the array of rhythm disorders, so that appropriate therapy can be administered.

When faced with a slow heart rhythm (Figs. 12.1 to 12.7), the key questions to address are: 1) Are P waves present? 2) What is the relationship between the P waves and the QRS complexes?

Differentiation of tachyarrhythmias requires assessment of: 1) the width of the QRS complex (normal or wide), 2) the morphology and rate of the P waves, 3) the relationship between the P waves and the QRS complexes, and 4) the response to vagal maneuvers (as indicated in Figure 12.9).

Each of the EKG texts listed at the end of Chapter 4 provides many examples of the common rhythm disorders presented in this chapter.

ADDITIONAL READING

Dreifus LS. Guidelines for implantation of cardiac pacemakers and antiarrhythmic devices: a report of the American College of Cardiology/American Heart Association Task Force on Assessment of Diagnostic and Therapeutic Cardiovascular Procedures. J Am Coll Cardiol 1991;18:1.

Ganz LI, Friedman PL. Supraventricular tachycardia. N Engl J Med 1995;332:162–173.

Josephson ME. Clinical Cardiac Electrophysiology. 2nd ed. Philadelphia: Lea & Febiger, 1993.

Kim YH, et al. Nonpharmacologic therapies in patients with ventricular tachyarrhythmias. Catheter ablation and ventricular tachycardia surgery. Cardiol Clin 1993;11:85.

Mandel WJ, ed. Cardiac Arrhythmias: Their Mechanisms, Diagnosis, and Management. 3rd ed. Philadelphia: JB Lippincott, 1995.

Waldo AL, Wit AL. Mechanisms of cardiac arrhythmias. Lancet 1993;341:1189–1193.

Waldo AL, Wit AL. Mechanisms of cardiac arrhythmias and conduction disturbances. In: Schlant RC, Alexander RW, eds. The Heart. New York: McGraw-Hill, 1994.

Zipes DP. Specific arrhythmias: diagnosis and treatment. In: Braunwald E, ed. Heart Disease: A Textbook of Cardiovascular Medicine. Philadelphia: WB Saunders, 1997:640–704.

Zipes DP, Jalife J, eds. Cardiac Electrophysiology: From Cell to Bedside. 2nd ed. Philadelphia: WB Saunders, 1995.

Acknowledgments   The first edition of this chapter was written by Wendy Armstrong, MD, Nicholas Boulis, MD, Elliott M. Antman, MD, and Leonard S. Lilly, MD.

Hypertension

Rahul Deshmukh, Allison Smith, and Leonard S. Lilly

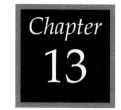

Chapter
13

More than 50 million Americans have hypertension—a blood pressure high enough to be a danger to their well-being. Hypertension can be implicated in as many as 800,000 deaths per year, as well as nonlethal myocardial infarctions, strokes, and permanent damage to the retina and kidney. Since an elevated blood pressure is usually asymptomatic until an acute cardiovascular event strikes, screening for hypertension is a very important aspect of preventive medicine.

Hypertension is also a scientific problem of unexpected complexity: In almost 95% of affected patients, the cause of the blood pressure elevation is unknown, a condition termed primary or **essential hypertension (EH)**. Evidence suggests that there are multiple, diverse causes for EH, and considerable insight into these factors can be achieved by studying the normal physiology of blood pressure control, as we will examine.

High blood pressure attributed to a *definable* cause is termed **secondary hypertension**. Although far less common than EH, conditions that cause secondary hypertension are very important because they are often amenable to permanent cure. Following the discussions of essential and secondary hypertension, this chapter considers the clinical consequences of an elevated blood pressure and approaches to treatment.

WHAT IS HYPERTENSION?

Blood pressure values vary widely in the population. Diastolic pressures follow the smooth bell-shaped distribution shown in Figure 13.1, and both systolic and diastolic pressures rise with increasing age as illustrated in Figure 13.2. The risk of complications of an elevated pressure increases progressively with higher values, so that the exact cutoff point for the definition of hypertension is somewhat arbitrary, but the currently established criteria are listed in Table 13.1. By these criteria, a diastolic pressure consistently at or above 90 mmHg, or a systolic pressure at or above 140 mmHg, establishes the diagnosis of hypertension. Those with "High Normal" blood pressure have an increased risk of developing definite hypertension and therefore need to be monitored closely. The definitions in Table 13.1 are based on studies that have examined the incidence of cardiovascular complications related to blood pressure values, and although the emphasis has historically been on the level of *diastolic* pressure, evidence suggests that the *systolic* pressure is

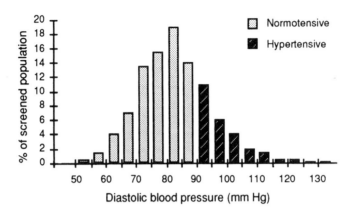

Figure 13.1.   Distribution of diastolic blood pressure values in the 30- to 69-year age group (n = 158,906). Hypertension is arbitrarily defined as a diastolic BP ≥ 90 mmHg. (Modified from Hypertension Detection and Follow-up Program. A progress report. Circ Res 1977;40(Suppl 1):106.)

equally important in predicting hypertensive complications.

HOW IS BLOOD PRESSURE REGULATED?

Blood pressure (BP) is the product of cardiac output (CO) and total peripheral vascular resistance (TPR):

$$BP = CO \times TPR$$

In turn, cardiac output is the product of cardiac stroke volume (SV) and heart rate (HR):

$$CO = SV \times HR$$

in which the stroke volume is largely determined by cardiac contractility and by the amount of venous return to the heart (i.e., the preload, as described in Chapter 9).

It follows that at least three systems are directly responsible for blood pressure regulation: the *heart*, which supplies the pumping pressure; *blood vessel tone*, which largely determines systemic resistance; and the *kidney*, which regulates intravascular volume. Figure 13.3 shows how these three systems contribute to the CO and TPR.

The renal component of blood pressure regulation deserves special mention, in light of the temptation to view hypertension as a "cardiovascular problem." No matter how high the cardiac output and how constricted the blood vessels, renal ex-

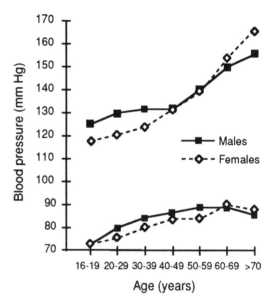

Figure 13.2.   The relationship between blood pressure and age (n = 1029). Systolic (upper curves) and diastolic (lower curves) values are shown. Note that by age 60, the average systolic pressure of women exceeds that of men. (Modified from Kotchen JM, McKean HE, Kotchen TA. Blood pressure trends with aging. Hypertension 1982;4(Suppl 3):111–129.)

cretion has the capacity to completely return blood pressure to normal levels by reducing intravascular volume. Therefore, the maintenance of chronic hypertension requires renal participation, even though the factors responsible may lie outside of the renal parenchyma. Examples of such

TABLE 13.1. Classification of Blood Pressure in Adults

Category	Systolic Pressure (mm/Hg)	Diastolic Pressure (mm/Hg)
Normal	< 130	< 85
High-normal	130–139	85–89
Hypertension[a]		
Stage 1 (mild)	140–159	90–99
Stage 2 (moderate)	160–179	100–109
Stage 3 (severe)	180–209	110–119
Stage 4 (very severe)	≥ 210	≥ 120

[a] When a patient's systolic and diastolic readings fall into different stages, the higher category should be applied
Modified from the Joint National Committee Report on Detection, Evaluation, and Treatment of High Blood Pressure. Arch Intern Med. 1993;153:154–183.

factors include reduced blood perfusion to the kidney because of restricted flow through the renal artery, or aberrant secretion of circulating hormones that enhance renal sodium retention, as described below.

ESSENTIAL HYPERTENSION

Almost 95% of hypertensive patients have blood pressures that are elevated for no readily definable reason; they are therefore said to suffer from essential hypertension. The diagnosis of EH is one of exclusion; it is the option left to the clinician after ruling out all of the causes of secondary hypertension described later in this chapter.

Essential hypertension is more a description than a diagnosis, indicating only that a patient manifests a specific physical finding (high blood pressure) for which no cause has been found. In all likelihood, different underlying defects are responsible for the elevated pressure in different subpopulations of patients. Because the exact nature of these defects is unknown, to understand EH is to understand the possibilities—what could go wrong with normal physiology to produce chronically elevated blood pressure?

Our discussion of EH therefore reflects what is currently known about its severity, epidemiology and genetics, experimental findings and natural history. The picture that will emerge is that essential hypertension likely results from the synergy of multiple defects of blood pressure regulation that interact with environmental stressors. The regulatory defects may be acquired or genetically determined, and may be independent of each other. As a result, EH patients exhibit varied combinations of regulatory defects and therefore have different physiologic bases for their elevated blood pressures.

Severity

Approximately 80% of EH patients have stage 1 hypertension; only 10% have either moderate or severe degrees. Although the cardiovascular danger of high blood pressure is greater for those with the higher pressures, it is the stage 1 and 2 hypertensive patients who, because of their sheer numbers, account for the vast morbidity and mortality attributable to EH.

Epidemiology

Heredity appears to play an important role in EH, but definite genetic markers have not yet been identified. There is clearly a higher rate of elevated blood pressures among first-degree relatives of hypertensives than in the general population. Concordance between identical twins is not complete, but is high, and is significantly greater than that for dizygotic twins. Hypothecized genetic abnormalities include defects in the renal excretion of sodium, abnormal sodium transport across cell membranes, and abnormally high autonomic nervous system response to exogenous stress. Of note, normotensive relatives of EH patients can often be shown to exhibit physiologic abnormalities of a type that, in conjunction with other regulatory defects, could lead to an elevated pressure (e.g., abnormalities of renal blood flow regulation).

A genetic component to EH is also suggested by the uneven distribution of hypertension among racial groups. For example, in most age distributions, blacks are significantly more likely to be hypertensive than

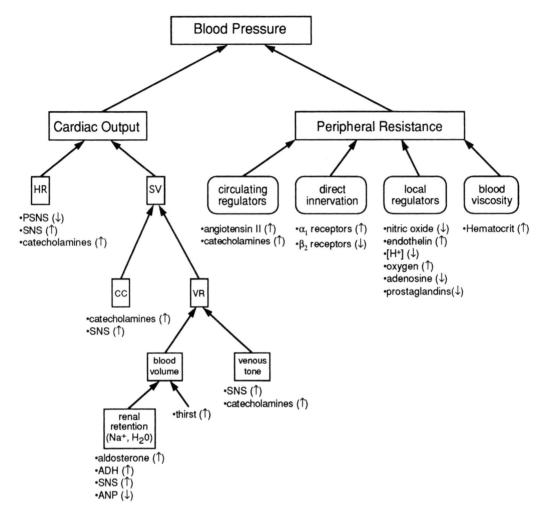

Figure 13.3.   Regulation of systemic blood pressure. The small arrows indicate whether there is a stimulatory (↑) or inhibitory (↓) effect on the boxed parameters. HR, heart rate; SV, stroke volume; PSNS, parasympathetic nervous system; SNS, sympathetic nervous system; CC, cardiac contractility; VR, venous return; ADH, antidiuretic hormone; ANP, atrial natriuretic peptide.

are individuals of other races. Environmental differences may also contribute to this disparity, as suggested by the concordance of blood pressures among spouses. Finally, age is an important factor, as there is an increased prevalence of hypertensives among older individuals.

Experimental Findings

Multiple defects of blood pressure regulation have been found in essential hypertensives and their relatives. By themselves, or in conjunction with one another, these

abnormalities might contribute to chronic BP elevation.

The *heart* can contribute to a high cardiac output-based hypertension, due to abnormal neural or catecholamine stimulation. For example, when tested under psychologically stressful conditions, hypertensive patients (and their first-degree relatives) often develop excessive heart rate acceleration compared with control subjects, suggesting an excessive sympathetic response.

The *blood vessels* can contribute to a peripheral vascular resistance-based hypertension, by constricting in response to: 1) malregulation of the sympathetic nervous system, 2) abnormal regulation of vascular tone by local factors, including nitric oxide (EDRF-NO), endothelin, and atrial natriuritic factor, or 3) ion channel defects in contractile vascular smooth muscle.

The *kidney* can induce a volume-based hypertension by retaining excessive sodium and water, due to: 1) failure to regulate renal blood flow appropriately, 2) ion channel defects (e.g., reduced basolateral Na^+/K^+-ATPase) directly causing sodium retention, or 3) inappropriate hormonal regulation. For example, the renin-angiotensin-aldosterone axis is an important hormonal regulator of peripheral vascular resistance (see below). Renin levels in EH patients (relative to normotensives) are subnormal in 30%, normal in 60%, and high in 10%. Since renin secretion should be *suppressed* by high blood pressure, even "normal" levels of renin secretion are inappropriate in hypertensive patients. Thus, abnormalities of renin regulation may play

a role in some individuals with essential hypertension.

Figure 13.4 highlights these and other potential mechanisms of essential hypertension. Note that although the heart, vessels, and kidneys are the organs ultimately responsible for producing the pressure, primary defects may be located elsewhere, as well (e.g., the central nervous system, arterial baroreceptors, and adrenal gland hormone secretion). Though abnormal regulation at these sites can contribute to elevated blood pressure, it is important to remember that without renal complicity, malfunction of other systems would not produce sustained hypertension, for the normal kidney is capable of eliminating sufficient volume to return the blood pressure to normal.

Recent research has shown that another potentially important factor in the development of EH relates to the hormone insulin. In many patients with hypertension, especially those who are obese or have type II diabetes mellitus, there is impaired insulin-

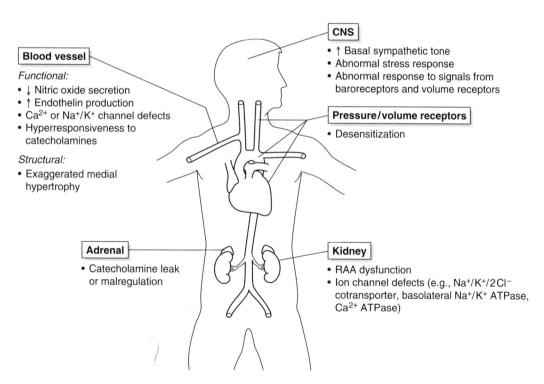

Figure 13.4.   Potential primary abnormalities in essential hypertension (EH). These defects are supported by experimental evidence, but their contribution to EH in an individual patient is unclear. CNS, central nervous system.

dependent transport of glucose into the peripheral tissues (termed *insulin resistance*). As a result, serum glucose levels rise, stimulating the pancreas to release greater amounts of insulin. Such hyperinsulinemia can theoretically raise arterial pressure by at least four mechanisms: 1) insulin stimulates renal sodium reabsorption, thereby increasing intravascular volume; 2) insulin increases sympathetic nervous system activity and raises the concentration of circulating catecholamines; 3) insulin is a mitogen that stimulates arterial vascular smooth muscle hypertrophy; and 4) insulin alters cell membrane ion transport that can lead to increased intracellular calcium and heightened vascular tone. Whether hyperinsulinemia truly plays an important role in the genesis of essential hypertension is not yet known, and remains a subject of ongoing laboratory investigations.

Natural History

Essential hypertension characteristically arises after young adulthood. Its prevalence increases with age such that more than 60% of Americans over age 60 have a diastolic pressure greater than 90 mmHg and an additional number have isolated elevation of systolic pressure (> 140 mmHg).

In addition, the hemodynamic characteristics of blood pressure elevation in EH tend to change over time (Fig. 13.5). In hypertensive patients younger than age 40, the BP tends to be driven by high cardiac output in the setting of normal total peripheral resistance (TPR), termed the "hyperkinetic" phase of EH. Eventually, however, the contribution by CO tends to decline, while TPR increases as the heart and vessels adapt to the prolonged stress. For example, the development of left ventricular hypertrophy in chronic hypertension compromises diastolic filling (which in turn reduces stroke volume and cardiac output), whereas medial hypertrophy of the arterioles reduces the lumen diameter and increases the resistance to forward blood flow. Thus, older hypertensive patients tend to have elevated TPR as the principal abnormality, with a normal or reduced CO. This progression from "high CO, normal TPR" to "normal CO, high TPR" occurs independent of whether the mean arterial pressure rises over time or remains unchanged.

Thus, essential hypertension is a clinical syndrome that may arise from many potential abnormalities, but it exhibits a characteristic hemodynamic profile and natural history. It is likely that multiple defects, separately inherited or acquired, acting together, chronically raise the blood pressure in affected individuals. Although we may not understand the precise underlying mechanism in any individual hypertensive patient, we can at least describe what kind of pathophysiology might be at fault. Es-

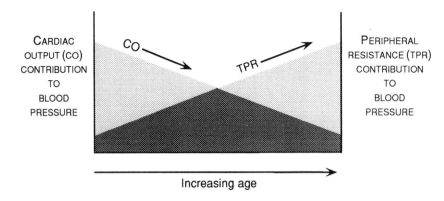

Figure 13.5. Hemodynamic progression of essential hypertension (EH). Schematic representation of the changing contribution of cardiac output (CO) and total peripheral resistance (TPR) as age increases in many patients with EH.

sential hypertension, though "idiopathic," is not entirely a black box.

SECONDARY HYPERTENSION

Although EH dominates the clinical picture, in 5% of patients with hypertension, there is a defined structural or hormonal cause. Though cases of such secondary hypertension are relatively uncommon, their identification is important because these conditions are often curable, and may require therapy different from that administered for EH. Moreover, if left uncontrolled, adaptive cardiovascular changes may develop analogous to those of long-standing EH, which could cause the elevated pressures to persist even after the underlying cause is corrected.

Although secondary forms should be considered in the work-up of all patients with hypertension, there are clinical clues that a given patient may have one of the correctable conditions (Table 13.2):

1. **Age**. If a patient develops hypertension younger than age 20 or older than age 50 (outside of the usual range of EH), secondary hypertension is more likely.
2. **Severity**. Secondary hypertension often causes the BP to rise into the stage 3 (severe) category, whereas most EH patients have stage 1 to 2 (mild to moderate) hypertension.
3. **Onset**. Secondary forms of hypertension

often present abruptly in a patient who was previously normotensive, rather than gradually progressing over years as is the usual case in EH.

4. **Associated signs and symptoms**. The process that induces the hypertension may give rise to other characteristic abnormalities, identified by the history and physical examination. For example, a renal artery "bruit" (swishing sound due to turbulent blood flow through a stenotic artery) may be heard on abdominal examination in a patient with renal artery stenosis.
5. **Family history**. EH patients often have hypertensive first-degree relatives, whereas secondary hypertension more commonly occurs sporadically.

The usual clinical evaluation of a patient with recently diagnosed hypertension begins with a careful history and physical examination, including a search for clues of secondary forms of hypertension. Examples of typical screening studies include: 1) a urinalysis and serum concentration of creatinine and blood urea nitrogen (abnormal in renal parenchymal disease), 2) the serum potassium level (abnormally low in renovascular hypertension or primary aldosteronism), and 3) a chest radiograph (abnormal in aortic coarctation). If no abnormalities are found, the patient is presumed to have EH and treated accordingly. If, however, the patient's blood pressure is refractory to usual therapy, then more de-

TABLE 13.2. Causes of Hypertension

Type	Percent of Hypertensives	Clinical Clues
"Essential"	95%	• Age of onset: 20–50
		• Family history of hypertension
		• Normal serum [K⁺], urinalysis
Chronic renal disease	2%–4%	• ↑ [Creatinine], abnormal urinalysis
Renovascular	1%	• Abdominal bruit
		• Sudden onset (especially if age > 50 or < 20)
		• ↓ Serum [K⁺]
Pheochromocytoma	0.2%	• Paroxysms of palpitations, diaphoresis & anxiety
		• Episodic hypertension in 1/3 of patients
Coarctation of the aorta	0.1%	• Blood pressure in arms > legs, or right arm > left arm
		• Midsystolic murmur between scapulae
		• CXR: aortic indentation, rib-notching owing to collaterals
Primary aldosteronism	0.1%	• ↓ Serum [K⁺]
Cushing's syndrome	0.1%	• "Cushingoid" appearance (e.g., central obesity, hirsutism)

tailed diagnostic testing is performed to search for other specific forms of secondary hypertension.

Exogenous Causes

A number of medications can elevate the blood pressure. For example, oral contraceptive pills may cause secondary hypertension in some women. The mechanism is likely related to increased activity of the renin-angiotensin system: Estrogens increase the hepatic synthesis of angiotensinogen, leading to greater production of angiotensin II (Fig. 13.6). Angiotensin II raises blood pressure by several mechanisms, most notably by direct vasoconstriction and by stimulating the adrenal release of aldosterone. The latter hormone causes renal sodium retention and therefore increased intravascular volume.

Other medications that can raise blood pressure include glucocorticoids, cyclosporine A (an antirejection drug used in patients with organ transplants), erythropoietin (a hormone that increases bone marrow red blood cell formation; elevation of BP is due to increased blood viscosity and reversal of local hypoxic vasodilatation),

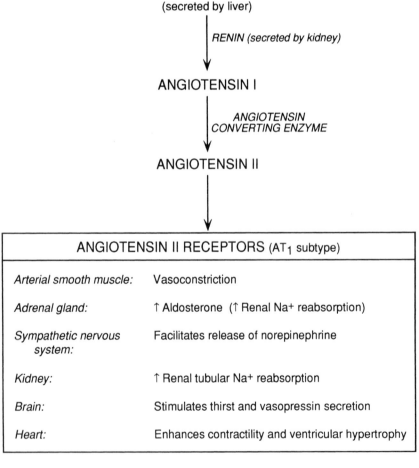

Figure 13.6. The Renin-Angiotensin-Aldosterone system. Liver-derived angiotensinogen is cleaved in the circulation by renin (of kidney origin) to form angiotensin I (AI). AI is rapidly cleaved in the circulation to the potent vasoconstrictor angiotensin II (AII) by angiotensin converting enzyme. AII also modulates the release of aldosterone from the adrenal cortex. Aldosterone in turn acts to reabsorb Na^+ from the distal nephron, resulting in increased intravascular volume. The other listed effects of AII receptor stimulation may also contribute to the development and maintenance of hypertension.

sympathomimetic drugs, and phenylpro-
panolamine (the latter two are common components in over-the-counter cold remedies).

Two other substances that may contribute to hypertension are the use of cocaine and chronic excessive ethanol consumption.

Renal Causes

Given the crucial role of the kidney in the
control of blood pressure, it is not surprising that renal dysfunction can lead to hypertension. In fact, renal disease contributes
to the two leading endogenous causes of
secondary hypertension: renal parenchymal disease, accounting for 2% to 4% of hypertensive patients, and renal arterial stenosis, which accounts for approximately 1%.

Renal Parenchymal Disease

Parenchymal damage to the kidney can
result from diverse pathologic processes.
The major mechanism by which injury
leads to elevated blood pressure is through
increased intravascular volume. Damaged
nephrons are unable to excrete normal
amounts of sodium and water, leading to a
rise in volume, elevated cardiac output, and
hence, increased blood pressure.

If renal function is only mildly impaired,
then the blood pressure may stabilize at a
level at which the higher systemic pressure
(and therefore renal perfusion pressure) enables sodium excretion to balance sodium intake. Conversely, if a patient has end-stage
renal failure, glomerular filtration rate (GFR)
is so greatly decreased that the kidney simply
cannot excrete sufficient volume, and malig-
nant-range blood pressures may follow.

Renal parenchymal disease may contribute to hypertension even if the GFR is
not greatly reduced, through the excessive
elaboration of renin.

Renovascular Hypertension (RH)

Stenosis of one or both renal arteries
leads to hypertension. Although emboli,

vasculitis, and external compression of the
renal arteries can result in RH, the two most
common causes are atherosclerosis and fibromuscular dysplasia of these arteries.
Atherosclerotic lesions arise from extensive
plaque formation either within the renal
artery or in the aorta at the origin of the renal artery. Atherosclerotic RH accounts for
about two-thirds of all cases of RH and occurs most commonly in elderly men. *Fibromuscular* lesions, in contrast, consist of discrete regions of fibrous or muscular
proliferation, generally within the arterial
media. Fibromuscular dysplasia accounts
for about one-third of cases of RH and characteristically occurs in young Caucasian
women.

The elevated blood pressure in RH arises
from reduced renal blood flow to the affected kidney, which responds to the lower
perfusion pressure by secreting renin. The
latter raises the blood pressure through the
subsequent actions of angiotensin II (vasoconstriction) and aldosterone (sodium retention), shown in Figure 13.6.

The diagnosis of RH is suggested by an
abdominal bruit, which can be identified in
40% to 60% of patients, or by the presence of
unexplained hypokalemia (owing to excessive renal excretion of potassium because of
the elevated aldosterone levels). RH is a correctable form of hypertension that is often
successfully treated by percutaneous balloon angioplasty or surgical reconstruction
of the stenosed vessel. Medical therapy,
particularly with angiotensin converting
enzyme (ACE) inhibitors, can also be effective initial therapy in patients with unilateral renal artery disease. ACE inhibitors
negate the effect of elevated circulating
renin in this situation by impeding the formation of angiotensin II (see Chapter 17).

Mechanical Cause

Coarctation of the Aorta

Coarctation is an infrequent congenital
narrowing of the aorta that most commonly
occurs just distal to the origin of the left subclavian artery (see Chapter 16). As a result

of the relative obstruction to flow, the blood pressure in the aortic arch, head, and arms is higher than that in the descending aorta and its branches and in the lower extremities. Sometimes the coarctation involves the origin of the left subclavian artery, so that the pressure of the left arm may be lower than that of the right.

Hypertension in this condition arises by two mechanisms. First, reduced blood flow to the kidneys stimulates the renin-angiotensin system, resulting in vasoconstriction (via angiotensin II). Second, high pressures proximal to the coarctation stiffen the aortic arch through medial hyperplasia and accelerated atherosclerosis, blunting the normal baroreceptor response to elevated intravascular pressure.

Clinical clues to the presence of coarctation include symptoms of inadequate blood flow to the legs or left arm, such as claudication or fatigue, or the finding of weakened or absent femoral pulses. A midsystolic murmur associated with the stenotic segment of the aorta may be auscultated, especially over the back, between the scapulae. The chest radiograph may show indentation of the aorta at the level of the coarctation. It may also demonstrate a notched appearance of the ribs secondary to the enlargement of collateral intercostal arteries, which shunt blood around the aortic narrowing. Treatment options include angioplasty or surgery to correct the stenosis. However, the hypertension may not abate completely after mechanical correction, possibly because of persistent desensitization of the arterial baroreceptors.

Endocrine Causes

Circulating hormones play an important role in the control of normal blood pressure, so that it is not surprising that endocrine diseases may cause hypertension. When suspected, the presence of such endocrine conditions is evaluated in four ways:

1. History of characteristic signs and symptoms
2. Measurement of hormone levels

3. Assessment of hormone secretion in response to stimulation or inhibition
4. Imaging studies to identify tumors secreting the excessive hormone

Pheochromocytoma

Pheochromocytomas are catecholamine-secreting tumors of neuroendocrine cells (usually in the adrenal medulla) that cause approximately 0.2% of cases of hypertension. The release of epinephrine and norepinephrine by the tumor results in intermittent or chronic vasoconstriction, tachycardia, and other sympathetic-mediated effects. A characteristic presentation consists of paroxysmal rises in blood pressure accompanied by "autonomic attacks" due to the increased catecholamine levels: severe throbbing headaches, profuse sweating, palpitations and tachycardia. Although some patients are actually normotensive between attacks, most have sustained hypertension. Ten percent of pheochromocytomas are malignant.

Determination of plasma catecholamine levels, or urine catecholamines and their metabolites (e.g., vanillylmandelic acid and metanephrine), obtained under controlled circumstances, are used to identify this condition. Because some pheochromocytomas secrete only episodically, diagnosis may require measurement of catecholamines immediately following an attack.

Pharmacologic therapy of pheochromocytomas includes the combination of an alpha-receptor blocker (e.g., phenoxybenzamine) combined with a beta-blocker. However, once the tumor is localized by computed tomography (CT), magnetic resonance imaging (MRI), or by angiography, the definitive therapy is surgical resection. For patients with inoperable disease, treatment consists of alpha and beta blockade, as well as drugs that inhibit catecholamine biosynthesis (e.g., alpha-methyltyrosine).

Adrenocortical Hormone Excess

Among the hormones produced by the adrenal cortex are mineralocorticoids and glucocorticoids. Excess of either of these can result in hypertension.

Mineralocorticoids, primarily aldosterone, increase blood volume by stimulating reabsorption of sodium into the circulation by the distal portions of the nephron. This occurs in exchange for potassium excretion into the urine, and the resulting hypokalemia is an important diagnostic marker of mineralocorticoid excess. *Primary aldosteronism,* found in approximately 0.1% of hypertensive patients, is generally the result of an adrenal adenoma, but may also result from bilateral hyperplasia of the adrenal glands. Clinically, the disease may be asymptomatic, so diagnosis relies on detection of hypokalemia, and is confirmed by measurement of excessive aldosterone secretion and suppressed plasma renin levels. Therapy includes either surgical removal of the adenoma or medical management with aldosterone receptor antagonists (e.g., spironolactone). *Secondary aldosteronism* can result from increased angiotensin II (AII) production by the very rare renin-secreting tumor.

Much more commonly, angiotensin II levels may be elevated in women taking oral contraceptive pills (which stimulate hepatic production of angiotensinogen, as indicated above), or because of decreased AII degradation in chronic liver diseases.

Glucocorticoids, such as cortisol, also elevate blood pressure when present in excess, likely via blood volume expansion and increased renin synthesis. Nearly 80% of patients with Cushing's syndrome, a disorder of glucocorticoid excess, have some degree of hypertension. These patients often present with classic "Cushingoid" features: characteristic rounded facial appearance, central obesity, proximal muscle weakness, and hirsutism. The primary lesion may be either a pituitary ACTH-secreting adenoma, a peripheral ACTH-secreting tumor (either of which causes adrenal cortical hyperplasia), or an adrenal cortisol-secreting adenoma.

Thyroid Hormone Abnormalities

Approximately one-third of *hyperthyroid* and one-fourth of *hypothyroid* patients have significant hypertension. Thyroid hormones exert their cardiovascular effects by: 1) inducing sodium-potassium ATPases in the heart and vessels, 2) increasing blood volume, and 3) stimulating tissue metabolism and oxygen demand, with secondary accumulation of metabolites that modulate local vascular tone. Hyperthyroid patients develop hypertension through cardiac hyperactivity and an increase in blood volume. Hypothyroid patients likely become hypertensive via a mechanism mediated through local control: as basal metabolic rate falls, so does the accumulation of local metabolites, such that relative vasoconstriction develops.

CONSEQUENCES OF HYPERTENSION

Whatever the cause of blood pressure elevation, the ultimate consequences are similar. High blood pressure itself is generally asymptomatic, but it can result in devastating effects on many organs, especially the blood vessels, heart, kidney, and retina.

Clinical Signs and Symptoms

In the past, "classic" symptoms of hypertension were considered to include headache, epistaxis (nose bleeds), and dizziness. The usefulness of these symptoms has been called into question, however, by studies that indicate that they are found no more frequently among hypertensive patients than in the general population. Yet some symptoms, such as flushing, sweating, and blurred vision, do seem more common in the hypertensive population. In general, however, the majority of hypertensive patients are asymptomatic, and are diagnosed simply by blood pressure measurement on routine physical examinations.

Several physical signs of hypertension discussed in the next section directly result from the elevated pressure, including left ventricular hypertrophy (LVH) and retinopathy. In addition, hypertension complicated by atherosclerosis can be manifest by arterial bruits, particularly in the carotid and femoral arteries.

Organ Damage Due to Hypertension

Target organ complications of hypertension reflect the degree of chronic blood pressure elevation. Such organ damage can be attributed to: 1) the increased workload of the heart, and 2) arterial damage due to the combined effects of the elevated pressure itself (weakened vessel walls) and accelerated atherosclerosis (Fig. 13.7). Abnormalities of the vasculature that result from elevated pressure include smooth muscle hypertrophy, endothelial cell dysfunction, and fatigue of elastic fibers. Chronic hypertensive trauma to the endothelium promotes atherosclerosis possibly by disrupting normal protective mechanisms such as the secretion of EDRF-NO and by initiating smooth muscle cell hypertrophy. Arteries lined by atherosclerotic plaque may thrombose, or may serve as a source of cholesterol emboli that occlude distal vessels, causing organ infarction (such as cerebrovascular occlusion, resulting in a stroke). In addition,

atherosclerosis of large arteries hinders their elasticity, resulting in systolic pressure spikes that can further traumatize endothelium, or provoke events such as aneurysm rupture.

The major target organs for the destructive complications of chronic hypertension are the heart, the cerebrovascular system, the aorta and peripheral vascular system, the kidney, and the retina (Table 13.3). Left untreated, approximately half of hypertensive patients die from coronary artery disease or congestive heart failure, a third from stroke, and 10% to 15% from renal failure.

Heart

The major cardiac effects of hypertension relate to the increased afterload against which the heart must contract, and accelerated atherosclerosis within the coronary arteries.

Left Ventricular Hypertrophy and Diastolic Dysfunction

The high arterial pressure (heightened afterload) increases the wall tension of the left ventricle, which compensates through hypertrophy. *Concentric hypertrophy* (with-

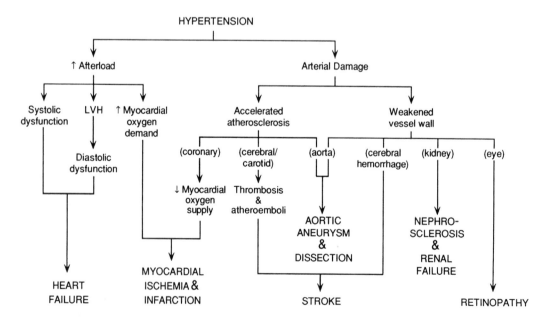

Figure 13.7. Pathophysiology of the major consequences of hypertension. LVH, left ventricular hypertrophy.

TABLE 13.3. Target Organ Damage in Hypertension

Organ System	Manifestations
Heart	• Left ventricular hypertrophy • Heart failure • Myocardial ischemia & infarction
Cerebrovascular	• Stroke
Aorta & peripheral vascular	• Aortic aneurysm and/or dissection • Arteriosclerosis
Kidney	• Nephrosclerosis • Renal failure
Retina	• Arterial narrowing • Hemorrhages, exudates, papilledema

out dilatation) is the normal pattern of compensation, although conditions that elevate blood pressure by virtue of increased circulating volume (e.g., primary aldosteronism) may instead develop *eccentric* hypertrophy with chamber dilatation (see Chapter 9). LVH results in increased stiffness of the left ventricle with diastolic dysfunction, manifest by elevation of LV filling pressure that can result in pulmonary congestion (see Chapter 9).

Physical findings of LVH may include a heaving left ventricular impulse on chest palpation, indicative of the increased muscle mass. It is frequently accompanied by a fourth heart sound (see Chapter 2), as the left atrium contracts into the stiffened left ventricle.

LVH has been shown to be one of the strongest predictors of cardiac morbidity in hypertensives. The degree of hypertrophy correlates with the development of congestive heart failure, angina, arrhythmias, myocardial infarction, and sudden cardiac death.

Systolic Dysfunction

Although LVH initially serves a compensatory role, later in the course of systemic hypertension, the increased left ventricular mass may be insufficient to balance the high wall tension caused by the elevated afterload. As LV contractile capacity deteriorates, findings of systolic dysfunction become evident (reduced cardiac output and pulmonary congestion). Systolic dysfunction is also provoked by the accelerated development of coronary artery disease with re-

sultant periods of myocardial ishemia and/or infarction.

Coronary Artery Disease

Chronic hypertension is a major contributor to the development of myocardial ischemia and infarction. These complications reflect the combination of accelerated coronary atherosclerosis (decreased myocardial oxygen supply) and the high systolic workload (increased oxygen demand). Not only is acute MI more common among hypertensives than normotensives, but the former also have a higher incidence of post-MI complications such as rupture of the ventricular wall, left ventricular aneurysm formation, and congestive heart failure. In fact, 60% of patients who die of transmural MIs have a history of hypertension.

Cerebrovascular System

Hypertension is the major modifiable risk factor in the prevention of strokes (cerebrovascular accidents, or CVAs). Although diastolic pressure is important, it is the magnitude of the systolic pressure that has been most closely linked to CVAs. The presence of isolated systolic hypertension more than doubles an individual's chance of this complication.

Hypertension-induced strokes can be hemorrhagic or, more commonly, atherothrombotic. *Hemorrhagic* CVAs result from rupture of microaneurysms induced in cerebral parenchymal vessels by longstanding hypertension. *Atherothrombotic*, or thromboembolic, CVAs arise when portions of atherosclerotic plaque within the carotids or major cerebral arteries, or thrombi that form on those plaques, break off and embolize to smaller distal vessels. Additionally, intracerebral vessels may directly occlude by local atherosclerotic plaque rupture and thrombosis.

Occlusion of small penetrating arteries can result in multiple tiny infarcts. As these lesions soften and are absorbed by phagocytic cells, small (≤ 3 mm diameter) cavities form, termed *lacunae*. Such lacunar infarctions are seen almost exclusively in patients with longstanding hypertension and are usually localized to the penetrating branches of the middle and posterior circulation of the brain.

The generalized arterial narrowing found in hypertensive patients reduces collateral flow to ischemic tissues, and also imposes structural requirements for higher perfusion pressure to maintain adequate tissue flow. This leaves the hypertensive patient vulnerable to cerebral infarcts in areas supplied by the distal ends of arterial branches ("watershed" infarcts) if the blood pressure should fall suddenly.

The stroke risk is effectively diminished by treating hypertension, which has contributed to the 50% reduction in mortality attributed to cerebrovascular events in the past two decades.

Aorta and Peripheral Vasculature

The accelerated atherosclerosis associated with hypertension may result in plaque formation and narrowing throughout the arterial vasculature. In addition to the coronary arteries, lesions most commonly appear within the aorta and the major arteries to the lower extremities, neck, and brain.

Chronic hypertension may lead to the development of aortic aneurysms, particularly of the abdominal aorta (see Chapter 15). An **abdominal aortic aneurysm** (AAA) is a fusiform dilatation of the aorta, usually located below the level of the renal arteries, caused by the mechanical stress of the high pressure on an arterial wall already weak-

ened by medial damage and atherosclerosis. Aneurysms > 6 cm in diameter have a very high likelihood of rupture within 2 years if not surgically corrected.

Another life-threatening vascular consequence of high blood pressure is **aortic dissection** (see Chapter 15). Elevated blood pressure, especially in the highest ranges, accelerates degenerative changes in the media of the aorta. When the weakened wall is further exposed to high pressure, the intima may tear, allowing blood to dissect into the aortic media and propagate in either direction within the vessel wall, "clipping off" and obstructing major branch vessels along the way (e.g., coronary or carotid arteries). The mortality rate of aortic dissection is greater than 90% unless treated emergently, usually by surgical repair if the proximal aorta is involved. Subsequent rigorous control of hypertension is essential.

Kidney

Hypertension-induced nephropathy (nephrosclerosis) is a leading cause of renal failure that results from damage to the renal vasculature. Histologically, the vessel walls become thickened with a hyaline infiltrate, known as hyaline arteriolosclerosis (Fig. 13.8). Higher levels of hypertension can induce smooth muscle hypertrophy and even necrosis of capillary walls, termed fibrinoid necrosis. These changes result in reduced vascular supply and subsequent ischemic atrophy of tubules and, to a lesser extent, glomeruli. Because intact nephrons can usually compensate for those damaged by patchy ischemia, mild hypertension rarely leads to renal insufficiency in the absence of other insults to the kidney. However, malignant levels of hypertension can inflict permanent damage to the point that dialysis becomes necessary.

One of the consequences of hypertensive renal failure is perpetuation of the elevated blood pressure. For example, progressive renal failure compromises the ability of the kidney to regulate blood volume, that further contributes to chronic blood pressure elevation.

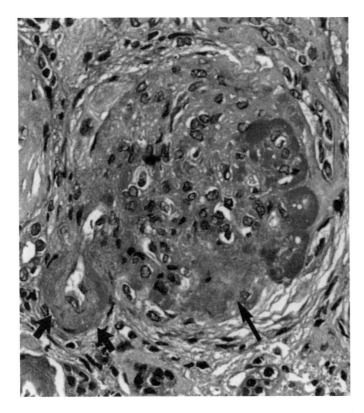

Figure 13.8. Histologic effects of chronic hypertension on the kidney. The arteriolar walls are thickened by hyaline infiltrate (short arrows). The glomeruli (long arrow) appear partially sclerosed because of reduced vascular supply. (Courtesy of Dr. Helmut G. Rennke, Brigham and Women's Hospital, Boston, Massachusetts.)

Retina

The retina is the only location where systemic arteries can be directly visualized by physical examination. High blood pressure induces abnormalities that are collectively termed **hypertensive retinopathy**. Although vision may be compromised when the damage is extensive, more commonly the changes serve as an asymptomatic clinical marker for the severity of hypertension and its duration.

Severe hypertension that is *acute in onset* (e.g., uncontrolled and/or malignant hypertension) may burst small retinal vessels, causing *hemorrhages, exudation of plasma lipids,* and areas of *local infarction* (Fig. 13.9C). If ischemia of the optic nerve develops, patients may describe generalized blurred vision. Retinal ischemia caused by hemorrhage leads to more patchy loss of vision. **Papilledema,** or swelling of the optic disc with blurring of its margins, may arise from high intracranial pressure when the blood pressure reaches malignant levels and cerebrovascular autoregulation begins to fail.

Chronically elevated blood pressure results in a different set of retinal findings (Fig. 13.9B): Papilledema is absent, but vasoconstriction results in arterial narrowing, and medial hypertrophy thickens the vessel wall, which "nicks" (indents) crossing veins. With more severe chronic hypertension, arterial sclerosis is evident as an increased reflection of light through the ophthalmoscope (termed "copper" or "silver" wiring). Although these changes are not in themselves of major functional import, they indicate that the patient has had long-standing, poorly controlled hypertension.

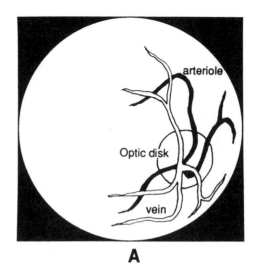

A

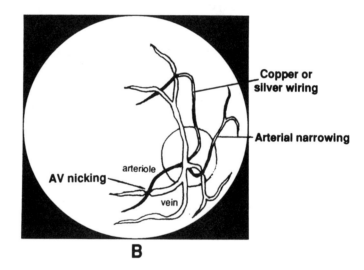

B

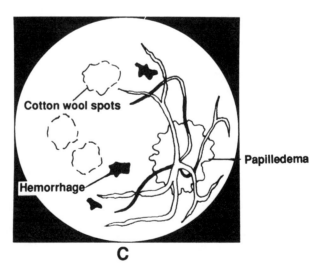

Figure 13.9.   Retinal abnormalities in acute and chronic hypertension. A. Normal retina. **B.** Chronic hypertension, demonstrating narrowed arteries, arteriovenous "nicking," copper and silver wiring (reflection off of sclerosed arteries). **C.** Malignant hypertension, characterized by hemorrhages, hard exudates (extravasated lipid), cotton-wool spots (infarcted zones), and papilledema.

C

HYPERTENSIVE CRISES

Hypertensive crises are medical emergencies characterized by a severe elevation of blood pressure. In the past, such elevations were usually a consequence of inadequate BP treatment. Now, hypertensive crises are more often because of acute hemodynamic insults (e.g., acute renal disease), superimposed on a chronic hypertensive state. As a result of rapid pathologic changes (fibrinoid necrosis) within the blood vessels and kidney, a spiraling increase in blood pressure evolves. Further volume expansion and vasoconstriction occur as renal perfusion drops and serum renin and angiotensin levels rise.

Severe BP elevation results in increased intracranial pressure, and patients may present with *hypertensive encephalopathy*, manifested by headache, blurred vision, confusion, somnolence, and sometimes coma. When hypertension results in acute damage to retinal vessels *accelerated-malignant hypertension* is said to be present. Funduscopic examination shows the effects of the rapid pressure rise as hemorrhages, exudates, and sometimes papilledema. The increased load on the left ventricle during hypertensive crises may precipitate angina (because of increased myocardial oxygen demand) or pulmonary edema.

Hypertensive crises require rapid therapy to reduce the blood pressure to prevent permanent vascular complications. Correction of the blood pressure is generally followed by reversal of the acute pathologic changes, including papilledema and retinal exudation, although renal damage often persists.

TREATMENT OF HYPERTENSION

The therapeutic approach to the hypertensive patient should be tempered by two considerations. First, a single elevated blood pressure measurement does not establish the diagnosis of hypertension, because blood pressure varies considerably throughout the day. Moreover, blood pressure measurement in the hospital or doctor's office may be affected by the "white coat" effect resulting from patient anxiety. The average of multiple readings taken on two or three separate office visits and/or in the home environment provides a more reliable basis for labeling a patient hypertensive.

Second, although mild hypertension is a major public health problem because so many people suffer from it, for the individual with stage 1 hypertension, the risk is small. For example, the additional risk of a stroke is approximately 1 in 850 per year. Hence, observation for a few months to see whether the low-level hypertension is persistent, or whether lifestyle changes can reduce the pressure, is a recommended alternative to immediate drug therapy. This is especially true in the absence of other cardiovascular risk factors such as smoking or high serum LDL cholesterol.

In the majority of hypertensive patients, drug therapy is ultimately the most effective way to prevent future complications, but that should not deter consideration of other beneficial lifestyle changes.

Nonpharmacologic Treatment

Weight Reduction

Studies have consistently found obesity and hypertension to be highly correlated with each other, especially when the obesity is of a central (abdominal) distribution. Furthermore, blood pressure reduction follows weight loss in a large portion of hypertensives who are more than 10% over ideal weight.

The explanation for the obesity-hypertension connection is not fully known. The blood pressure drop accompanying weight loss may be partly due to reduced circulating catecholamine levels, and therefore a lower TPR. Another link may relate to serum insulin levels. Obesity is often associated with resistance to the activity of insulin and secondary hyperinsulinemia. Hyperinsulinemia leads to other hormonal, ionic and trophic actions that may contribute to an elevated blood pressure, as described above.

Exercise

Sedentary normotensive people have a 20% to 50% higher risk of developing hypertention than their more active peers. Regular aerobic exercise, such as walking, jogging or bicycling, has been shown to contribute to blood pressure reduction over and above any resulting weight loss. A hypertensive patient who becomes physically conditioned manifests a lower resting heart rate and reduced levels of circulating catecholamines than before training, suggesting a fall in sympathetic tone.

Diet

In addition to caloric restriction for weight loss, changes in the composition of a patient's diet may be important for blood pressure reduction.

Sodium

Salt restriction for people with high blood pressure is a controversial issue, but there are several epidemiological and clinical trials that support moderation of sodium intake in hypertensives. In normotensive individuals, excess sodium intake is simply excreted by the kidneys, but about 50% of essential hypertensives are found to have blood pressures that vary with sodium intake, suggesting a defect in natriuresis. Sensitivity to sodium levels is more common in black and elderly hypertensive patients. Because low-salt diets tend to increase the effectiveness of antihypertensive medications in general, the current recommendation is for moderation in salt intake, to < 6 g sodium chloride (or < 2.3 g sodium) per day , which is one-third less than the average American consumption.

Potassium

Total body potassium content tends to be decreased by a diet low in fruits and vegetables, or in individuals who take potassium-wasting diuretics. Potassium deficiency has several theoretical effects that may raise blood pressure, and dietary supplements to replete low potassium levels are routinely recommended. Thus far however, there is no solid evidence that adding potassium supplements to the diet of a normokalemic hypertensive will lower the blood pressure.

Alcohol

The chronic intake of alcoholic beverages correlates with high blood pressure and resistance to antihypertensive medications. Moreover, experimental evidence shows that blood pressure (especially systolic) may rise acutely following alcohol consumption. The reason for this link remains incompletely understood, but decreases in chronic alcohol intake have been shown to lower blood pressure.

Other

Low calcium intake, magnesium depletion, and high dietary intake of saturated fats have all been associated with elevated blood pressure, but the responsible mechanisms and the implications for therapy are unclear. Caffeine ingestion transiently increases blood pressure (as much as 5 to 15 mmHg after two cups of coffee), but routine use does not seem to produce chronic pressure elevation.

Smoking

Cigarette smoking transiently increases blood pressure, probably via a nicotine effect on autonomic ganglia. Although smoking increases cardiovascular risk overall, smokers are actually found to have a *lower* incidence of hypertension than are nonsmokers. Moreover, smoking cessation is often accompanied by a small increase in blood pressure. Both phenomena may be linked to body weight, because smokers tend to be leaner than nonsmokers and may gain weight after they quit. The atherogenic effect of smoking does make renovascular hypertension (of the atherosclerotic type) more common in smokers than in nonsmokers. Cigarette usage is associated with many other health hazards, and all patients should be discouraged from smoking.

Relaxation Therapy

Blood pressure frequently rises under conditions of stress. In addition, essential hypertensive patients and their relatives often show higher than normal basal sympathetic tone and exaggerated autonomic responses to mental stress. Hence, relaxation techniques have been advocated as a method to control hypertension. Available methods include biofeedback and meditation. The effectiveness of such therapy depends on patient attitude and long-term compliance.

In summary, nonpharmacologic therapy offers a wide range of options that do not have the expense and potential side effects of prescribed drug use. The effectiveness of these therapies should come as no surprise, given the extent to which environmental factors play a role in hypertension. Therefore, such behavior-based interventions are recommended as first-line therapy in individuals whose hypertension is not an immediate danger to life and well-being.

Pharmacologic Treatment

Antihypertensive medications are the standard means to lower chronically elevated blood pressure, and are indicated if nonpharmacologic treatment proves inadequate. More than 100 drug preparations are available to treat hypertension, but the most commonly used medications fall into four classes: diuretics, sympatholytics, vasodilators, and drugs that interfere with the renin-angiotensin system (Table 13.4). The individual actions of these groups on the physiologic abnormalities in hypertension are shown in Figure 13.10. The pharmacology of many of the antihypertensive drug groups is described in greater detail in Chapter 17.

Diuretics have been used for many years as treatment for hypertension. They reduce circulatory volume, cardiac output, and mean arterial pressure, and are most effective in patients with mild to moderate hypertension who have normal renal function.

TABLE 13.4. Classes of Antihypertensive Medications

Drug Class	Types (see Chapter 17)
Diuretics	Thiazides
	Aldosterone-antagonists
Sympatholytics	Central α_2-agonists
	Peripheral α_1-blockers
	β-blockers
	Combined α-β-blockers
Vasodilators	Calcium channel blockers
	Direct vasodilators (e.g., hydralazine, minoxidil)
Renin-angiotensin system antagonists	Converting-enzyme inhibitors
	Angiotensin II receptor blockers

They are especially effective in black and in elderly hypertensives, who tend to be salt-sensitive. Diuretics have been among drugs used in long-term clinical trials shown to reduce the morbidity and mortality associated with hypertension, and are inexpensive compared with other available agents. Thiazide diuretics (e.g., hydrochlorothiazide) and potassium-sparing diuretics (e.g., spironolactone) promote Na^+ and Cl^- excretion in the nephron. Loop diuretics (e.g., furosemide) are generally too potent, and their actions too short-lived for use as antihypertensive agents.

Diuretics may result in adverse metabolic side effects, including elevation of serum glucose, cholesterol, and triglyceride levels. In addition, hypokalemia, hyperuricemia, and decreased sexual function are common side effects. However, when diuretics are prescribed in low dosage, it is often possible to accrue the desired antihypertensive effect while minimizing the adverse complications.

Sympatholytic agents block peripheral vasoconstriction and reduce heart rate and contractility (see Chapter 17). *Centrally acting* α-2 adrenergic agonists, such as methyldopa and clonidine, reduce sympathetic outflow to the heart, blood vessels, and kidneys. These are rarely used today, owing to their high frequency of side effects. *Systemic* adrenoceptor antagonists used in hypertension fall into two classes: those that block peripheral α_1-receptors and those that block β-receptors. α_1 antag-

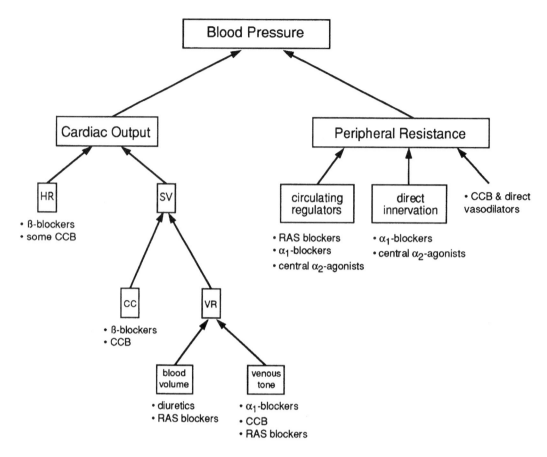

Figure 13.10. Physiologic effects of antihypertensive medications. Note that some antihypertensives work at multiple sites. HR, heart rate; SV, stroke volume; CC, cardiac contractility; VR, venous return; CCB, Ca^{++} channel blockers; RAS blockers, renin-angiotensin system blockers (i.e., angiotensin converting enzyme inhibitors and angiotensin II receptor antagonists).

onists, such as prazosin, cause a decrease in TPR through relaxation of vascular smooth muscle. β-blockers, such as propranolol, reduce CO through a decrease in heart rate and mild decrease in contractility; these agents also decrease the secretion of renin (and therefore angiotensin II), causing a decrease in total peripheral resistance. Adverse effects of β-blockers include fatigue, impotence, and hyperglycemia. They may also adversely alter lipid metabolism; most β-blockers cause a rise in serum triglycerides and a reduction of "good" HDL cholesterol (note that beta-blockers with intrinsic sympathomimetic activity (see Chapter 17), or those with combined α-blocking properties do not adversely effect HDL levels).

Commonly used peripheral **vasodilators**

include Ca^{++} channel blockers, hydralazine, and minoxidil. Ca^{++} channel blockers reduce the influx of calcium responsible for cardiac and vascular smooth muscle contraction (see Chapter 17). Long-acting (i.e., sustained-release drug taken once a day) Ca^{++} channel blockers are frequently used to treat hypertension. The shorter acting Ca^{++} channel blocker preparations are no longer used for this purpose. They are less convenient (must be taken 2–3 times per day) and have recently been implicated in adverse cardiovascular outcomes (i.e., a possible heightened occurence of myocardial infarction in individuals treated with the short-acting forms). Hydralazine and minoxidil directly relax vascular smooth muscle of precapillary resistance vessels. Their use in treating hypertension has waned with the advent of newer agents with fewer side effects.

Drugs that interfere with the renin-angiotensin system include angiotensin converting enzyme (ACE) inhibitors and angiotensin II receptor antagonists. **ACE inhibitors** decrease blood pressure by blocking the conversion of angiotensin I to angiotensin II (Fig. 13.6), thereby reducing the vasopressor activity of AII and also the secretion of aldosterone. Thus, there is a reduction in TPR, as well as of sodium retention by the kidney. An additional antihypertensive effect of the ACE inhibitors is to increase the concentration of the circulating vasodilator bradykinin (see Chapter 17). ACE inhibitors are generally well-tolerated and have gained much popularity in the past several years. They have been shown to reduce mortality in patients following an acute MI and also among patients with chronic symptomatic systolic heart failure (see Chapter 9). They also slow the deterioration of renal function in patients with diabetic nephropathy. The most common side effect of ACE inhibitors in clinical experience is the development of a reversible dry cough (likely related to the increased bradykinin effect); hyperkalemia and azotemia may also occur , as described in Chapter 17.

Angiotensin II receptor antagonists are the newest class of antihypertensive agents. The action of this group is to block the binding of angiotensin II to its receptors (i.e., subtype AT_1 receptors) in blood vessels and other targets (Fig. 13.6). By inhibiting the effects of angiotensin II (and thereby causing vasodilation and reduced secretion of aldosterone), the blood pressure falls. In clinical trials, the antihypertensive efficacy of this group is similar to that of ACE inhibitors. However, a potential advantage is that unlike the ACE inhibitors, this class does not produce cough as a side effect.

Given the large number of antihypertensive drugs available, the choice of which drug to use as initial therapy in an individual patient can seem daunting. The first-line drugs recommended by the Joint National Committee on Detection, Evaluation, and Treatment of High Blood Pressure include diuretics, β-blockers, ACE inhibitors, Ca^{++} channel antagonists, α_1-receptor blockers, and combined α-β-receptor blockers. However, that committee has urged that a diuretic or β-blocker be tried first, as these drugs have been associated with reduced long-term morbidity and mortality in clinical trials, and are less costly than other antihypertensives. This recommendation has caused considerable controversy because other groups of drugs are often better tolerated than diuretics and beta-blockers. As therapy is likely to continue for many years, consideration of adverse effects and impact of drug therapy on the patient's quality of life are very important.

There are some other guiding principles. First, the chosen drug regimen should conform to the patient's specific needs. For example, an anxious young patient in the throes of the "hyperkinetic" phase of EH might be best treated with a β-blocker, while a better choice for the same patient many years later, after the pressure becomes more dependent on peripheral vascular resistance, could be a vasodilator (e.g., long-acting Ca^{++} channel blocker).

Another helpful principle of antihypertensive drug therapy concerns the use of multiple agents. The effects of one drug, acting at one physiologic control point, can be defeated by natural compensatory mechanisms. For example, the drop in renal perfusion by hydralazine (a direct vasodilator) can activate the renin-angiotensin system, prompting the kidney to retain more volume, thereby blunting the antihypertensive benefit. Combination drug therapy is aimed at preventing such an action, by utilizing agents acting at different complimentary sites. In this example, a direct vasodilator is often paired with a low-dose diuretic to avoid the undesired volume expansion effect.

In conclusion, hypertension emerges as a fascinating clinical problem, important because of its prevalence and devastating consequences, and interesting because of its usually obscure cause(s). The work-up and treatment of a patient with hypertension requires methodical consideration of the ways in which normal cardiovascular physiology can go astray. Because most patients still fall unsatisfyingly into the idiopathic category of essential hypertension, there is still much room for creative thought and research in this area.

SUMMARY

1. Hypertension is defined as a chronic diastolic blood pressure (BP) of $\geq$ 90 mmHg or a systolic BP $\geq$ 140 mmHg.
2. Hypertension is of unknown cause in 95% of patients ("essential hypertension"). Secondary hypertension may arise from many causes, including: 1) renal parenchymal disease, 2) renovascular hypertension, 3) pheochromocytoma, 4) coarctation of the aorta, and 5) primary aldosteronism.
3. Most hypertensive patients remain asymptomatic until complications arise. Complications include: 1) stroke, 2) myocardial infarction, 3) heart failure, 4) aortic aneurysms and dissection, 5) renal damage, and 6) retinopathy.
4. Treatment of hypertension includes lifestyle and dietary changes, followed by pharmacologic therapy. The first-line antihypertensive drugs used today include diuretics, β-blockers, ACE inhibitors, long-acting Ca^{++} channel antagonists, and α_1-receptor blockers.

ADDITIONAL READING

Goodfriend TL, Elliott ME, Catt KJ. Angiotensin receptors and their antagonists. N Engl J Med 1996; 334:1649–1654.

Hollenberg NK. Hypertension: mechanisms and therapy. In: Braunwald E, ed. Atlas of Heart Diseases. St. Louis: CV Mosby, 1995.

Hunt SC, Hopkins PN, Williams RR. Hypertension: genetics and mechanisms. In: Fuster V, Ross R, Topol EJ, eds. Atherosclerosis and Coronary Artery Disease. Philadelphia: Lippincott-Raven, 1996:209–236.

Joint National Committee on Detection, Evaluation, and Treatment of High Blood Pressure. The fifth report of the Joint National Committee on Detection, Evaluation, and Treatment of High Blood Pressure (JNC V). Arch Intern Med 1993;153:154–183.

Kannel WB. Blood pressure as a cardiovascular risk factor. JAMA 1996;275:1571–1576.

Kaplan NM. Clinical Hypertension. 6th ed. Baltimore: Williams & Wilkins, 1994.

Oliverio MI, Coffman TM. Angiotensin-II receptors: New targets for antihypertensive therapy. Clin Cardiol 1997;20:3–6.

Sytkowski PA, D'Agostino RB, Belanger AJ, et al. Secular trends in long-term sustained hypertension. long-term treatment, and cardiovascular mortality. Circulation 1996;93:697–703.

Acknowledgments   The previous edition of this chapter was written by Rajesh S. Magrulkar, MD, Peter A. Nigrovic, MD, and Thomas J. Moore, MD.

Diseases of the Pericardium

*Thomas G. Roberts
and Leonard S. Lilly*

Diseases of the pericardium form a spectrum that ranges from benign, self-limited pericarditis to life-threatening cardiac tamponade. The clinical manifestations of these disorders, and approaches to their management, can be predicted from an understanding of pericardial anatomy and pathophysiology, as presented in this chapter.

ANATOMY AND FUNCTION

The pericardium is a two-layered sac that encircles the heart. The inner serosal layer (*visceral pericardium*) adheres to the outer wall of the heart and is reflected back upon itself, at the level of the great vessels, to join the tough fibrous outer layer (*parietal pericardium*). A thin film of pericardial fluid slightly separates the two layers and decreases the friction between them.

The pericardium appears to serve three functions: 1) it fixes the heart within the mediastinum and limits its motion, 2) it prevents extreme dilatation of the heart during sudden rises of intracardiac volume, and 3) it may function as a barrier to limit the spread of infection from the adjacent lungs. However, patients with complete absence of the pericardium (either congenitally, or after surgical removal) are generally asymptomatic, casting doubt on its actual importance in normal physiology. Yet like the unnecessary appendix, the pericardium can become diseased and cause great harm.

In the healthy heart, intrapericardial pressure varies during the respiratory cycle from −5 cm (during inspiration) to +5 cm water (during expiration) and nearly equals the pressure within the pleural space. However, pathologic changes in pericardial stiffness or the accumulation of fluid within the pericardial sac may profoundly increase this pressure.

ACUTE PERICARDITIS

The most common affliction of the pericardium is acute pericarditis, which refers to inflammation of its layers. Many disease states and etiologic agents produce this syndrome (Table 14.1), the most common of which are described here.

TABLE 14.1. Most Common Causes of Acute Pericarditis

Infectious
  Viral
  Tuberculosis
  Pyogenic bacteria
Noninfectious
  Postmyocardial infarction
  Uremia
  Neoplastic disease
  Radiation-induced
  Connective-tissue diseases
  Drug-induced

Etiology

Infectious

Idiopathic and Viral Pericarditis

Acute pericarditis is most often of "idiopathic" origin, meaning that the actual cause is unknown. However, epidemiologic studies have demonstrated that many such episodes are actually caused by viral infection, especially by echovirus or Coxsackie virus group B. Although a viral origin could be confirmed in infected patients by comparing antiviral titers of acute and convalescent serum, this is rarely done in the clinical setting because the patient has usually recovered by the time those results would be available. Thus, "idiopathic" and viral pericarditis are considered similar clinical entities, and the terms are used interchangeably.

Other viruses known to cause pericarditis include those responsible for influenza, varicella, mumps, hepatitis B, and infectious mononucleosis. Pericarditis has been found with increased frequency among patients with AIDS, possibly related to HIV itself, but often due to superimposed tuberculous or other bacterial infections in this immunocompromised population.

Tuberculous Pericarditis

Although tuberculosis remains a worldwide problem, its incidence in the United States is low. It is, however, an important cause of pericarditis in immunosuppressed individuals, such as those with AIDS. Tuberculous pericarditis arises from reactivation of the organism in mediastinal lymph nodes, with spread into the pericardium. It can also extend directly from a site of tuberculosis within the lungs, or the organism can arrive at the pericardium by hematogenous dissemination.

Nontuberculous Bacterial Pericarditis (Purulent Pericarditis)

Bacterial pericarditis has also been rare since the advent of antibiotics. The pneumococcus and staphylococci are responsible most frequently, whereas Gram-negative infection occurs less often. Common mechanisms by which bacterial invasion of the pericardium develops include: 1) perforating trauma to the chest (e.g., stab wound), 2) contamination during chest surgery, 3) extension of an intracardiac infection (i.e., infective endocarditis), 4) extension of pneumonia or a subdiaphragmatic infection, and 5) hematogenous spread from a remote infection. Bacterial pericarditis is a fulminant illness, but is rare in otherwise healthy individuals; it is most likely to occur in immunocompromised states, including those with severe burns, malignancies, and AIDS.

Noninfectious

Pericarditis Following Myocardial Infarction

There are two forms of pericarditis associated with acute myocardial infarction (MI). The early form occurs within the first few days of MI, affecting 10% to 15% of patients. It likely results from epicardial inflammation extending from the injured myocardium, and is therefore most common in patients with transmural infarctions. The prognosis following acute MI is not affected by the presence of pericarditis; its major importance is in distinguishing it from the pain of recurrent myocardial ischemia. The incidence of this form of pericarditis has been declining since the introduction of thrombolytic therapy for acute MI, likely because of the associated reduction in infarct size.

The second form is known as *Dressler's syndrome*, which develops 2 weeks to several months following an acute MI. Its cause is unknown, but is thought to be of autoimmune origin, possibly directed against antigens released from necrotic myocardial cells. A clinically similar form of pericarditis may occur weeks to months following heart surgery (termed *postpericardiotomy pericarditis*).

Uremic Pericarditis

Pericarditis is a serious complication of chronic renal failure, but its pathogenesis is unknown. Studies have shown no correlation between the plasma level of nitrogen waste products and the incidence of this form of pericarditis, and it may even develop in patients during the first few months of dialysis therapy.

Neoplastic Pericarditis

Tumor within the pericardium most commonly results from metastatic spread or local invasion by cancer of the lung, breast, or lymphoma. Primary tumors of the pericardium are rare. Neoplastic effusions are usually large and hemorrhagic, and frequently lead to cardiac tamponade, a severe complication described below.

Radiation-Induced Pericarditis

Pericarditis may complicate previous radiation therapy to the thorax (e.g., administered for the treatment of certain tumors), especially if the cumulative dose has exceeded 4000 rads. Radiation-induced damage causes a local inflammatory response that can result in pericardial effusions and fibrosis. Cytologic examination of the pericardial fluid helps to distinguish radiation-induced pericardial damage from that of tumor invasion.

Pericarditis Associated With Connective Tissue Diseases

Pericardial involvement is common in many connective tissue diseases, including systemic lupus erythematosus (SLE), rheumatoid arthritis, and progressive systemic sclerosis. For example, 20%–40% of patients with SLE experience clinically detectable pericarditis during the course of their disease. Customary treatment of the underlying connective tissue disease usually ameliorates the pericarditis as well.

Drug-Induced Pericarditis

Many pharmaceutical agents can result in pericarditis, often by inducing a systemic lupus-like syndrome. Drugs that most commonly induce this syndrome include the antiarrhythmic *procainamide* and the vasodilator *hydralazine*. This form of pericarditis usually abates when the causative drug is discontinued.

Pathogenesis

Similar to other inflammatory processes, pericarditis is characterized by three stages: 1) local *vasodilation* with transudation of protein-poor, cell-free fluid into the pericardial space, 2) *increased vascular permeability*, with leak of protein into the pericardial space, and 3) *leukocyte exudation*, initially by neutrophils, followed later by mononuclear cells.

The leukocytes are of critical importance because they help contain or eliminate the offending infectious or autoimmune agent. However, metabolic products released by these cells may prolong inflammation, cause pain and local cellular damage, and mediate somatic symptoms such as fever. Therefore, the immune response to pericardial injury may significantly contribute to tissue damage and symptomatology.

Pathology

The pathologic appearance of the pericardium depends on the underlying cause and severity of inflammation. **Serous pericarditis** is characterized by scant polymorphonuclear leukocytes, lymphocytes, and histiocytes. The exudate is a thin fluid secreted by the mesothelial cells lining the serosal surface of the pericardium. This likely represents the early inflammatory response common to all types of acute pericarditis.

Serofibrinous pericarditis is the most commonly observed morphologic pattern in patients with pericarditis. The pericardial exudate contains plasma proteins, including fibrinogen (which may be converted into fibrin), yielding a grossly rough and shaggy appearance (termed "bread and butter" pericarditis). Portions of the visceral and parietal pericardium may become thickened and fused. Occasionally, this process leads to a dense scar that restricts movement and diastolic filling of the cardiac chambers (constrictive pericarditis), as described below.

Suppurative (or purulent) pericarditis is an intense inflammatory response associated most commonly with bacterial infection. The serosal surfaces are erythematous and coated with purulent exudate.

Hemorrhagic pericarditis refers to a grossly bloody form of pericardial inflammation and is most often due to tuberculosis or neoplasm.

Clinical Features

History

The most frequent symptoms of acute pericarditis are *chest pain* and *fever* (Table 14.2). The pain may be severe and most often localizes to the retrosternal area and left precordium; it may radiate to the back and ridge of the left trapezius muscle. What differentiates it from myocardial ischemia or infarction is that the pain of pericarditis is typically sharp and *pleuritic* (it is aggravated by inspiration and coughing) and *positional:* sitting and leaning forward, for example, often lessen the discomfort. *Dyspnea* is common during acute pericarditis, but is not exertional, and probably results from a reluctance of the patient to breathe deeply, because of the pleuritic pain.

Patients with idiopathic or viral pericarditis are typically young and previously healthy. Pericarditis of other causes should be suspected in individuals with the underlying diseases in Table 14.1 who develop the typical sharp, pleuritic chest pains and fever.

Physical Examination

A scratchy pericardial *friction rub* is common in acute pericarditis and is produced by the movement of the inflamed pericardial layers against one another. Auscultation of the rub is best heard using the diaphragm of the stethoscope with the patient leaning forward, while exhaling (which brings the pericardium closer to the chest wall and stethoscope). In its full form, the rub consists of three components, corresponding to the phases of greatest cardiac movement: ventricular contraction, ventricular relaxation, and atrial contraction. Characteristically, the pericardial rub is evanescent, so that it may come and go from one examination to the next.

Diagnostic Approach

The presence of pleuritic, positional chest pain and the characteristic pericardial friction rub implicate the presence of acute pericarditis. However, certain laboratory studies are helpful to confirm the diagnosis, and to assess any impending complications.

The *electrocardiogram* is abnormal in 90% of patients with acute pericarditis, and helps to distinguish it from other forms of cardiac disease, such as an acute MI. The most important EKG pattern, which reflects inflammation of the adjacent myocardium, consists of *diffuse ST-segment elevation* in most of the EKG leads, usually with the exception of aV_R and V_1 (Fig. 14.1). In addition, *PR segment depression* is often evident, reflecting abnormal atrial repolarization related to the inflammatory process. These abnormalities are in contrast to the EKG of acute MI, in which the ST segments are elevated only in the leads overlying the region of infarction.

Further testing in acute pericarditis often includes *echocardiography* to evaluate for the presence and hemodynamic significance of an effusion. Additional data that may be useful in individual cases to define the cause of pericarditis include: 1) PPD skin test for tuberculosis, 2) serologic tests (ANA and rheumatoid factor) to screen for connective tissue diseases, and 3) a careful search for malignancy, especially of the lung and breast (physical examination supplemented by chest radiograph and mam-

---

TABLE 14.2. Clinical Features of Acute Pericarditis

1. Pleuritic chest pain
2. Fever
3. Pericardial friction rub
4. EKG abnormalities

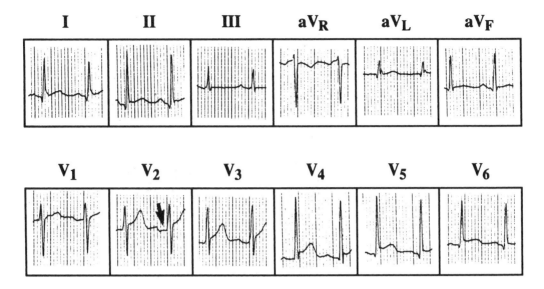

Figure 14.1. Electrocardiogram in acute pericarditis. Diffuse ST segment elevation is present. Also note depression of the PR segment (arrow).

mogram). The yield of diagnostic pericardiocentesis (removal of pericardial fluid through a needle) in uncomplicated acute pericarditis is low, and should be reserved for patients with very large effusions or evidence of cardiac chamber compression, as discussed below.

Treatment

Idiopathic or viral pericarditis is a self-limited disease that usually runs its course in 1 to 3 weeks. Management consists of *rest*, to reduce the interaction of the inflamed pericardial layers, and *pain relief* by analgesic and anti-inflammatory drugs (aspirin and other nonsteroidal anti-inflammatory agents). Oral corticosteroids are often effective for severe or recurrent pericardial pain, but should *not* be used in uncomplicated cases, because of potentially devastating side effects, and because even gradual withdrawal of this form of therapy often leads to recurrent symptoms of pericarditis.

The forms of pericarditis that follow myocardial infarction are treated in a similar fashion, with rest and aspirin. To reduce the risk of intrapericardial hemorrhage, anticoagulants, otherwise often used in the setting of acute MI, are relatively contraindicated.

Purulent pericarditis requires more aggressive treatment, including catheter drainage of the pericardium and intensive antibiotic therapy, but even with such therapy, the mortality rate is very high. Tuberculous pericarditis requires prolonged multidrug antituberculous therapy. Pericarditis in the setting of uremia often resolves following intensive dialysis. Neoplastic pericardial disease usually indicates widely metastatic cancer, and therapy is unfortunately only palliative, using radiation or chemotherapy.

PERICARDIAL EFFUSION

Etiology

The normal pericardial space contains 15 to 50 ml of pericardial fluid, a plasma ultrafiltrate secreted by the mesothelial cells that line the serosal layer. However, a larger volume of fluid may accumulate in association with any of the forms of acute pericarditis discussed above.

In addition, noninflammatory serous effusions may result from conditions of: 1) increased capillary permeability (e.g., severe hypothyroidism), 2) increased capillary hydrostatic pressure (e.g., congestive heart failure), or 3) decreased plasma oncotic pressure (e.g., cirrhosis or the nephrotic syndrome). Chylous effusions may occur in the presence of lymphatic obstruction of pericardial drainage, due most commonly to neoplasms and tuberculosis.

Pathophysiology

Because the pericardium is a relatively stiff structure, the relationship between its internal volume and pressure is not linear (Fig. 14.2, curve A). Note that the initial portion of this curve is nearly flat, indicating that at the low volumes normally present within the pericardium, a small increase in volume leads to only a small rise in pressure. However, when the intrapericardial volume expands beyond a critical level (arrow), a dramatic increase in pressure is incited by the nondistensible sac. At that point, even a minor increase in volume can translate into an enormous compressive force on the heart.

Three factors determine whether a pericardial effusion remains clinically silent, or whether symptoms of cardiac compression ensue: 1) the *volume* of fluid, 2) the *rate* at which the fluid accumulates, and 3) the *compliance* characteristics of the pericardium.

A *sudden* increase of pericardial volume,

as may occur with chest trauma with intrapericardial hemorrhage, results in marked elevation of pericardial pressure (Fig. 14.2, steep portion of curve A), and the potential for severe cardiac chamber compression. Even smaller amounts of fluid may cause marked elevation of pressure if the pericardium is pathologically noncompliant and stiff, as may occur in the presence of tumor or fibrosis of the sac. In contrast, if the pericardial effusion accumulates *slowly*, over weeks to months, the pericardium gradually stretches, such that the volume-pressure relationship curve shifts toward the right (Fig. 14.2, curve B). With this adaptation, the pericardium can accommodate larger volumes (e.g., 1 to 2 *liters*) without marked elevation of intrapericardial pressure.

Clinical Features

There is a spectrum of possible symptoms associated with pericardial effusions. For example, the patient with a large effusion may be asymptomatic, may complain of a dull constant ache in the left side of the chest, or present with symptoms of cardiac tamponade, described below. In addition, the effusion may cause symptoms due to compression of adjacent structures, such as dysphagia (difficult swallowing because of esophageal compression), dyspnea (shortness of breath resulting from lung compres-

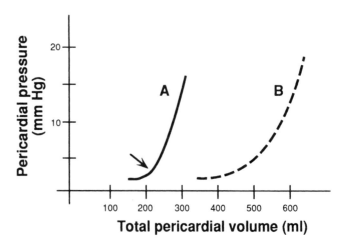

Figure 14.2. Schematic representation of the volume-pressure relationship of the normal pericardium (A). At the very lowest levels, a small rise in volume results in a small rise in pressure. However, when the limits of pericardial stretch are reached (arrow), the curve becomes very steep, and a further small rise in intrapericardial volume results in markedly increased pressure. B. Chronic slow accumulation of volume allows the pericardium to gradually stretch over time, so that the curve shifts to the right, and much larger volumes are accommodated at lower pressures. (Modified from Freeman GL, LeWinter MM. Pericardial adaptations during chronic dilation in dogs. Circ Res 1984;54:294.)

TABLE 14.3. Clinical Features of Large Pericardial Effusion

1. Soft heart sounds
2. Reduced intensity of friction rub
3. Ewart's sign (dullness over posterior left lung)

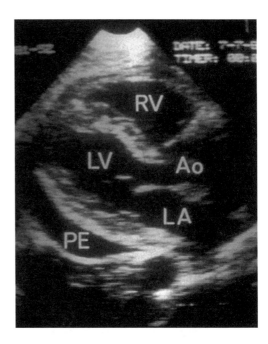

Figure 14.3. Two-dimensional echocardiogram (parasternal long axis view) of a small pericardial effusion (PE) posterior to the left ventricle (LV). Ao, aortic root; LA, left atrium; RV, right ventricle.

sion), hoarseness (due to recurrent laryngeal nerve compression), or hiccups (because of phrenic nerve stimulation).

On examination (Table 14.3), a large pericardial fluid "insulates" the heart from the chest wall, and the heart sounds may be muffled. In fact, a friction rub that had been present during the acute phase of pericarditis may disappear if a large effusion separates the inflamed layers widely from one another. Dullness to percussion of the left lung over the angle of the scapula may occur, known as "Ewart's sign," and is due to compressive atelectasis by the enlarged pericardial sac.

Diagnostic Studies

The *chest radiograph* may be normal if only a small pericardial effusion is present. However, if more than approximately 250 ml has accumulated, the cardiac silhouette is enlarged in a globular, symmetric fashion. In large effusions, the *electrocardiogram* may demonstrate reduced voltage of the complexes because of the insulation effect of the surrounding fluid. In the presence of extremely large effusions, the height of the QRS complex may vary from beat to beat (electrical alternans); this results from a constantly changing electrical axis, as the heart swings from side-to-side within the large pericardial volume.

The most useful laboratory test in the evaluation of an effusion is the *echocardiogram* (Fig. 14.3), which can identify pericardial collections as small as 20 ml. This noninvasive technique can quantify the volume of pericardial fluid, determine whether ventricular filling is compromised, and when necessary, help direct the placement of a pericardiocentesis needle.

Treatment

If the cause of the effusion is known, then therapy is directed toward the underlying disorder (e.g., intensive dialysis for uremic effusion). If the cause is not evident, the clinical state of the patient determines whether pericardiocentesis (removal of pericardial fluid) should be undertaken. An asymptomatic effusion, even of large volume, can be observed for months or years, without specific intervention. However, if serial examination demonstrates a precipitous rise in pericardial volume, or hemodynamic compression of the cardiac chambers becomes evident, then pericardiocentesis should be performed for therapeutic drainage, and for analysis of the pericardial fluid.

CARDIAC TAMPONADE

At the opposite end of the spectrum from the asymptomatic pericardial effusion is cardiac tamponade. In this condition, pericardial fluid accumulates under high pressure, compresses the cardiac chambers, and severely limits filling of the heart. As a result, ventricular stroke volume and cardiac output decline, potentially leading to hypotensive shock and death.

Etiology

Any etiology of acute pericarditis (Table 14.1) can progress to cardiac tamponade, but the most common causes are neoplastic, postviral, and uremic pericarditis. Acute hemorrhage into the pericardium is also an important cause of tamponade, which can result from: 1) blunt or penetrating chest trauma, 2) rupture of the LV free wall following myocardial infarction (see Chapter 7), or 3) as a complication of a dissecting aortic aneurysm (see Chapter 15).

Pathophysiology

As a result of the surrounding tense pericardial fluid, the heart is compressed, and *the diastolic pressure within each chamber becomes elevated and equal to the pericardial pressure.* The pathophysiologic consequences of this are illustrated in Figure 14.4. Because filling of the heart chambers is impaired, the systemic and pulmonary venous pressures become elevated, as normal return of blood to the heart cannot be accommodated. The increase of systemic venous pressure results in signs of right-sided heart failure (jugular venous distension, hepatomegaly, peripheral edema), whereas elevated pulmonary venous pressure can lead to pulmonary congestion. In addition, reduced filling of the ventricles during diastole decreases the systolic stroke volume, and the cardiac output declines.

These derangements trigger compen-

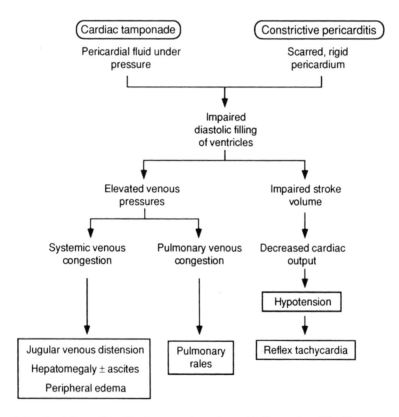

Figure 14.4. Pathophysiology of cardiac tamponade and constrictive pericarditis. The symptoms and signs (boxes) arise from impaired diastolic filling of the ventricles in the absence of systolic contractile dysfunction.

satory mechanisms aimed at maintaining tissue perfusion, initially through activation of the sympathetic nervous system (see Chapter 9). Nonetheless, failure to evacuate the effusion leads to inadequate perfusion of vital organs, shock, and ultimately death.

Clinical Features

Cardiac tamponade should be suspected in any patient with known pericarditis, pericardial effusion, or chest trauma who develops signs and symptoms of systemic vascular congestion and decreased cardiac output (Table 14.4). The key physical findings include: 1) jugular venous distension, 2) systemic hypotension, and 3) a small, quiet heart on physical examination, due to the insulating effects of the effusion. Other signs include sinus tachycardia and pulsus paradoxus (described below). Dyspnea and tachypnea reflect pulmonary congestion, as well as decreased oxygen delivery to peripheral tissues.

If tamponade develops suddenly, symptoms of profound hypotension are evident, including confusion and agitation. However, if the effusion develops more slowly, over a period of weeks, then fatigue (low cardiac output) and peripheral edema (right-sided heart failure) may be the presenting complaints.

Pulsus paradoxus is an important physical sign in cardiac tamponade that can be measured at the bedside using a blood pressure cuff. It refers to a cyclical *decrease of systolic blood pressure (> 10 mmHg) during normal inspiration.*

Pulsus paradoxus is not really "paradoxical"; it is just an exaggeration of ap-

propriate cardiac physiology. Normally, expansion of the thorax during inspiration causes the intrathoracic pressure to become more negative, compared with the expiratory phase. This facilitates systemic venous return to the chest, and augments filling of the right ventricle (RV). The transient increase in RV size shifts the interventricular septum toward the left, which slightly diminishes *left* ventricular (LV) filling. Thus, normally, LV stroke volume and systolic blood pressure decline slightly following inspiration.

In cardiac tamponade, this situation is exaggerated as both ventricles share a reduced, fixed volume due to external compression by the tense pericardial fluid. In this case, the inspiratory increase of right ventricular volume and bulging of the interventricular septum toward the left have a proportionally greater effect on the impairment of LV filling. Thus, in tamponade there is a more substantial reduction of LV stroke volume (and therefore systolic blood pressure) following inspiration.

Pulsus paradoxus is not diagnostic of tamponade because it may be present in other conditions in which inspiration is exaggerated, including severe asthma and chronic obstructive airways disease.

Diagnostic Approach

Echocardiography is the most useful noninvasive technique in evaluating whether pericardial effusion has led to cardiac tamponade. An important indicator of high-pressure pericardial fluid is evidence of compression of the right ventricle and right atrium during diastole (see Fig. 3.12). In addition, echocardiography can differentiate between cardiac tamponade and other causes of low cardiac output, such as systolic ventricular dysfunction.

The definitive diagnostic procedure for cardiac tamponade is cardiac catheterization with intracardiac and intrapericardial pressure measurements, usually combined with therapeutic pericardiocentesis, as described in the next section.

TABLE 14.4. Clinical Features of Cardiac Tamponade

1. Jugular venous distension
2. Hypotension with pulsus paradoxus
3. Quiet precordium on palpation
4. Sinus tachycardia

Treatment

Removal of the high-pressure pericardial fluid is the only measure that reverses the abnormal, life-threatening physiology in this condition. Pericardiocentesis is best performed in the cardiac catheterization laboratory, where the hemodynamic effect of fluid removal is assessed. The patient is positioned head up at a 45° angle to promote pooling of the effusion, and a needle is inserted into the pericardial space, just below the xiphoid process, in order to avoid trauma to the coronary arteries. A catheter is then threaded into the pericardial space and connected to a transducer for pressure measurement. Another catheter is threaded from a systemic vein into the right side of the heart, and simultaneous recordings of intracardiac and intrapericardial pressures are compared. In tamponade, the pericardial pressure is elevated and *equal* to the diastolic pressures within the cardiac chambers; all of the latter are elevated to the same degree because of the surrounding compressive force of the effusion.

In addition, the right atrial pressure tracing, which is equivalent to the jugular venous pressure on physical examination, is abnormal (Fig. 14.5): In a normal individual, during early diastole, as the right ventricular (RV) pressure falls and the tricuspid valve opens, blood quickly flows from the right atrium into the RV, such that there is a rapid decline in RA pressure ("y" descent). In tamponade, however, the pericardial fluid compresses the RV, and prevents its rapid expansion. Thus the RA cannot empty quickly, and *the y descent is blunted.*

Following successful pericardiocentesis, the pericardial pressure returns to normal (approximately 0 mmHg), and is no longer equal to the pressures within the heart chambers, which also decline to their normal levels. In addition, a normal y descent returns to the RA tracing. After initial aspiration of fluid, the pericardial catheter may be left in place for a day or two to allow more complete drainage.

When obtained, pericardial fluid should be stained and cultured for bacteria, fungi, and acid fast bacilli (tuberculosis), and cy-

tologic examination should be performed to evaluate for malignancy. If a large effusion or cardiac tamponade recurs, repeat pericardiocentesis may be performed; a more definitive procedure to prevent recurrent tamponade in some cases is surgical removal of part, or all, of the pericardium.

CONSTRICTIVE PERICARDITIS

The other major complication of pericardial disease is known as constrictive pericarditis. This is a condition not often encountered, but important to understand, because it can masquerade as other, more common disorders. In addition, it is an affliction that may be very symptomatic, yet fully treatable if recognized.

Etiology and Pathogenesis

Earlier in this century, tuberculosis was the major cause of pericardial constriction, but that is much less common today in industrialized societies. The most common cause now is "idiopathic" (i.e., months to years following presumed idiopathic/viral acute pericarditis). However, any cause of pericarditis (Table 14.1) can lead to this complication.

Pathology

Following an episode of acute pericarditis, any developed pericardial effusion usually undergoes gradual resorption. However, in patients who later develop constrictive pericarditis, the fluid undergoes organization, with subsequent fusion of the pericardial layers, followed by fibrous scar formation. In some patients, calcification of the adherent layers ensues, further stiffening the pericardium.

Pathophysiology

The pathophysiologic abnormalities in constrictive pericarditis occur during dias-

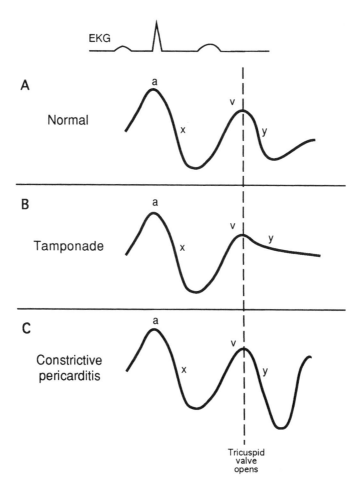

Figure 14.5.   Schematic diagrams of right atrial (or jugular venous) pressure recordings. A. Normal. The initial "a" wave represents atrial contraction. The "v" wave reflects passive filling of the atria during systole, when the tricuspid and mitral valves are closed. After the tricuspid valve opens, the right atrial pressure falls ("y" descent) as blood empties into the right ventricle. **B.** Cardiac tamponade. High-pressure pericardial fluid compresses the heart, impairing right ventricular filling, so that the y descent is blunted. **C.** Constrictive pericarditis. The *earliest* phase of diastolic filling is not impaired so that the y descent is not blunted. The y descent appears accentuated because it descends from a higher than normal right atrial pressure. The right atrial "c" wave (described in Chapter 2) is not shown.

tole; systolic contraction of the ventricles is normal. In this condition, a rigid, scarred pericardium encircles the heart and *inhibits normal filling of the cardiac chambers.* In diastole, as blood passes from the right atrium into the right ventricle, the RV size expands and quickly reaches the limit imposed by the constricting pericardium. At that point, further filling is suddenly arrested, and venous return to the right heart ceases. Thus, systemic venous pressure rises, and signs of right-sided heart failure ensue. In addition, the impaired filling of the left ventricle causes a reduction in stroke volume, cardiac output, and therefore blood pressure.

Clinical Features

The symptoms and signs of constrictive pericarditis usually develop over months to years. They result from: 1) reduced cardiac output (fatigue, hypotension, reflex tachycardia), and 2) elevated systemic venous pressures (jugular venous distension, hepatomegaly with ascites, and peripheral edema).

Because the most impressive physical findings are often the insidious development of hepatomegaly and ascites, such patients are often mistakenly thought to suffer from hepatic cirrhosis or an intra-abdominal tumor. It is only after careful inspection of the jugular veins that a cardiac source of the problem is identified, and the correct diagnosis of constrictive pericarditis ultimately made.

On cardiac examination, an early diastolic "knock" may follow S_2 (see Chapter 2) in patients with severe calcific constriction. It represents the sudden cessation of ventricular diastolic filling imposed by the rigid pericardial sac.

Unlike cardiac tamponade, pericardial constriction does not usually result in pulsus paradoxus (inspiratory fall in systemic blood pressure). Recall that in tamponade, that sign reflects inspiratory augmentation of right ventricular filling, at the expense of LV filling. However, in constrictive pericarditis, the negative intrathoracic pressure generated by inspiration is not transmitted through the rigid pericardial shell to the right-sided heart chambers; therefore, inspiratory augmentation of right ventricular filling does not occur. Rather, when a patient with severe pericardial constriction inhales, the negative intrathoracic pressure draws blood toward the thorax, where it cannot be accommodated by the constricted right-sided cardiac chambers. Thus, the increased venous return accumulates in the intrathoracic systemic veins, causing the jugular veins to become more distended during inspiration (**Kussmaul's sign**). This is the opposite of normal physiology, in which inspiration results in a *decline* in jugular venous pressure, as venous return is drawn into the heart. The usual effect of respiration in pericardial disease is summarized as follows:

	Constrictive pericarditis	Cardiac tamponade
Pulsus paradoxus	−	+
Kussmaul's sign	+	−

Diagnostic Approach

The *chest radiograph* in constrictive pericarditis shows a normal or mildly enlarged cardiac silhouette. Calcification of the pericardium is detected in up to 50% of patients. The *EKG* generally shows only nonspecific ST and T wave abnormalities, although atrial arrhythmias are common.

Echocardiographic evidence of constriction is subtle: the pericardium, if well-imaged, is thickened; the ventricular cavities are small and contract vigorously, and diastolic ventricular filling terminates abruptly in early diastole, as the chambers reach the limit imposed by the rigid shell.

CT or *MRI* is superior to echocardiography in the assessment of pericardial anatomy and thickness. The presence of normal pericardial thickness by these modalities is generally a reliable indication that constrictive pericarditis is *not* present.

The diagnosis of constrictive pericarditis is confirmed by *cardiac catheterization*. There are three key features: 1) elevation and equalization of the diastolic pressures in each of the cardiac chambers, 2) the right and left ventricular tracings show an early diastolic "dip and plateau" configuration (Fig. 14.6)—this pattern reflects blood flow into the ventricles at the very onset of diastole, just after the tricuspid and mitral valves open, followed by sudden cessation of filling as further expansion of the ventricles is arrested by the surrounding rigid shell, and 3) the right atrial pressure tracing shows a prominent y descent (Fig. 14.5): After the tricuspid valve opens, the right atrium quickly empties into the RV during the very brief period before filling is arrested. This is in contrast to cardiac tamponade, in which the external compressive force throughout the cardiac cycle *prevents* rapid ventricular filling, even in early diastole, such that the y descent is blunted.

The clinical and hemodynamic findings of constrictive pericarditis can be similar to those of restrictive cardiomyopathy (see Chapter 10), another not-very-common condition. Distinguishing between these two syndromes is important, however, because pericardial constriction is correctable, whereas most cases of restrictive cardiomyopathy are not. An endomyocardial biopsy is sometimes necessary to distinguish between these (biopsy is normal in constric-

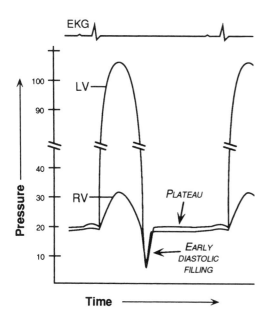

Figure 14.6. Schematic tracings of left (LV) and right (RV) ventricular pressures in constrictive pericarditis. Early diastolic ventricular filling abruptly halts as the volume in the ventricles quickly reaches the limits imposed by the constricting pericardium (the "plateau"). Throughout most of diastole, the LV and RV pressures are abnormally elevated and equal.

tion, but usually abnormal in restrictive cardiomyopathy).

Treatment

The only effective treatment of severe constrictive pericarditis is surgical removal of the pericardium. Symptoms and signs of constriction may not resolve immediately because of the associated stiffness of the neighboring outer walls of the heart, but eventual symptomatic improvement is expected in 90% of patients who undergo this procedure.

SUMMARY

1. Acute pericarditis is most often of idiopathic/viral cause, and is usually a self-limited illness. More serious forms of pericarditis arise from the conditions listed in Table 14.1.

2. Common findings in acute pericarditis include: 1) pleuritic chest pain, 2) fever, 3) pericardial friction rub, and 4) diffuse ST segment elevation on the EKG (often accompanied by PR depression).

3. Complications of pericarditis include cardiac tamponade (accumulation of pericardial fluid under high pressure, which compresses the cardiac chambers), and constrictive pericarditis (restricted filling of the heart because of surrounding rigid pericardium).

ADDITIONAL READING

Baim D, Grossman W. Cardiac Catheterization, Angiography, and Intervention. Baltimore: Williams & Wilkins, 1996:801–821.

Brockington G, Zebede J, et al. Constrictive pericarditis. Cardiol Clin 1990;8:645.

Fowler N. Constrictive pericarditis: its history and current status. Clin Cardiol 1995;18:341.

Guberman B, Fowler N, et al. Cardiac tamponade in medical patients. Circulation 1981;64:633.

Lorell BH. Pericardial diseases. In: Braunwald E, ed. Heart Disease: A Textbook of Cardiovascular Medicine. 5th ed. Philadelphia: WB Saunders, 1997: 1478–1534.

McGregor M. Current concepts in pulsus paradoxus. N Engl J Med 1979;301:48.

Reddy PS, Curtiss E, et al. Cardiac tamponade: hemodynamic observations in man. Circulation 1978;58: 265.

Shabetai R. Diseases of the pericardium. Cardiol Clin 1990;8:579.

Singh S, Wann S, et al. Right ventricular and right atrial collapse in patients with cardiac tamponade—a combined echocardiographic and hemodynamic study. Circulation 1984;70:966.

Spodick DH. Macrophysiology, microphysiology, and anatomy of the pericardium: a synopsis. Am Heart J 1992;124:1046–1051.

Watkins MW. Physiologic role of the normal pericardium. Annu Review Med 1993;44:171–180.

Acknowledgments   The previous edition of this chapter was written by Angela Fowler, MD, Kathy Glatter, MD, Alan Braverman, MD, and Leonard S. Lilly, MD.

Diseases of the Peripheral Vasculature

Chapter 15

C. Geoffrey McDonough and Mark A. Creager

Peripheral vascular disease is an umbrella term that includes a number of diverse pathologic entities that affect arteries, veins, and lymphatics. While this terminology makes a distinction between the "central" coronary and "peripheral" systemic vessels, the vasculature as a whole comprises a dynamic, integrated, and multifunctional organ system that does not naturally comply with this semantic division.

Blood vessels serve many critical functions. First, they regulate the differential distribution of blood to tissues. Second, blood vessels actively synthesize and secrete vasoactive substances that regulate vascular tone, and antithrombotic substances that maintain the fluidity of blood and vessel patency (see Chapters 5 and 6). Third, the vessels play an integral role in the transport and distribution of immune cells to traumatized or infected tissues. Disease states of the peripheral vasculature interfere with these essential functions.

Peripheral vascular diseases result from many pathophysiologic processes that can be grouped into three categories: 1) *structural changes in the vessel wall* secondary to degenerative diseases, infection, or inflammation that lead to aneurysm, dissection, or rupture; 2) *narrowing of the vascular lumen* due to atherosclerosis, thrombosis or inflammation; and 3) *spasm* of vascular smooth muscle. These processes can occur in isolation, or they can potentiate one another.

DISEASES OF THE AORTA

The aorta is the largest conductance vessel of the vascular system. In adults, its diameter is approximately 3 cm at its origin at the base of the heart. The **ascending aorta,** 5 to 6 cm in length, leads to the **aortic arch,** from which arise three major branches: the brachiocephalic (which bifurcates into the right common carotid and subclavian arteries), the left common carotid, and the left subclavian arteries. As the **descending aorta** continues beyond the arch, its diameter narrows to approximately 2.0–2.5 cm in normal adults. As the aorta pierces the diaphragm, it becomes the **abdominal aorta,** which provides arteries to the abdominal viscera before bifurcating into the left and right common iliac arteries, which supply the pelvic organs and lower extremities.

The aorta, like other arteries, is composed of three layers, as diagrammed in Chapter 5, Figure 5.1. At the luminal surface, the intima is composed of endothelial cells overlying the internal elastic lamina. The endothelial layer is a functional interface between the vasculature and the circulating systems of coagulation, of complement, and of humoral and cell-mediated immunity. The media is comprised of smooth muscle cells, and of a matrix that includes collagen and elastic fibers. Collagen provides tensile strength, a stiffness that allows the vessels to withstand high pressure loads. Elastin, capable of stretching to 250% of its original length, confers a distensible quality on vessels that allows them to recoil under pressure. The adventitia is made up primarily of collagen fibers, perivascular nerves, and vasa vasorum. The latter is a rich vascular network that supplies oxygenated blood to the layers of the thoracic aorta. The abdominal aorta, however, is devoid of vasa vasorum, which may account for its increased susceptibility to dilation and aneurysm formation.

The predominance of elastin in the media (2:1 over collagen) allows the aorta to expand during systole, and then to recoil during diastole. This recoil against the closed aortic valve contributes to the distal propagation of blood flow during the phase of left ventricular relaxation. With advancing age, the elastic component of the aorta and its branches degenerates, collagen becomes more prominent, and the arteries stiffen. Systolic blood pressure therefore tends to rise with age since less energy is dissipated into the aorta during left ventricular contraction. The aorta is subject to injury from mechanical trauma because it is continuously exposed to high pulsatile pressure and shear stress.

Diseases of the aorta most commonly appear as one of three clinical conditions: aneurysm, dissection, or obstruction.

Aortic Aneurysms

An aneurysm is an abnormal, localized dilatation of an artery. In the aorta, aneurysms are distinguished from *diffuse ectasia*, which is a generalized, yet lesser increase of the aortic diameter. Ectasia develops in older individuals as elastic fibers fragment, smooth muscle cells decrease in number, and acid mucopolysaccharide ground substance accumulates within the vessel wall.

The term aneurysm is applied when the diameter of a portion of the aorta has increased by 50% or more, or if a portion of the abdominal aorta has enlarged to greater than 3.5–4.0 cm in diameter. A **true aneurysm** represents a dilatation of all three layers of the aorta, creating a large bulge of the vessel wall. True aneurysms are characterized as either *fusiform* or *saccular*, depending on the extent of the vessel's circumference within the aneurysm (Fig. 15.1). A fusiform aneurysm, the more common type, is one in which the entire circumference of a segment of the aorta is dilated, whereas a saccular aneurysm is a localized outpouching involving only a portion of the circumference.

In distinction, a **pseudoaneurysm,** or **false aneurysm,** is a contained *rupture* of the vessel wall that may mimic the appearance of a true aneurysm. A pseudoaneurysm develops when blood leaks out of the vessel lumen through a hole in the intimal and medial layers and is contained merely by the layer of adventitia or perivascular organized thrombus (Fig. 15.1). Such a lesion may develop at sites of vessel injury caused by infection or trauma, such as puncture of the vessel during surgery or percutaneous catheterization. Pseudoaneurysms are very unstable lesions that are prone to rupture.

Aneurysms may be confined to the abdominal aorta (most common), the thoracic aorta, or may involve both locations. They may also appear in peripheral and cerebral arteries.

Etiology and Pathogenesis of True Aortic Aneurysms

The etiology of aortic aneurysm formation is multifactorial, and may vary depending on the location of the lesion. Atherosclerosis is an important contributor, implicated in approximately 90% of abdominal aortic aneurysms (Fig. 15.2). Within the thoracic aorta, atherosclerotic aneurysms are more common in the descending, compared with the ascending, portions. Atherosclerotic aneurysms rarely develop before age 50, they are more common in men, and their development is accelerated by other risk factors that predis-

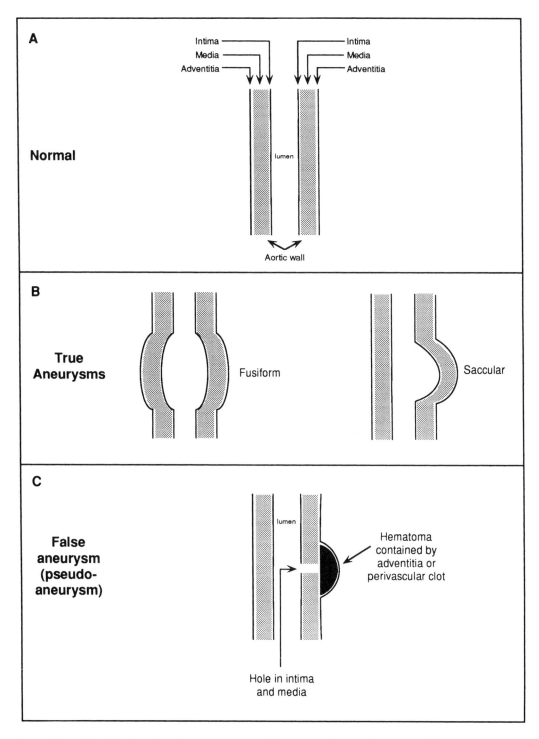

Figure 15.1. Classification of aortic aneurysms. A. The normal arterial wall consists of three layers: the intima, media, and adventitia. **B.** True aneurysms represent localized dilatation of all three layers of the arterial wall. Fusiform aneurysms involve the entire circumference of the aorta, whereas saccular aneurysms are a localized bulge of only a portion of the circumference. **C.** A false aneurysm (or pseudoaneurysm) is actually a hole in the intima and media, with hematoma contained by a thin layer of adventitia or perivascular clot.

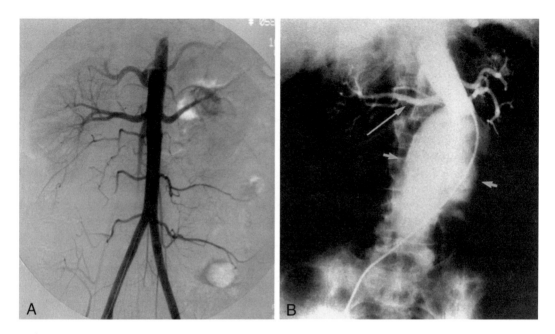

Figure 15.2. **A.** Angiogram of the abdominal aorta in a normal individual (vascular structures appear black in this digital subtraction image). Note the renal arteries and the outline of the kidneys. **B.** Angiographic demonstration of an abdominal aortic aneurysm (short arrows). The aorta is dilated below the level of the renal arteries (long arrow). Blood vessels containing the injected contrast agent appear *white* on this conventional angiogram.

pose to atherosclerosis (i.e. smoking, hypertension, dyslipidemia).

Aneurysms of the ascending thoracic aorta are *uncommonly* atherosclerotic in origin. Rather, degenerative changes in the media appear to play an important role. This process, termed **cystic medial degeneration** (or **cystic medial necrosis**) involves the degeneration and fragmentation of elastic fibers, with subsequent accumulation of collagenous and mucoid material within the medial layer. When present, cystic medial degeneration of the aortic media often affects the ascending aorta because it is subjected to the greatest pulsatile expansion and shear stress during systole. Medial degeneration may occur in association with connective tissue disorders (e.g., Marfan's syndrome, Ehlers–Danlos syndrome), or in response to hypertension and aging.

Less common causes of aortic aneurysms are included in Table 15.1. For

example, weakness of the media and aneurysm formation may result from certain infections, such as syphilis or spread from bacterial endocarditis. Recently, an increasing number of genetic defects in the connective tissue fibers that make up the medial layer of the arterial wall have been observed in patients with aortic aneurysms, suggesting a familial basis for the disease. Approximately 5%–10% of patients have a first-degree relative in whom aortic aneurysm has been diagnosed.

Clinical Presentation and Diagnosis

Aortic aneurysms are often asymptomatic, but occasionally patients are aware of a pulsatile mass, particularly when the abdominal aorta is involved. More often, when symptoms occur, it is because of compression of neighboring structures by the expanding aneurysm. For example, erosion

TABLE 15.1. Some Causes of True Aortic Aneurysms

- Atherosclerosis
- Cystic medical necrosis
    Idiopathic
    Marfan syndrome
    Ehlers-Danlos syndrome
- Infectious aortitis
    Syphilitic aortitis
    Mycotic aneurysms (primary or embolic
        infection of vessel wall)
- Vasculitis
    Takayasu's arteritis
    Giant cell arteritis
- Congenital aneurysms

of vertebrae by a large abdominal aneurysm may cause back pain. Compression of the esophagus or trachea by a thoracic aneurysm may cause dysphagia, hemoptysis, or respiratory symptoms such as dyspnea, wheezing, or cough. Enlargement of the aorta may also stretch the left recurrent laryngeal nerve as it passes around the ligamentum arteriosum (the embryonic remnant of the ductus arteriosus, located between the pulmonary artery and distal aortic arch), resulting in hoarseness. Aneurysms of the ascending thoracic aorta may dilate the aortic ring, resulting in aortic regurgitation, with subsequent symptoms of heart failure.

Aortic aneurysms are often first suspected when aortic dilatation is observed as an incidental finding on chest or abdominal radiographs, particularly if the aneurysmal walls are calcified. Aneurysms of the abdominal aorta or of the large peripheral arteries may also come to attention because of careful palpation during physical examination. Confirmation of aortic aneurysms is achieved by ultrasonography, computed tomography (CT), magnetic resonance imaging (MRI), or conventional arteriography.

The most devastating consequence of aortic aneurysms is rupture, which is often fatal. An aneurysm may rupture suddenly, or it may leak slowly — extravasating blood into the vessel wall, causing pain and local tenderness. Thoracic aortic aneurysms may rupture into the pleural space, mediastinum, or bronchi. Abdominal aortic aneurysms may rupture into the retroperi-

toneal space or abdominal cavity, or they may erode into the intestines, resulting in massive gastrointestinal bleeding. Natural history studies have shown that the risk of rupture is related to the size of the aneurysm, as predicted by the law of LaPlace (i.e., wall tension is proportional to the product of pressure and radius). The 5-year risk of rupture of an abdominal aortic aneurysm < 5 cm in diameter is 1%–2%. Conversely, the risk is 20%–40% if the aneurysm exceeds 5 cm in diameter.

Treatment

Treatment of an aortic aneurysm usually involves surgical repair with placement of a prosthetic graft. Surgery is recommended for most abdominal aortic aneurysms exceeding 4.5–5cm in diameter, or for those expanding in diameter at a rate exceeding 1 cm per year. It is generally recommended that thoracic aortic aneurysms be surgically repaired if they exceed 6 cm in diameter, or if symptoms are present due to compression of adjacent structures. In patients with the Marfan syndrome, however, in whom the complication rate of aneurysms is high, surgical repair is often recommended when thoracic aortic aneurysms are greater than 5 cm in diameter.

Aortic Dissection

Aortic dissection is a life-threatening condition in which a blood-filled channel divides the medial layers of the aorta, splitting (or "dissecting") the intima from the adventitia along various lengths of the vessel.

Etiology, Pathogenesis, and Classification

Aortic dissection is thought to arise from a tear in the intimal layer of the vessel wall that allows blood from the lumen, under the driving force of the systemic pressure, to enter into the media and propogate along the plane of the muscle layer. Another postulated origin of aortic dissection relates to rupture of vasa vasorum with hemorrhage into the media (forming an intramural hematoma), that subsequently tears through the intima and into the vessel's lumen.

Any condition that interferes with the normal integrity of the elastic or muscular components of the medial layer can predispose to aortic dissection. Such degeneration may arise from chronic hypertension, aging, and/or cystic medial degeneration (a feature of certain hereditary connective tissue disorders, such as the Marfan and Ehlers-Danlos syndromes). In addition, traumatic insult to the aorta (e.g., blunt chest trauma, or accidental vessel damage during intra-arterial catheterization or cardiac surgery) can also incite dissection.

Aortic dissection is most common in the sixth and seventh decades, and occurs more frequently in men. More than two-thirds of patients have a history of hypertension.

Dissection most commonly involves the ascending thoracic aorta (65%) and descending thoracic aorta (20%), while the aortic arch (10%) and abdominal aortic (5%) segments are less commonly affected.

Dissections are commonly classified into two types (types A and B), depending on their location and extent (Fig. 15.3). Type A, or proximal dissections, are those in which the ascending aorta is involved. They may be confined to the ascending aorta, or extend into the arch and descending portion of the vessel. Type B, or distal dissections, do not involve the ascending aorta or arch, and are confined to the descending thoracic and abdominal aorta. This distinction is important, since treatment strategies and prognosis are determined by location. Proximal aortic involvement tends to be the more devastating form due to its potential for extension into the coronary and arch vessels, into the support structures of the aortic valve, or into the pericardial space. Approximately two-thirds of dissections are type A, and one-third type B.

Clinical Presentation and Diagnosis

The most common symptom of aortic dissection is sudden, severe pain with a "tearing" or "ripping" quality in the anterior chest (typical of type A dissections) or between the scapulae (in type B dissec-

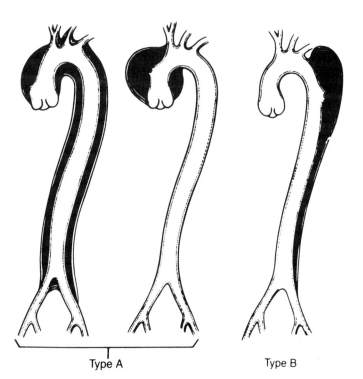

Figure 15.3. Aortic dissection.
Type A involves the ascending aorta, whereas type B does not. (Reprinted with permission from Cotran RS, Kumar V, Robbins SL. Robbin's pathologic basis of disease. Philadelphia: WB Saunders, 1989.)

Type A   Type B

tions). Classically, this pain then travels as the dissection propagates along the aorta. Other symptoms relate to the catastrophic complications that can occur at the time of presentation or thereafter (Table 15.2) and include: 1) rupture through the adventitia anywhere along the aorta (often into the left pleural space or pericardium), 2) occlusion of major branches of the aorta by the propagating hematoma within the vessel wall, which compresses the lumen and can result in myocardial infarction (coronary artery involvement), stroke (carotid artery involvement), or loss of pulse in an extremity, and 3) extension into the aortic root with disruption of the aortic valve support apparatus causing aortic regurgitation.

As a result, several important physical findings may be present. Hypertension is frequently detected, either as an underlying cause of dissection or because of the sympathetic nervous system response to severe pain. However, if the dissection has occluded flow to one of the subclavian arteries, a difference in systolic blood pressure between the arms is noted. Neurologic deficits may accompany dissection into the carotid vessels. If a type A dissection results in aortic regurgitation, an early diastolic murmur is present on auscultation. Leakage from a type A dissection into the pericardial sac may produce signs of cardiac tamponade (see Chapter 14).

The diagnosis of aortic dissection must not be delayed, because catastrophic complications or death may rapidly ensue. The confirmatory imaging techniques most useful in detecting dissection include transesophageal echocardiography, magnetic resonance imaging, and contrast angiography. In many hospital settings, transesophageal echocardiography is the initial diagnostic test because of its availability, excellent sensitivity and specificity, and reasonable cost.

Treatment

Treatment of aortic dissection is designed to arrest progression of the dissecting channel. Immediate therapy is directed at reduction of systolic blood pressure and decreasing the force of left ventricular contraction, in order to lower the aortic wall shear stress. Useful pharmacologic agents in this regard include β-blockers (to reduce the force of contraction and heart rate, and to lower blood pressure) and vasodilators such as sodium-nitroprusside (to rapidly reduce blood pressure). In proximal (type A) dissections, early surgical correction has been shown to improve outcome compared with medical therapy alone. Surgical therapy involves repair of the intimal tear, suturing the edges of the false channel, and if necessary, insertion of a synthetic aortic graft.

Conversely, patients with uncomplicated type B dissections are initially managed with aggressive medical therapy alone; early surgical intervention does not result in improved outcome in such patients compared with medical therapy. These patients are brought to surgery, however, if there is clinical evidence of propagation of the dissection, compromise of major branches of the aorta, impending rupture, or continued pain.

TABLE 15.2. Complications of Aortic Dissection

Rupture
- Pericardial tamponade
- Hemomediastinum
- Hemothorax (usually left-sided)

Occlusion of aortic branch vessels
- Carotid (stroke)
- Coronary (MI)
- Splanchnic (organ infarction)
- Renal (acute renal failure)

Distortion of aortic annulus
- Aortic regurgitation

DISEASES CAUSING ARTERIAL OCCLUSION

Arterial occlusion may result from atherosclerosis, thromboembolism, or vasculitis (inflammation of the vessel wall). The clinical presentation of these disorders results from decreased perfusion to the affected limb or organs.

Arteriosclerosis Obliterans

Etiology and Pathogenesis

Arteriosclerosis obliterans is a chronic occlusive disease resulting from the formation
of atherosclerotic plaques in large and
medium-sized arteries, leading to progressive stenosis and obstruction. This disorder
is often referred to as peripheral arterial occlusive disease (PAOD). It is the most prevalent vascular disorder, with a symptomatic
incidence of 0.3% of the entire population
and of 5.2% of individuals over the age of 70.
The pathology of PAOD is identical to that
seen in atherosclerotic coronary artery disease, and the major coronary risk factors
(e.g., cigarette smoking, dyslipidemia, diabetes mellitus, and hypertension) are also
risk factors for PAOD. Approximately 45%
of patients with symptomatic PAOD also
have clinically significant CAD, and it is not
uncommon for patients with PAOD to suffer episodes of myocardial ischemia and to
succumb to myocardial infarction.

The pathophysiology of PAOD is also
similar to that of CAD (as described in Chapter 6). Ischemia of the affected region occurs
when there is an imbalance between oxygen
supply and demand: Exercise raises the demand for blood flow in the tissues, and a narrowed artery is unable to provide adequate
flow. The fatigue, pain, and weakness of the
affected extremity that results from intermittent ischemia is termed **claudication**. The
symptoms of claudication are temporary
and resolve with rest, as the balance between
oxygen supply and demand is restored.

In severe PAOD, patients may experience ischemic pain *at rest*, usually affecting
the feet or toes. The chronically reduced
blood flow in this case predisposes the extremity to ulceration, infection, and skin
necrosis (Fig. 15.4). Patients with diabetes
mellitus and those who smoke are at a
higher risk of these complications.

Clinical Presentation and Diagnosis

PAOD commonly affects the aorta, the iliac, femoral, popliteal, and tibioperoneal ar-

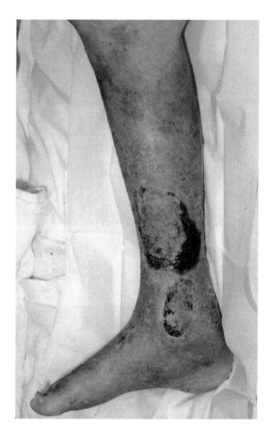

**Figure 15.4. Vascular insufficiency ulceration
near the medial malleolus of the right leg.** Note the
irregular borders, superficial character, and
pigmentation of surrounding skin.

teries (Fig. 15.5). Therefore, intermittent
claudication of the lower extremities is a
frequent presenting symptom. Such patients develop calf, thigh, or buttock discomfort precipitated by walking and relieved by rest. The location of claudication
corresponds to the diseased artery, with the
femoral and popliteal arteries being the
most common site (Table 15.3). The arteries
of the upper extremities are less frequently
affected, but brachiocephalic or subclavian
artery disease can cause arm claudication.
As the disease progresses, reduced blood
flow may occur at rest, causing pain and
paresthesias in the most distal parts of the
extremity. Such "rest pain" is often maximal when the patient lies flat, and relieved
somewhat by placing the involved extremities in a dependent position.

Physical examination generally reveals

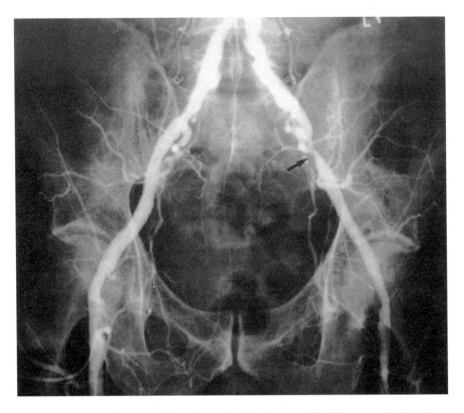

Figure 15.5. **An angiogram demonstrating atherosclerotic disease of the iliac vessels.** Note the severe stenosis of the left external iliac artery.

TABLE 15.3. Relation of Stenotic Site to Claudication Symptoms

Site	Location of Claudication Symptoms
Distal aorta or iliac arteries	Buttocks, hips, thighs, or calves
Femoral-popliteal arteries	Calves
Subclavian or axillary arteries	Arms

loss of pulses distal to the stenotic segment. Bruits (swishing sound auscultated over a region of turbulent blood flow) may be audible in the abdomen (because of stenoses within the mesenteric or renal arteries) or over iliac, femoral, or subclavian arterial stenoses. In patients with chronic severe ischemia, the lack of blood perfusion results in muscle atrophy, pallor, cyanotic discoloration, hair loss, and occasionally gangrene and necrosis of the foot and digits.

In the evaluation of PAOD, it is helpful to measure the ratio of blood pressure in the ankles to that in the arms (termed the ankle-brachial index (ABI)) using sphygmomanometer cuffs and a Doppler instrument to detect blood flow. A normal ABI is ≥ 1.0 (i.e., the ankle pressure is equal to or slightly greater than that in the arms). An index < 0.9 is associated with symptoms of claudication, whereas an index < 0.5 is often observed in patients with rest pain and severe arterial compromise of the affected extremity.

Treatment

The goal of medical treatment is directed at decreasing the risk factors that contribute to PAOD, and at increasing exercise capacity. Exercise, particularly walking, often improves endurance. Conversely, vasodilator drugs have not been shown to improve symptoms of claudication. Agents that affect the rheologic properties of blood (e.g., pentoxiphylline) have been useful in some patients. Revascularization is indicated for patients with disabling claudication or severe limb ischemia. Surgical procedures include bypass operations to circumvent the occluded arteries using prosthetic or saphenous vein grafts. Nonsurgical revascularization can be performed on selected patients using percutaneous transluminal angioplasty.

Acute Arterial Occlusion

Acute arterial occlusion is caused either by embolization from a cardiac or vascular site or by thrombus formation in situ. The origin of arterial emboli is most often the heart, usually due to disorders in which there is intracardiac stasis of flow (Table 15.4). Emboli may also originate from thrombus or atheromatous material overlying an atherosclerotic segment of the aorta itself. Rarely, arterial emboli may originate from the *venous* circulation: If a venous clot travels to the right-heart chambers and is able to pass through an abnormal intracardiac communication (e.g., an atrial septal defect), it would then enter into the systemic arterial circulation (a condition known as a **paradoxical embolism**). Primary arterial thrombus formation may appear at sites of endothelial damage or atherosclerotic stenoses, or within bypass grafts.

The extent of tissue damage from throm-

TABLE 15.4. Origins of Arterial Emboli

- Cardiac origin
  - Stagnant left atrial flow (e.g., atrial fibrillation, mitral stenosis)
  - Left ventricular mural thrombus (e.g., dilated cardiomyopathy, myocardial infarction, ventricular aneurysm)
  - Valvular lesions (endocarditis, mitral stenosis, thrombus on prosthetic valve)
  - Left atrial myxoma (mobile tumor in left atrium)
- Aortic origin
  - Thrombus material overlying atherosclerotic segment
- Venous origin
  - Paradoxical embolism travels through intra-cardiac shunt

---

boembolism relates to the site of the occluded artery and the degree of collateral circulation serving the tissue beyond the obstruction. Common symptoms and signs that may develop from reduced blood supply include pain, pallor, paralysis, parasthesia, and pulselessness (termed the "five P's"). A sixth "P," poikilothermia (coolness) is also often manifest.

Therapy includes an anticoagulant agent, such as intravenous heparin, to prevent propagation of the clot and to reduce the likelihood of additional embolic events. A fibrinolytic agent (e.g., urokinase or tissue plasminogen activator) is used in selected cases to lyse acute thrombi. Surgical techniques to improve severely compromised blood flow include removal of the thrombus or arterial bypass surgery.

Vasculitic Syndromes

Vasculitis (inflammation of the vessel wall) results from immune complex deposition or from cell-mediated immune reactions directed against the vessel wall. Immune complexes activate the complement cascade with subsequent release of chemoattractants and anaphylotoxins that direct neutrophil migration to the vessel wall and increase vascular permeability. Neutrophils injure the vessel by releasing their lysozomal contents and by producing toxic oxygen-derived free radicals. In cell-mediated immune reactions, T lymphocytes bind to vascular antigens and release lymphokines, which attract additional lymphocytes and macrophages to the vessel wall. These inflammatory processes can cause end-organ ischemia because of either vascular necrosis or local thrombosis.

The cause of most of the vasculitic syndromes is unknown, but they often can be distinguished from one another by the pattern of vessels involved and by histologic characteristics (Table 15.5).

Polyarteritis nodosa (PAN) is a necrotizing systemic vasculitis of small and medium-sized arteries. The name is derived from the many nodules that are found along the course of these vessels. It has a preva-

TABLE 15.5. Vasculitic Syndromes

Type	Arteries Commonly Affected	Histology
Polyarteritis nodosa	Small-medium size (especially renal, coronary, hepatic, skeletal muscle)	PMN infiltration, acute fibrinoid necrosis, aneurysmal dilatation
Takayasu's arteritis	Aorta and its branches	Granulomatous arteritis with fibrosis; marked luminal narrowing
Temporal arteritis (Giant cell arteritis)	Medium-large size (especially cranial vessels, aortic arch and its branches)	Lymphocyte infiltration, intimal fibrosis, granuloma formation
Thromboangiitis obliterans (Buerger's disease)	Small size (especially arteries of the distal extremities)	Inflammation and thrombosis without necrosis

PMN, polymorphonuclear leucocytes

lence of approximately 6 per 100,000 and a male-to-female ratio of 1.6:1. Histologic examination of affected arteries reveals polymorphonuclear infiltration in all three vessel layers, intimal proliferation and degeneration, and fibrinoid necrosis with occlusion of the lumen. The vessel wall and elastic lamina are disrupted, leading to aneurysmal dilatation of the vessel. PAN may be idiopathic, but can also be seen in the setting of hepatitis B infection (30% of PAN cases). The resultant ischemia distal to the involved vessel damages tissues and visceral organs, the most commonly affected of which are the kidney, heart, and liver. Patients may experience generalized inflammatory symptoms such as fever, malaise, and musculoskeletal pains. Alternatively, symptoms may relate to decreased organ blood flow. For example, the presentation may be one of hypertension due to reduced flow into the renal arteries with subsequent activation of the renin-angiotensin system (see Chapter 13).

The presence of antineutrophil cytoplasmic antibodies (ANCAs) in the circulation is highly suggestive of necrotizing vasculitis, but the diagnosis of polyarteritis nodosa is established by biopsy of involved vessels. The prognosis is poor if the disease remains unrecognized: The 5-year survival rate for untreated patients is as low as 15%, but may improve to 80% if the diagnosis is established and therapy with prednisone and other immunosuppressive agents is instituted.

Takayasu's arteritis is a disease of unknown cause that targets the aorta and its major branches. It most often occurs in women younger than age 40. The majority of cases have been reported from Asia and Africa, but it occurs worldwide. General symptoms include malaise and fever, but focal symptoms are related to inflammation of the affected vessel and include cerebrovascular ischemia (brachiocephalic or carotid artery), myocardial ischemia (coronary artery), or arm claudication (brachiocephalic or subclavian artery). The carotid and limb pulses are diminished or absent in nearly 85% of patients at the time of diagnosis; hence, this condition is often termed "pulseless" disease. Histologic examination of affected vessels reveals infiltration of plasma cells and lymphocytes into the media and adventitia, giant cells, intimal proliferation, disruption of the elastic lamina, and fibrosis. Steroid and cytotoxic drugs may alleviate symptoms of Takayasu's arteritis, but their effect on survival has not been established. Surgical bypass of obstructed vessels may be helpful in severe cases.

Temporal arteritis (also termed **giant cell arteritis**) is a disease of medium-sized to large arteries that most commonly involves the cranial vessels, the aortic arch, and its branches. It is an uncommon disease, with an incidence of 24 per 100,000. In distinction to polyarteritis nodosa, renal, hepatic, and coronary vessels are usually spared in this condition. It occurs most often in patients older than 55, and 65% of patients are female. Histologic findings in infected vessels include lymphocyte infiltration, intimal fibrosis, and focal necrosis, as well as granuloma formation containing multinucleated giant cells.

Symptoms of temporal arteritis relate to the distribution of affected arteries, and may include prominent headache (temporal artery) or facial pain and claudication of the jaw while chewing (facial artery). Nearly 50% of patients suffer visual impairment due to involvement of the ophthalmic artery; a severe complication that can develop is irreversible blindness because of occlusion of branches of that vessel. In temporal arteritis, the erythrocyte sedimentation rate is invariably elevated and the diagnosis is confirmed by biopsy of an involved vessel, usually a temporal artery. Temporal arteritis usually runs a self-limited course of 1 to 5 years. High-dose steroid treatment is effective at treating vasculitis and preventing visual complications.

Thromboangiitis obliterans (Buerger's disease) is an inflammatory disease of medium-sized arteries involving the distal vessels of the upper and lower extremities. It has a very strong association with cigarette smoking, and is most common in men under the age of 40. Less than 2% of patients are female. There is an increased incidence of HLA-A9 and HLA-B5 in affected individuals, and allergy to tobacco may play a role in some cases. Biopsy specimens of affected vessels (Fig. 15.6) reveal segmental arteritis or phlebitis with neutrophil infiltration, but without necrosis, and there is preservation of the internal elastic lamina. The diagnosis can be established by angiography and tissue biopsy.

The clinical presentation is often characterized by a triad of symptoms and signs: distal arterial occlusion, Raynaud's phenomenon (described below), and migrating superficial vein thrombophlebitis. As a result of arterial occlusion, patients develop arm and foot claudication, as well as ischemia of the digits. There is no specific treatment, but smoking cessation often prevents progression of the disease and its complications.

DISEASE CAUSING ARTERIAL SPASM: RAYNAUD'S PHENOMENON

Raynaud's phenomenon is a vasospastic disease of the digital arteries (most often the fingers) that occurs in susceptible individuals when exposed to cool temperatures, and

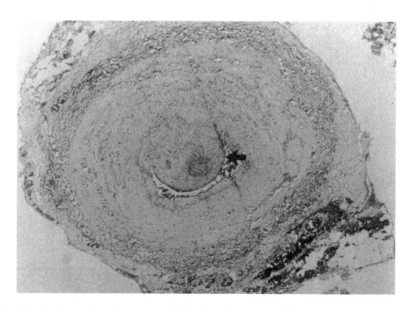

Figure 15.6. Histologic section of an artery displaying thromboangiitis obliterans. There is endothelial cell and fibroblast proliferation in the vessel wall, and thrombus is present in the vessel lumen (arrow).

sometimes by emotional stress. Typically, episodes of vasospasm are characterized by a triphasic color response: First, the fingers and/or toes blanch to a distinct white color as blood flow is interrupted (Fig. 15.7). The second phase is characterized by cyanosis, related to local accumulation of desaturated hemoglobin, followed by the third phase: a ruddy color as blood flow begins to resume. Accompanying the color response may be numbness, paresthesias, or pain of the affected digits.

This condition may occur as an isolated disorder, termed *primary Raynaud's phenomenon* or *Raynaud's disease*. Such patients are predominantly female, and between the ages of 20 and 40. Genetic factors do not appear to play a role in the disease. Primary Raynaud's phenomenon most often manifests in the fingers, but 40% of patients also have involvement of their toes. The prognosis of primary Raynaud's phenomenon is relatively benign, with only 16% of patients reporting a worsening of their symptoms over time.

Secondary Raynaud's phenomenon may also appear as a component of other conditions such as connective tissue diseases (e.g., scleroderma, systemic lupus erythematosus), arterial occlusive disorders, blood dyscrasias, or the thoracic outlet syndrome.

The transient vasospasm that occurs in Raynaud's phenomenon is a nonphysiologic constriction of blood vessels that can result in tissue ischemia. Peripheral blood flow is normally regulated by intrinsic vascular tone, sympathetic nervous system activity, rheologic factors such as blood viscosity, and a number of circulating hormonal substances. The fingers are a special case because they contain only sympathetic vasoconstrictor fibers, whereas other regional circulations have both constrictor and dilator fibers. In patients with Raynaud's phenomenon, vasoconstriction develops in response to cooling, possibly because of exaggerated reflex sympathetic tone, or through a heightened local vascular responsiveness to sympathetic stimuli.

Treatment of Raynaud's phenomenon involves avoiding cold environments or us-

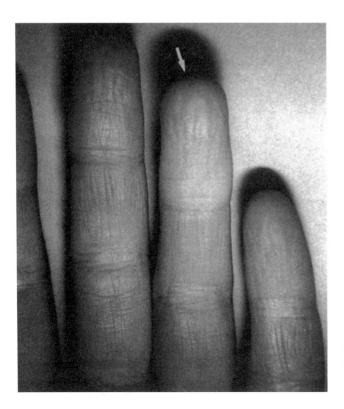

Figure 15.7. Raynaud's phenomenon of the upper extremity. The fourth digit (arrow) is blanched (phase 1 of the tricolor response).

ing insulated gloves during such exposure. There has also been some success in preventing vasospasm with pharmacologic agents that relax vascular tone, including calcium channel blockers and alpha$_1$-adrenergic blockers (described in Chapter 17).

VENOUS DISEASE

Veins are high-capacitance vessels that contain more than 70% of the total blood volume. In contrast to the muscular structure of arteries, the subendothelial layer of veins is thin, and the tunica media comprises fewer, smaller bundles of smooth muscle cells intermixed with reticular and elastic fibers. While veins of the extremities do possess intrinsic vasomotor activity, transport of blood back to the heart relies greatly on external compression provided by the surrounding skeletal muscles and on a series of one-way endothelial valves.

Veins of the extremities can be classified as either deep or superficial. In the lower ex-

tremity, where most peripheral venous disorders occur, the deep veins generally course along the arteries, whereas the superficial veins are located subcutaneously. The superficial veins are dependent upon drainage into deeper structures via a series of perforating connectors for return of blood to the right atrium.

Varicose Veins

Varicose veins (Fig. 15.8) are dilated, tortuous superficial vessels that often develop in the lower extremities. Clinically apparent varicose veins occur in 10%–20% of the general population. They affect women two to three times more frequently than men, and roughly half of patients have a family history of this condition. Varicosities can occur in any vein in the body, but are most common in the saphenous veins of the leg and their tributaries. They may also develop in the anorectal area (hemorrhoids), in the lower esophageal veins (esophageal

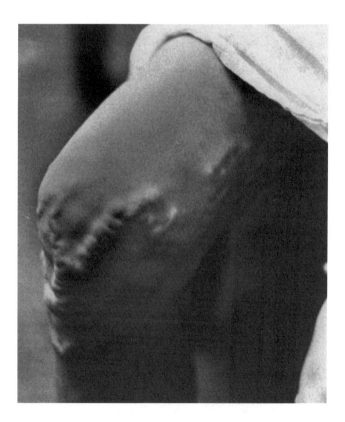

Figure 15.8. A patient with extensive venous varicosities of the right leg.

varices), and in the spermatic cord (varicocele).

Varicosity is thought to result from intrinsic weakness of the vessel wall, from increased intraluminal pressure, or from congenital defects in the structure and function of the valves that severely reduce antegrade (toward the heart) venous flow. Varicose veins in the lower extremity can be classified as either primary or secondary. *Primary* varicose veins originate in the superficial system, and factors that contribute to their development include pregnancy, prolonged standing, and obesity. During pregnancy or prolonged standing, the high venous pressure within the legs promotes the development of varicosity in individuals with inherent weakness of the venous walls. Adipose tissue surrounding vessel walls in obese patients offers less structural support to veins than lean mass. *Secondary* varicose veins occur when an abnormality in the deep venous system is the cause of superficial varicosities. These may develop in the setting of deep venous insufficiency or occlusion, or when the perforating veins are incompetent. In such cases, deep venous blood is shunted retrograde via perforating channels into superficial veins, increasing intraluminal pressure and volume in these vessels and causing dilatation and varicosity formation.

Many individuals with varicose veins are asymptomatic but seek treatment for cosmetic reasons. When symptoms do develop, they include a dull ache or pressure sensation in the legs after prolonged standing, usually relieved by elevation of the limb. Superficial venous insufficiency may result when venous valves are unable to function normally in the dilated veins. This can cause swelling and skin ulceration that is particularly severe near the ankle. Relative stasis of blood within varicose veins can promote superficial vein thrombosis. Varicosities can rupture, causing a hematoma at the site of hemorrhage.

Varicose veins are usually treated conservatively. Patients should elevate their legs while supine, avoid prolonged standing, and wear external compression stockings which counterbalance the increased venous hydrostatic pressure. Small symptomatic varicose veins are sometimes treated by injection of a sclerosing solution into the vein. Surgical therapy includes vein ligation and removal and is reserved for patients who are very symptomatic, suffer recurrent superficial vein thrombosis, or develop skin ulcerations.

Venous Thrombosis

The terms venous thrombosis or thrombophlebitis are used to describe thrombus within a superficial or deep vein and the inflammatory response in the vessel wall that it incites. Thrombi in the lower extremities are classified by location as either deep venous thrombi or superficial venous thrombi.

Initially, the venous thrombus is composed principally of platelets and fibrin. Later, red blood cells become interspersed within the fibrin, and the thrombus tends to propagate in the direction of blood flow. The changes in the vessel wall can be minimal, or they can involve granulocyte infiltration, loss of endothelium, and edema. Thrombi may diminish or obstruct vascular flow, or they may dislodge and form emboli.

Deep Venous Thrombosis

Epidemiology, Etiology, and Pathogenesis

Deep venous thrombosis (DVT) occurs most commonly in the veins of the calves, but it may also develop initially in more proximal veins such as the popliteal, femoral, and iliac vessels. If left untreated, 20%–30% of the DVTs that occur in the calves may propagate to these proximal veins. The two major consequences of deep vein thrombosis are pulmonary embolism, and the postphlebitic syndrome. Pulmonary embolism can supervene when a clot, most often from a DVT in the proximal veins of the lower extremities, dislodges and travels through the inferior vena cava and right heart chambers, finally reaching and obstructing a portion of the pulmonary vasculature (Fig. 15.9). Pulmonary embolism is common (incidence of approximately 600,000 per year in the United States) and is often fatal, with an untreated mortality of 30%–40%.

Postphlebitic syndrome, or chronic deep venous insufficiency, results from valvular damage and/or persistent occlusion by deep venous thrombosis. This may lead to chronic leg swelling, stasis pigmentation, and skin ulcerations.

In 1856, Virchow described a triad of factors that predispose to venous thrombosis: 1) stasis of blood flow, 2) hypercoagulability, and 3) vascular damage.

Stasis disrupts laminar flow and brings platelets into contact with the endothelium. This allows coagulation factors to accumulate and retards the influx of clotting inhibitors. Factors that slow venous flow and induce stasis include immobilization (e.g.,

prolonged bed rest after surgery, sitting in a car or an airplane for a long trip), cardiac failure, and hyperviscosity syndromes (Table 15.6).

A variety of clinical disorders cause systemic hypercoagulability, including resistance of factor V to activated protein C, and inherited deficiencies of antithrombin III, protein C, and protein S (see Chapter 7). Pancreatic, lung, stomach, breast, and genitourinary tract adenocarcinomas are associated with a high prevalence of venous thrombosis. This is thought to occur in part because necrotic tumor cells release thrombogenic factors. Hypercoagulability may also be present in other disease states, including systemic lupus erythematosus (antiphopholipid antibody syndrome), myeloproliferative diseases, dysfibrinogenemia, and disseminated intravascular coagulation.

Vascular damage either by external injury or by intravenous catheters can denude

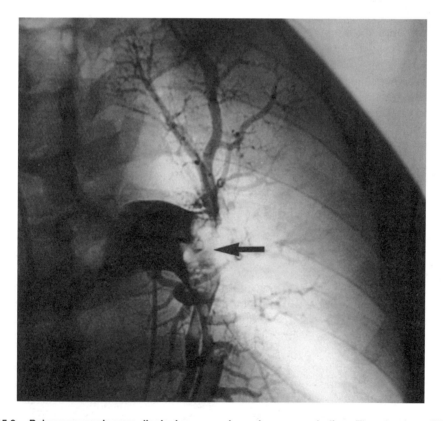

Figure 15.9. Pulmonary angiogram displaying a massive pulmonary embolism. There is a large filling defect in the left main pulmonary artery (arrow), additional filling defects in the lower pulmonary artery branches, and a paucity of vessels in the left midlung region (due to obstructed flow).

TABLE 15.6. Conditions That Predispose to DVT

Stasis of blood flow
- Prolonged inactivity (following surgery, long travel by car, air)
- Immobilized extremity (following bone fracture)
- Heart failure (with systemic venous congestion)
- Hyperviscosity syndromes (e.g., polycythemia vera)

Hypercoagulable states
- Inherited disorders of coagulation
  Antithrombin III deficiency
  Deficiency of protein C or protein S
  Resistance to activated protein C (Factor V Leiden)
  Antiphospholipid antibodies ("lupus anticoagulant")
- Neoplastic disease (e.g., pancreatic, lung, stomach, breast cancers)
- Pregnancy and oral contraceptive use (or other high estrogen states)
- Myeloproliferative diseases
- Smoking

Vascular damage
- Instrumentation (e.g., intravenous catheters)
- Trauma

the vascular endothelium and expose subendothelial collagen. Exposed collagen acts as a substrate for the binding of von Willebrand's factor and platelets, and can serve in this setting as the initiator of the clotting cascade. Less dramatic damage to the vascular endothelium that causes dysfunction rather than denudation can also favor thrombosis. This is because the endothelium actively secretes both vasodilator factors and platelet inhibitors such as endothelium derived relaxing factor (EDRF-NO) and prostacyclin (PGI_2), and antithrombotic molecules such as thrombomodulin and heparan sulfate. When the vascular endothelium is damaged, synthetic function is diminished and thrombosis is favored.

The risk of venous thrombosis is particularly high after fractures of the spine, pelvis, and bones of the lower extremities. The risk following bone fracture may be related to stasis of blood flow, increased coagulability, and possibly traumatic endothelial damage. In addition, venous thrombosis occurs frequently in patients undergoing surgical procedures, particularly major orthopedic operations.

During late pregnancy and the early postpartum period, women have a several-fold increase in the incidence of venous thrombus formation. In the third trimester, the fetus compresses the inferior vena cava and can cause stasis of blood flow, and a hypercoagulable state may be induced by high levels of circulating estrogens. Oral contraceptives and other pharmacologic estrogen products may also predispose to thrombus formation.

Clinical Presentation

Patients with DVT may be asymptomatic. Symptomatic patients often describe calf or thigh discomfort, particularly upon standing or walking, or report unilateral leg swelling. The physical signs of proximal DVT include edema of the involved leg and occasionally localized warmth and erythema. Tenderness may be present over the course of the phlebitic vein, and a deep venous cord (induration along the thrombosed vessel) is occasionally palpable. Calf pain produced by dorsiflexion of the foot (Homan's sign) is a nonspecific and unreliable sign of DVT.

Diagnosis

Laboratory tests used to diagnose DVT include contrast venography, duplex venous ultrasonography, and magnetic resonance venography. Contrast venography is an invasive imaging technique that remains the definitive diagnostic modality for both asymptomatic and symptomatic DVT. Radiocontrast material is administered into a foot vein, and images are obtained as the contrast ascends through the venous system of the leg. DVT is diagnosed if a filling defect is present (Fig. 15.10). A noninvasive technique, duplex venous ultrasonography is 97% sensitive and 97% specific for the diagnosis of symptomatic DVT in a proximal vein, but it is less sensitive for diagnosing calf vein thrombi. This technique uses real-time ultrasound scanning to image the vein, and pulsed Doppler ultrasound to assess blood flow within it. Criteria used for diagnosis of DVT with duplex ultrasonography include the inability to compress the vein with direct pressure (suggesting the pres-

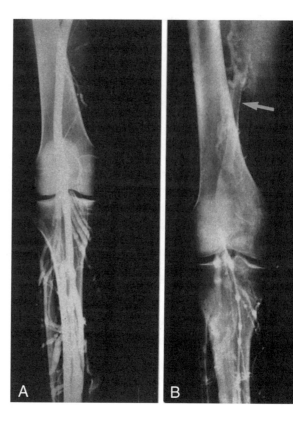

Figure 15.10. **A.** Normal venogram. Contrast material was injected into a foot vein, and fills the leg veins in this radiograph. **B.** Venogram demonstrating extensive thrombosis of the deep calf veins, popliteal vein, and superficial femoral vein. Arrows indicate filling defects in the superficial femoral vein (which is a deep vein) due to the presence of thrombus. The deep calf veins are filled with thrombus and cannot be visualized.

ence of an intraluminal thrombus), direct visualization of the thrombus, and absence of blood flow within the vein. Duplex venous ultrasonography is readily available and less expensive than contrast venography, and is now used more commonly.

Treatment

The most important reason for treating patients with proximal DVT is to prevent pulmonary embolism. Elevation of the affected extremity above the level of the heart is implemented to help reduce edema and tenderness, and anticoagulation is begun to prevent extension of the thrombus. Heparin is administered intravenously for at least 5 days to prevent additional clot formation. Warfarin, an oral anticoagulant, is prescribed for long-term management and is usually continued for several months, depending on the underlying precipitant of DVT. In patients with proximal DVT who cannot be treated with anticoagulant medication because of a bleeding disorder, an

intravascular filter can be inserted into the inferior vena cava to prevent emboli from reaching the lungs.

Treatment of patients with calf vein thrombosis is more controversial because pulmonary emboli from that site are uncommon. Some physicians advocate serial noninvasive monitoring to determine if the thrombus propagates into proximal veins. Others treat such thrombosis with intravenous heparin followed by warfarin for 3 to 6 months.

Prophylaxis against DVT is mandatory in clinical situations in which the risk of deep venous thrombosis is high, such as during bed rest following surgery. Prophylactic measures include subcutaneous heparin administration, low-dose oral warfarin, compression stockings and/or intermittent external pneumatic compression of the legs to prevent venous stasis. Recently, low molecular weight heparin (see Chapter 17) has been shown to be even more effective than conventional heparin for prevention of DVT after hip surgery, and this agent is being studied as DVT prophylaxis in other settings as well.

Superficial Thrombophlebitis

Much less serious than DVT, this is a benign disorder associated with inflammation and thrombosis of a superficial vein, just below the skin. Superficial thrombophlebitis may occur, for example, as a complication of an indwelling intravenous catheter. It is characterized by erythema, tenderness, and edema over the involved vein. Treatment consists of local heat and rest of the involved extremity. Aspirin or other anti-inflammatory medications may relieve the associated discomfort. Unlike DVT, superficial thrombophlebitis does not result in subsequent pulmonary embolization.

SUMMARY

1. Aortic aneurysms are of two types: true aneurysms and false (pseudo) aneurysms. True aneurysms are most commonly related to atherosclerosis, especially in the abdominal and descending thoracic aorta. In the ascending aorta, cystic medial necrosis is an important contributor to true aneurysm formation. A false aneurysm is actually a hole in the arterial intima and media, contained by a layer of adventitia or perivascular clot.

2. Symptoms of aortic aneurysms relate to compression of adjacent structures (back pain, dysphagia, respiratory symptoms) or blood leakage. The most severe consequence is aneurysm rupture.

3. Aortic dissections result from a splitting apart of a weakened medial layer of the aorta, often in the setting of advanced age, hypertension, or other causes of medial degeneration (cystic medial necrosis). Type A (proximal) aortic dissections involve the ascending aorta, whereas Type B dissections are confined to the descending aorta. The former are more common, more devastating, and require surgical treatment. Type B dissections may often be managed by medical therapy alone.

4. Arteriosclerosis obliterans is a common disease of large and medium-large arteries, often resulting in claudication of the limbs.

5. Acute arterial occlusion results from thrombus formation in situ or from arterial embolism. The latter arises from thrombus within the heart, from proximal arterial sites, or sometimes paradoxically from the systemic veins if an intracardiac shunt (e.g., patent foramen ovale or atrial septal defect) is present.

6. Vasculitic syndromes are inflammatory diseases of blood vessels that impair arterial blood flow and result in localized and systemic symptoms. They are distinguished from one another by the pattern of vessel involvement and morphologic findings (Table 15.5).

7. Raynaud's phenomenon is an episodic vasospasm of arteries that supply the digits of the upper and lower extremities. It may be a primary condition (Raynaud's disease) or appear in association with other disorders such as connective tissue diseases or blood dyscrasias.

8. Varicose veins are dilated tortuous vessels, which may present cosmetic problems. Occasionally they cause discomfort, become thrombosed, or lead to venous insufficiency.

9. Venous thrombosis results from stasis of blood flow, hypercoagulability, and vascular damage. The major complication of deep venous thrombosis is pulmonary embolism. A chronic complication is venous insufficiency causing chronic leg swelling and skin ulceration.

ADDITIONAL READING

Cigarroa JE, Isselbacher EM, DeSanctis RW, et al. Diagnostic imaging in the evaluation of suspected aortic dissection. Old standards and new directions. N Engl J Med 1993;328:35–43.
Coffman JD. Raynaud's phenomenon. An update. Hypertension 1991;17:593–602.
Creager MA, Dzau VJ. Vascular diseases of the extremities. In: Wilson JD, Braunwald E, Isselbacher

KJ, et al., eds. Harrison's Principles of Internal Medicine. 14th ed. New York: McGraw-Hill, 1997.

Dzau VJ, Creager MA. Diseases of the aorta. In: Wilson JD, Braunwald E, Isselbacher KJ, et al., eds. Harrison's Principles of Internal Medicine. 14th ed. New York: McGraw-Hill, 1997.

Fuster V, Halperin JL. Aortic dissection: a medical perspective. J Card Surg 1994;9:713–728.

Ginsberg JS. Management of venous thromboembolism. N Engl J Med 1996;335:1816–1828.

Greenhalgh RM, Mannick JA, eds. The Cause and Management of Aneurysms. Philadelphia: WB Saunders, 1990.

Loscalzo J, Creager MA, Dzau VJ, eds. The Textbook of Vascular Medicine and Biology. Boston: Little, Brown & Co., 1996.

Nienaber CA, von Kodolitsch Y, Nicolas V, et al. The diagnosis of thoracic aortic dissection by noninvasive imaging procedures. N Engl J Med 1993;328: 1–9.

Robicsek F, Thubrikar MJ. Hemodynamic considerations regarding the mechanism and prevention of aortic dissection. Ann Thorac Surg 1994;58:1247–1253.

Wienmann EE, Salzman EW. Deep vein thrombosis. N Engl J Med 1994;331:1630–1641.

Acknowledgments The previous edition of this chapter was written by Michael Diminick, MD, Stuart Kaplan, MD, Jesse Salmeron, MD, and Mark A. Creager, MD.

Congenital Heart Disease

Douglas W. Green,
Raymond Tabibiazar,
and Michael Freed

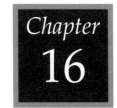

Congenital heart diseases are cardiac abnormalities present at birth that result in an alteration in heart function. Cardiac malformations are the most common type of congenital structural anomaly, affecting 8 out of every 1000 infants. Some of these abnormalities are severe and require immediate medical attention, but many are less pronounced and have minimal physiologic consequences. Although congenital heart defects are present at birth, milder defects may not become evident until days, weeks, or months later. On occasion, a congenital cardiac abnormality may even escape detection until adulthood.

The past half-century has seen tremendous growth in the understanding of the pathophysiology of congenital heart disease and in our ability to evaluate and treat those afflicted. However, there is as yet no clear understanding of the etiology of most of these heart disorders. Single gene defects, environmental factors, maternal ingestion of toxic substances, and viral exposures have all been shown to contribute to cardiac malformations, but in the majority of cases the specific cause remains unknown.

The survival of children with congenital heart disease has improved substantially in recent decades, due in large part to improved diagnostic and surgical techniques. However, more than 20% of children presenting with severe disease in the first month of life will not live beyond 1 year of age.

The cardiovascular system first appears during the third week of embryonic development as a cluster of angiogenic cells in the rostral end of the developing fetus. These cells grow and divide to form a primitive hollow tube that will ultimately evolve into the familiar four-chambered heart. During this process, the embryo develops a unique circulation that allows it to grow and develop within the uterus, using the placenta as the primary organ of gas, nutrient, and waste exchange. At birth, the placenta becomes unnecessary as the fetal lungs inflate and become functional. At the same time, several significant changes occur in the flow patterns through the newborn's cardiovascular system that allow the neonate to adjust to life outside the womb.

From this brief sketch, one can begin to appreciate the remarkable complexity of cardiogenesis, as well as envision some of the ways in which malformations could arise. This chapter begins with an overview of fetal cardiovascular development and then describes the most common forms of congenital heart disease.

NORMAL DEVELOPMENT OF THE CARDIOVASCULAR SYSTEM

By the middle of the third week of gestation, the nutrient and gas exchange needs of the rapidly growing embryo can no longer be met by diffusion alone; the tissues come instead to rely on the developing cardiovascular system, the first functioning organ system in the embryo, to deliver these substances over long distances.

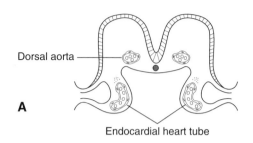

Development of the Heart Tube

At approximately day 17 of embryogenesis, mesenchymal cells ventral to the pericardial coelom begin to proliferate, eventually forming two longitudinal cell clusters known as angioblastic cords. These cords canalize, becoming paired endothelial heart tubes (Fig. 16.1). Lateral embryonic folding gradually opposes these two tubes, allowing them to fuse in the ventral midline, forming a single endocardial tube by day 22. The tube is continuous rostrally with the aortic arch system and caudally with the vessels of the venous system. Following tubal fusion and later overgrowth of splanchnic mesoderm to form myocardium, the primitive heart begins to beat, causing blood to circulate by the end of the third week. The pericardial coelom overlying the cardiogenic area will eventually become the pericardial cavity, housing the future heart.

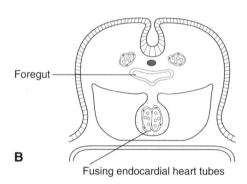

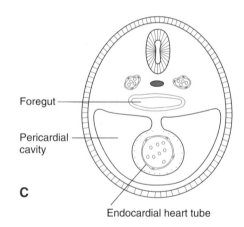

Formation of the Heart Loop

As the tubular heart grows and elongates, it develops a series of alternate constrictions and dilations, creating the first sign of the primitive heart chambers—the truncus arteriosus, bulbus cordis, ventricle, atrium, and sinus venosus (Fig. 16.2). Continued growth and elongation within the confined pericardial cavity necessitates bending of the heart tube upon itself, eventually forming a U-shaped loop pointing ventrally and to the right of the embryo. The end result of this looping is placement of the atrium and sinus venosus above and behind the truncus arteriosus, bulbus cordis, and ventricle (Fig 16.3). At this point, neither definitive septa between the developing chambers nor definitive valvular tissue

Figure 16.1. Embryonic transverse sections illustrating fusion of the two heart tubes into a single endocardial heart tube. A. 18 days. **B.** 21 days. **C.** 22 days.

have formed. The connection between the primitive atrium and ventricle is termed the **atrioventricular canal**. Continued development will see the atrioventricular canal become two separate canals, one housing the tricuspid valve and the other housing the mitral valve. The sinus venosus will eventually be incorporated into the right atrium, forming both the coronary sinus and a portion of the right atrial wall.

Septation

Septation of the developing atrium, atrioventricular canal, and ventricle begins in the middle of the fourth week, and continues through the fifth week. These events are described separately here. However, it is important to keep in mind that all three processes occur simultaneously.

Septation of the Atria

The primary atrial septum, also known as the **septum primum,** begins as a ridge of tissue on the roof of the common atrium that grows downward into the atrial cavity (Fig. 16.4). As the septum primum advances, it creates a large opening known as the **ostium primum** between the crescent-shaped leading edge of the septum and the endocardial cushions (masses of mesenchymal tissue) surrounding the atrioventricular canal. The ostium primum allows passage of blood between the forming atria. Eventually, the septum primum fuses with the superior aspect of the endocardial cushions, obliterating the ostium primum. Before the closure of the ostium primum is completed, however, small perforations appear in the center of the septum primum that ultimately coalesce to form the **ostium secundum,** preserving a pathway for blood flow between the atria (Fig. 16.4). Following closure of the ostium primum, a second crescentic membrane, the **septum secundum,** begins to develop immediately to the right of the superior aspect of the septum primum. This second septum grows downward, and in so doing overlaps the ostium

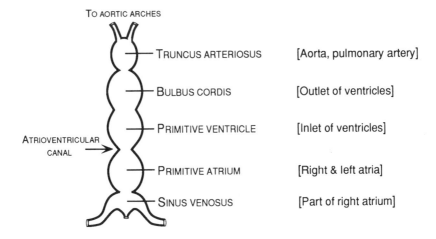

TO AORTIC ARCHES

TRUNCUS ARTERIOSUS   [Aorta, pulmonary artery]

BULBUS CORDIS   [Outlet of ventricles]

PRIMITIVE VENTRICLE   [Inlet of ventricles]

ATRIOVENTRICULAR
CANAL

PRIMITIVE ATRIUM   [Right & left atria]

SINUS VENOSUS   [Part of right atrium]

Figure 16.2.   The straight heart tube at approximately 22 days. The structures that will ultimately form from each segment are listed in brackets.

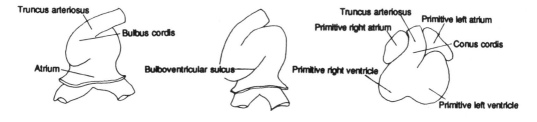

Truncus arteriosus

Bulbus cordis

Atrium

Bulboventricular sulcus

Truncus arteriosus

Primitive right atrium

Primitive left atrium

Conus cordis

Primitive right ventricle

Primitive left ventricle

Figure 16.3.   Left, middle. By day 24 continued growth and elongation within the confined pericardial space necessitates bending of the heart tube upon itself, forming a U-shaped loop that points ventrally and to the right. **Right.** Looping eventually places the atria above and behind the primitive ventricles.

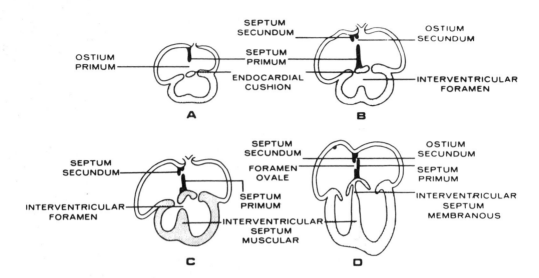

Figure 16.4.   Atrial septal formation at A, 30 days, B, 33 days, C, 37 days of development, and in D, the newborn. As the septum primum grows toward the ventricles, the opening between it and the atrioventricular canal is the ostium primum. Before the ostium primum completely closes, perforations within the upper portion of the septum primum form the ostium secundum. A second ridge of tissue, the septum secundum, grows downward to the right of the septum primum, partially covering the ostium secundum. The foramen ovale is an opening of the septum secundum that is covered by the "flap-valve" of the lower septum primum. (Modified from Moss AJ, Adams FH. Heart Disease in Infants, Children, and Adolescents. Baltimore: Williams & Wilkins, 1968:16.)

secundum. The septum secundum eventually fuses with the endocardial cushions, although in only a partial fashion, leaving an opening known as the **foramen ovale**. The superior edge of septum primum then gradually regresses, leaving the lower edge to act as the flap-type valve of the foramen ovale. The valve allows only right-to-left flow of blood between the atria; any rise in left atrial pressure would force the septum primum against the septum secundum, preventing left-to-right atrial passage of blood (Fig. 16.5). During gestation, blood passes from the right atrium to the left atrium through the foramen ovale because of the pressure gradient that exists between the atria (the pressure in the fetal right atrium is higher than that of the left atrium). This gradient changes direction postnatally, causing the valve to close, as described below.

Septation of the Atrioventricular Canal

Growth of the **endocardial cushions** contributes to the septal formation of the atria, and as described later, to the mem-

branous portion of the interventricular septum. The majority of endocardial cushion tissue growth, however, is in the horizontal plane, resulting in septation of the atrioventricular canal through the continued growth of the right, left, superior, and inferior endocardial cushions (Fig. 16.6). Septation creates separate right and left canals that will give rise to the tricuspid and mitral orifice, respectively.

Septation of the Ventricles and Ventricular Outflow Tracts

At the end of the fourth week, the primitive ventricle begins to grow and dilate, leaving a median muscular ridge, the primitive interventricular septum. The majority of the early increase in height of the interventricular septum is due to dilation of the two new ventricles forming on either side of it, and only later does new cell growth in the septum contribute to its size. The free edge of the muscular interventricular septum does not fuse with the endocardial cushions; the opening that remains and allows communication between the right and left ventricles is known as the interventricular foramen (Fig. 16.7). This foramen remains open until the seventh week of gestation, at which time fusion of tissue from the right and left bulbar ridges (see below) and the endocardial cushions forms the membranous portion of the interventricular septum.

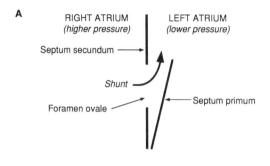

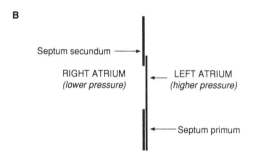

Figure 16.5. Diagramatic depiction of the flap-type valve of the foramen ovale. A. Before birth, the valve permits only right-to-left flow of blood from the higher-pressured right atrium (RA) to the lower-pressured left atrium (LA). **B.** Following birth, the pressure in the LA becomes greater than that in the RA, causing the septum primum to close firmly against the septum secundum. (Modified from Moore KL, Persaud TVN. The Developing Human. Philadelphia: WB Saunders, 1993:318.)

During the fifth week, mesenchymal proliferation taking place in the bulbus cordis and truncus arteriosus creates a pair of protrusions known as the bulbar ridges (Fig. 16.8). These ridges fuse in the midline, forming the aorticopulmonary septum. The formation of this septum results in the division of the bulbus cordis and the truncus arteriosus into two separate arterial channels, the pulmonary artery and the aorta, the former now continuous with the right ventricle and the latter continuous with the left ventricle. At the end of development, the bulbous cordis is incorporated into the right ventricle to form the infundibulum, which acts as the right ventricular outflow tract. As alluded to above, tissue from the endocardial cushions extends and merges with the aorticopulmonary septum rostrally and the muscular interventricular septum caudally to create the membranous interventricular foramen.

Development of the Cardiac Valves

Semilunar Valve Development (Aortic and Pulmonary Valves)

The semilunar valves begin to develop just prior to the completion of the aorticopulmonary septum. The process begins when three outgrowths of subendocardial mesenchymal tissue begin to form around both the aortic and pulmonary orifices. These growths are ultimately shaped and excavated by the joint action of programmed cell death and blood flow to cre-

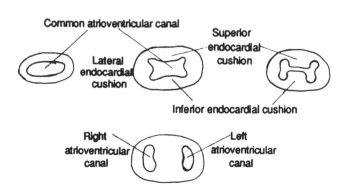

Figure 16.6. The progression of septal formation in the atrioventricular canal through successive stages. The septum forms through growth of the superior, inferior, and lateral endocardial cushions. The endocardial cushions are masses of mesenchymal tissue that surround the atrioventricular canal and aid in the formation of the orifices of the mitral and tricuspid valves, as well as the formation of the upper interventricular septum and lower interatrial septum.

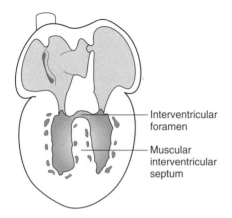

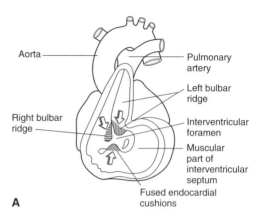

A

Figure 16.7.   The interventricular septum and the interventricular foramen. (Modified from Moore KL, Persaud TVN. The Developing Human. Philadelphia: WB Saunders, 1993:325.)

ate the three familiar, thin-walled cusps of both the aortic and pulmonary valves.

Atrioventricular Valve Development (Mitral and Tricuspid Valves)

After the endocardial cushions fuse to form the septa between the right and left atrioventricular canals, the subendocardial mesenchymal tissue that surrounds each canal begins to proliferate, developing similar outgrowths as in semilunar valve development. Soon afterward, programmed cell death occurs in the myocardial tissue on the ventricular surface of the nascent leaflets. This process leaves behind only a few, fine muscular strands to connect the valves to the ventricular wall (Fig.16.9). These muscular strands eventually degenerate and are replaced by strands of dense connective tissue, the chordae tendineae.

FETAL AND TRANSITIONAL CIRCULATIONS

The fetal circulation is elegantly designed to serve the needs of *in utero* development. At the time of birth, the circulation automatically undergoes modifications that establish the normal blood flow pattern of a newborn infant.

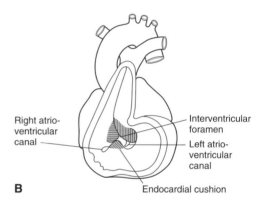

B

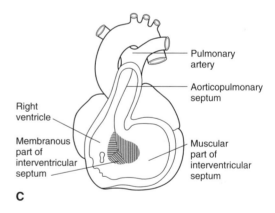

C

Figure 16.8.   Formation of the aorticopulmonary septum occurs via fusion of the bulbar ridges, resulting in division of the bulbus cordis and truncus arteriosus into the aorta and pulmonary artery (A, five weeks; B, six weeks; C, seven weeks). The bulbus cordis becomes the right ventricular outflow tract. Fusion of tissue from the endocardial cushions, the aorticopulmonary septum, and the muscular interventricular septum creates the membranous interventricular septum. (Modified from Moore KL, Persaud TVN. The Developing Human. Philadelphia: WB Saunders, 1993:322.)

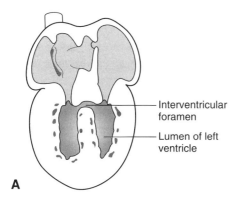

A

Interventricular foramen

Lumen of left ventricle

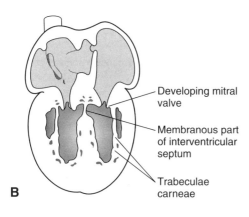

B

Developing mitral valve

Membranous part of interventricular septum

Trabeculae carneae

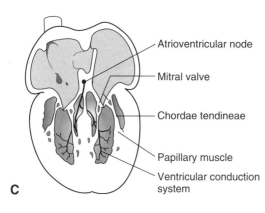

C

Atrioventricular node

Mitral valve

Chordae tendineae

Papillary muscle

Ventricular conduction system

Figure 16.9.   Proliferation of mesenchymal tissue surrounding the atrioventricular canals forms the atrioventricular valves. Degeneration of myocardium and replacement by connective tissue forms the chordae tendineae; their muscular attachments to the ventricular wall are the papillary muscles. (Modified from Moore KL, Persaud TVN. The Developing Human. Philadelphia: WB Saunders, 1993:325.)

Fetal Circulation

In the fetus, oxygenated blood leaves the placenta through the single umbilical vein (Fig. 16.10). Approximately half of the umbilical blood is shunted through the fetal **ductus venosus,** bypassing the hepatic vasculature and proceeding directly into the inferior vena cava. The remaining blood passes through the portal vein to the liver and then into the inferior vena cava through the hepatic veins. Inferior vena caval blood is therefore composed of a mixture of *oxygenated* umbilical venous blood and the blood of *low oxygen tension* returning from the systemic veins of the fetus. Because of this mixture, the oxygen tension of inferior vena caval blood is higher than that of blood returning to the fetal right atrium from the superior vena cava. This distinction is important because these two streams of blood are largely separated within the right atrium and ultimately follow different circulatory paths. The consequence of this separation is that the fetal brain and myocardium receive blood of relatively high oxygen content, whereas the more poorly oxygenated blood is diverted to the placenta (via the descending aorta and umbilical arteries) for subsequent oxygenation.

The majority of the inferior vena caval blood entering the right atrium is directed to the left atrium through the foramen ovale. This intracardiac shunt of relatively well-oxygenated blood is facilitated by the inferior border of the septum secundum, termed the crista dividens, which is positioned such that it overrides the opening of the IVC into the RA. This shunted blood then mixes with the small amount of poorly oxygenated blood returning to the left atrium through the fetal pulmonary veins (remember that the lungs are not ventilated *in utero;* the developing pulmonary tissues actually *remove* oxygen from the blood, rather than contribute to it). From the left atrium, blood flows into the left ventricle and is then pumped into the ascending aorta. From the aorta, this well-oxygenated blood is distributed primarily to three territories: 1) approximately 9% of the LV out-

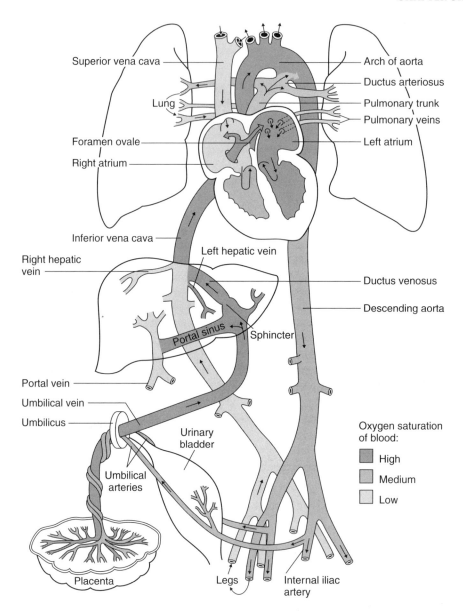

Figure 16.10.   The fetal circulation, as described in the text. Arrows indicate the direction of blood flow. Three shunts (ductus venosus, foramen ovale, and ductus arteriosus) allow the majority of the blood to bypass the lungs and liver during fetal life, but cease to function shortly after birth. (Modified from Moore KL, Persaud TVN. The Developing Human. Philadelphia: WB Saunders, 1993:344.)

put enters the coronary arteries and perfuses the myocardium, 2) 62% travels in the carotid and subclavian vessels to the upper body and brain, and 3) 29% passes into the descending aorta and is distributed throughout the rest of the fetal body.

The remaining well-oxygenated inferior vena caval blood entering the right atrium mixes with poorly oxygenated blood from the superior vena cava and passes into the right ventricle. In the fetus, the right ventricle is the "workhorse" of the heart, providing two-thirds of the total cardiac output. This output flows into the pulmonary artery, and from there, through either the **ductus arteriosus** into the descending aorta (88% of RV output), or through the pulmonary arteries and into the lungs (12% of

RV output). This unequal distribution of RV outflow is actually quite efficient: bypassing the lungs is desired because the fetal lungs are filled with amniotic fluid and are incapable of gas exchange. The low oxygen tension of the fluid in the lungs causes constriction of the pulmonary vessels, increasing pulmonary vascular resistance. The increase in pulmonary resistance facilitates the shunt of blood through the ductus arteriosus to the systemic circulation, ultimately directing the majority of the cardiac output into the descending aorta. From the descending aorta, there is distribution of blood flow to the lower body, and to the umbilical arteries, leading back to the placenta for gas exchange.

Transitional Circulation

Immediately following birth, the neonate rapidly adjusts to life outside of the womb. The newly functioning lungs replace the placenta as the organ of gas exchange, and the three shunts (ductus venosus, foramen ovale, and ductus arteriosus) that operated during gestation close. This shift in the site of gas exchange and the resulting changes in cardiovascular architecture allow the newborn to survive independently.

As the umbilical cord is clamped, or constricts naturally, the low-resistance placental flow is removed from the system, resulting in an increase in systemic vascular resistance. There is also an accompanying fall in pulmonary vascular resistance for two reasons: 1) the mechanical inflation of the lungs after birth stretches the lung tissues, causing pulmonary artery expansion and wall thinning, and 2) vasodilatation of the pulmonary vasculature ensues, thought to result from the rise in blood oxygen tension accompanying aeration of the lungs. The reduction in pulmonary resistance results in a dramatic increase in pulmonary blood flow. The fall in pulmonary vascular resistance is most marked within the first 24 hours after birth, but continues to decline for the next 2 to 6 weeks until adult levels of pulmonary resistance are achieved.

As the pulmonary resistance falls and more blood travels to the lungs via the pulmonary artery, it follows that venous return from the pulmonary veins to the LA also increases, such that the LA pressure rises. At the same time, cessation of umbilical flow and constriction of the ductus venosus cause a fall in the pressure in the inferior vena cava and right atrium. As a result of these pressure alterations in the atria (LA pressure now exceeds that in the RA), the valve of the foramen ovale is forced against the septum secundum, eliminating the previous flow between the atria (Fig. 16.5).

With oxygenation now occurring in the newborn lungs, the ductus arteriosus becomes superfluous, and it begins to constrict. This constriction is believed to be due to a local reaction of ductal tissue to the increased oxygen tension following birth, possibly mediated via changing levels of bradykinin or prostaglandins released from the lungs during their initial aeration. That is, during fetal life, a high circulating level of prostaglandin E_2 (PGE_2) is generated in response to relative hypoxia, and causes the ductus arteriosus to relax. After birth, PGE_2 levels decline and the ductus constricts. The responsiveness of the ductus to vasoactive substances depends on the gestational age of the fetus: the ductus often fails to constrict in premature infants, resulting in a congenital anomaly, patent ductus arteriosus, to be discussed later.

With the anatomic separation of the circulatory paths of the right and left sides of the heart now complete, the cardiac output of the left ventricle increases, while that of the right ventricle decreases such that the output of each becomes equal. The increased pressure and volume load this places on the left ventricle induces the myocardial cells of the LV to hypertrophy, while the decreased pressure and volume load on the right ventricle results in regression of the hypertrophic RV wall thickness.

COMMON CONGENITAL HEART LESIONS

Congenital heart defects are generally well tolerated before birth. *In utero,* the fetus benefits from shunting of blood through the ductus arteriosus and the foramen ovale, allowing flow to bypass most defects. It is only after birth, when the neonate has been separated from the maternal circulation and the oxygenation it provides, and the fetal shunts have closed, that congenital heart defects usually become manifest.

Congenital heart lesions can be categorized in a number of different ways. For example, they may be described as either "cyanotic" or "acyanotic" abnormalities. Cyanosis refers to a blue-purple discoloration of the skin and mucous membranes due to an elevated concentration of deoxygenated hemoglobin in the blood. In the context of congenital heart disease, cyanosis results from hypoxemia secondary to defects that allow poorly oxygenated blood from the right side of the heart to be shunted to the left side, bypassing the lungs.

Acyanotic lesions include those that result in either *left-to-right*-sided shunting of blood, or congenital intracardiac or vascular stenoses, or valvular regurgitation. Large left-to-right shunts at the atrial, ventricular, or great vessel level (all described below) cause the pulmonary artery volume and pressure to increase, sometimes associated with the later development of pulmonary arteriolar hypertrophy and increased resistance to flow. This process can lead to pulmonary hypertension, a major contributor to the clinical manifestations and prognosis of the underlying congenital defect. Over time, the elevated pulmonary resistance may force the direction of the original shunt to reverse, i.e., causing *right-to-left* flow, accompanied by the physical findings of hypoxemia and cyanosis.

The development of pulmonary hypertension due to chronic volume overload by a large left-to-right shunt is known as **Eisenmenger's syndrome**. Histologically in this condition, the pulmonary arteriolar media hypertrophies and the intima proliferates, encroaching upon the lumen and reducing the cross-sectional area of the pulmonary bed. Ultimately the vessels become thrombosed with obliteration of arterioles, and a plexiform network of collateral vessels develops around the occluded vessels. The underlying mechanism(s) by which this form of pulmonary vascular obstructive disease develops in patients with chronic left-to-right shunts is unknown. The only effective long-term treatment for Eisenmenger's syndrome is a lung or heart-lung transplant.

Acyanotic Lesions

Atrial Septal Defect

An atrial septal defect (ASD) is an opening in the atrial septum after birth that allows direct communication between the left and right atria. ASDs are relatively common, accounting for 5%–10% of congenital heart disease with a male to female ratio of about 1:2. They can occur anywhere along the atrial septum, but the most common site is at the midportion of the interatrial septum, in the region of the fossa ovalis, termed an *ostium secundum* ASD (Fig. 16.11). This defect arises from excessive resorption or inadequate development of the septum primum. Less commonly, an ASD appears in the atrioventricular canal portion of the atrial septum, adjacent to the atrioventricular valves (*ostium primum* defect), or in the superior portion of the atrial septum near the entry of the superior vena cava (*sinus venosus* ASD). Ostium primum defects are often associated with abnormal development of the mitral and tricuspid valves, whereas the sinus venosus ASD is often accompanied by anomalous drainage of pulmonary veins from the right lung into the right atrium.

Pathophysiology

Atrial septal defects are classified among the acyanotic congenital heart diseases since, in the uncomplicated case, oxygenated blood from the left atrium is shunted into the right atrium, but not vice versa. Flow through the atrial defect is a function of the size of the defect, the diastolic filling properties (compliance) of the two ventricles, and the relative impedance of the pul-

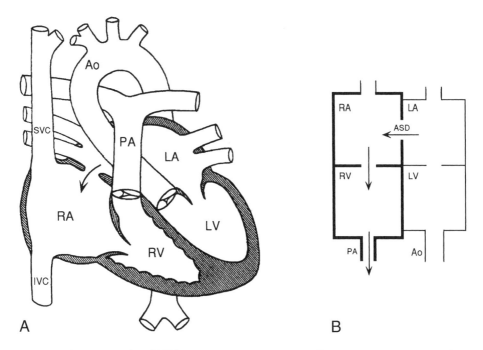

Figure 16.11. Atrial septal defect (ASD), ostium secundum type. A. The arrow indicates shunted flow from the left atrium (LA) toward the right atrium (RA). **B.** Schematic representation of blood flow through an uncomplicated ASD, resulting in enlargement of the RA, right ventricle and pulmonary artery.

monary and systemic circulations. Normally after birth, the RV wall is thinner than that of the LV and its compliance is greater, facilitating a left-to-right shunt. This results in right-sided volume overload and enlargement (Fig. 16.11B). If the right ventricular compliance decreases over time (because of the excessive load), the left-to-right shunt may become less. If pulmonary hypertension (i.e., Eisenmenger's syndrome) develops, the direction of the shunt of blood may actually *reverse* (i.e., right-to-left flow), such that desaturated blood enters the systemic circulation, resulting in systemic hypoxemia and cyanosis.

Symptoms

Most infants with ASD are asymptomatic. Frequently, their condition is detected by a murmur when they become school-age. However, if the defect is very small, the individual may remain asymptomatic for most of his or her life. The most common symptom in adults is the development of palpitations related to atrial ar-

rhythmias, as a result of right atrial enlargement.

Physical Examination

A prominent systolic impulse may be palpated along the lower left sternal border, resulting from the contraction of the dilated RV. The second heart sound demonstrates a widened, fixed splitting pattern (see Chapter 2). The increased blood volume pumped across the pulmonary valve creates a crescendo-decrescendo (ejection-type) systolic murmur. In addition, a mid-diastolic murmur may also be present at the lower left sternal border because of the increased flow across the tricuspid valve. Blood flow across the ASD itself does not produce a murmur because there is no significant pressure gradient between the two atria.

Laboratory Studies

On *chest radiographs,* the heart is usually enlarged due to right atrial and right ventricular enlargement, and there is prominence of the pulmonary artery with increased pulmonary vascular markings in the lung fields. The *EKG* shows RV hypertrophy and sometimes right atrial enlargement. Incomplete or complete right bundle branch block is common in all types of ASD, related to RV enlargement. In patients with the ostium primum type ASD, left axis deviation is also common. *Echocardiography* demonstrates right atrial and ventricular enlargement; the ASD may be visualized, or its presence implied by the demonstration of a transatrial shunt by Doppler flow interrogation. Transesophageal echocardiography may be performed for clarification if the diagnosis is uncertain.

Given the high sensitivity of the noninvasive techniques, it is rarely necessary to perform cardiac catheterization to confirm the presence of an ASD. However, catheterization may be useful in certain cases to quantify the volume of shunted blood, to accurately determine the degree of pulmonary hypertension or to assess for concurrent coronary disease in patients of advanced age. In a normal individual undergoing cardiac catheterization, the oxygen saturations measured in the right atrium and superior vena cava are approximately equal, but in the presence of an ASD, the oxygen saturation of the RA is greater, because of shunting of oxygenated left atrial blood into the right atrium.

Most patients with an ASD remain active and asymptomatic. If a significant shunt is detected, however, surgical closure is recommended to prevent the development of pulmonary hypertension in adulthood.

Ventricular Septal Defect

A ventricular septal defect (VSD) is an abnormal opening in the ventricular septum (Fig 16.12) that can occur as an isolated lesion, or in combination with other congenital heart abnormalities. VSDs are common defects, accounting for approximately 30% of congenital heart diseases, with an incidence of 0.1%–0.2% in the general population. They may occur anywhere along the

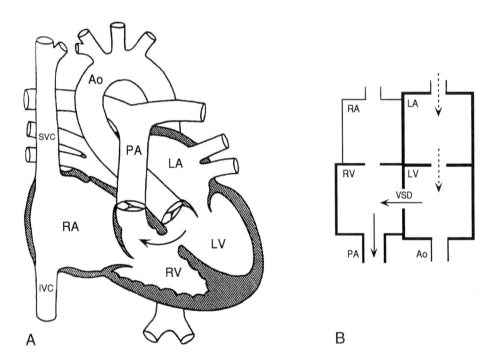

Figure 16.12. Ventricular septal defect (VSD). A. The arrow indicates shunted flow from the left ventricle (LV) toward the right ventricular (RV) outflow tract. **B.** Schematic representation of blood flow through an uncomplicated VSD. The dashed lines represent increased blood return to the left side of the heart as a result of the shunt, which causes enlargement primarily of the left atrium (LA) and ventricle (LV).

interventricular septum, but are most commonly located in the membranous portion of the septum.

Pathophysiology

The hemodynamic changes that accompany VSDs depend on the size of the defect and the relative resistances of the pulmonary and systemic vasculatures. For example, in small VSDs, the defect itself offers more resistance to flow than the pulmonary or systemic vasculature, so that the magnitude of the shunt depends largely on the size of the hole. Conversely, with larger "nonrestrictive" defects, the volume of the shunt is determined by the relative pulmonary and systemic vascular resistances. In the perinatal period, the high pulmonary vascular resistance is nearly equal to that of systemic vascular resistance. Therefore, minimal shunting occurs between the two ventricles. After birth however, the pulmonary vascular resistance gradually falls, which results in an increased left-to-right shunt through the defect. When the left-to-right shunt is large, pulmonary artery flow increases. As a result, left atrial blood return is also augmented (consisting of normal pulmonary venous return plus the left-to-right shunted flow), such that left atrial enlargement develops. Initially, the increased blood return to the left ventricle augments LV stroke volume (via the Frank-Starling mechanism), but over time, a large left-to-right shunt can result in systolic dysfunction and symptoms of heart failure. In addition, large left-to-right shunts can result in pulmonary hypertension and pulmonary vascular obstruction (Eisenmenger's syndrome) early in life. As pulmonary vascular resistance increases, the intracardiac shunt may reverse its direction (i.e., right-to-left shunt) with the development of systemic hypoxemia and cyanosis.

Symptoms

Symptoms associated with VSDs depend on the size of the defect and the degree of pulmonary hypertension. A small ventricular septal defect may remain asymptomatic. Conversely, infants with large VSDs may develop symptoms of congestive heart failure due to left-heart volume overload. Patients with VSDs complicated by pulmonary hypertension and reversed shunts may present with dyspnea and cyanosis. Bacterial endocarditis can develop regardless of the size of the VSD, related to the turbulent blood flow through the defect.

Physical Examination

The most common physical finding is a harsh holosystolic murmur heard loudest at the left sternal border. The smaller the defect, the more turbulent the blood flow through it, and the louder the murmur tends to be. A systolic thrill can commonly be palpated in the region of the murmur. If pulmonary hypertension develops, the holosystolic murmur diminishes (since there is less flow between the ventricles). In these patients, a loud pulmonic closure sound (P_2) and cyanosis may become evident.

Laboratory Studies

On *chest radiographs*, the heart silhouette may be normal in patients with small defects, but in those with large shunts, it is common to observe prominent pulmonary vascular markings, left atrial and left ventricular enlargement, and sometimes right ventricular enlargement (if pulmonary hypertension has developed). The *EKG* tracing may be normal if the defect is small. Left atrial enlargement and left ventricular hypertrophy are observed if there is volume-overload without pulmonary hypertension. With the development of pulmonary hypertension, right ventricular hypertrophy becomes evident. *Echocardiography* and Doppler studies can accurately determine the location of the VSD, and identify the direction and magnitude of the shunt. Cardiac catheterization of VSD patients with left-to-right shunts demonstrates an increase in oxygen saturation in the right ventricle compared with the right atrium, due to shunting of highly oxygenated blood from the left ventricle into the RV.

Treatment

At least 25% of small and moderate-sized ventricular septal defects undergo partial or complete spontaneous closure during childhood. Surgical correction of the defect is recommended in the first few months of life for children with congestive heart failure and failure to thrive. For children with pulmonary hypertension, surgical repair is recommended by 1 year of age in order to prevent irreversible pulmonary vascular changes. Moderate-sized ventricular septal defects without pulmonary hypertension, but with significant volume overload, are corrected later in childhood. Medical management includes endocarditis antibiotic prophylaxis for all patients with VSDs.

Patent Ductus Arteriosus

The ductus arteriosus is a vessel that connects the pulmonary artery to the descending aorta during fetal life. Patent ductus arteriosus (PDA) results when the ductus fails to close after birth, resulting in a persistent connection between the great vessels (Figure 16.13). This condition can occur as an isolated lesion or may accompany other, more complex abnormalities. It accounts for 6% of congenital heart diseases with a female to male ratio of 3:1. Premature infants, especially those weighing less than 1500 grams, have a higher risk of developing this condition.

Pathophysiology

Normally, the ductus arteriosus constricts after birth due to the sudden rise in blood oxygen tension and a reduction in circulating vasodilating prostaglandins. Over the next several weeks, intimal proliferation and fibrosis result in permanent closure of this embryonic vessel. Failure of the ductus to close after birth results in a persistent shunt between the ascending aorta and pulmonary artery, and the magnitude of flow through the shunt depends on the size of the ductus and the relative resistances of the systemic and pulmonary vasculatures. Prenatally, when the pulmonary vascular resistance is high, the blood is diverted away from the immature lung to the aorta. As the

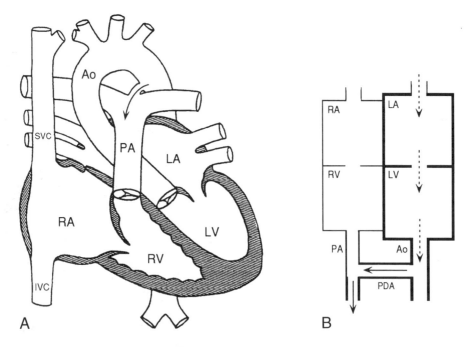

Figure 16.13. Patent ductus arteriosus (PDA). A. The arrow indicates shunted flow from the descending aorta (Ao) toward the pulmonary artery (PA). **B.** Schematic representation of blood flow through an uncomplicated PDA. The dashed lines represent increased blood return to the left side of the heart as a result of the shunt, which causes enlargement of the left atrium (LA), left ventricle (LV), and aorta.

pulmonary resistance drops postnatally, the shunt reverses and blood flows from the aorta into the pulmonary artery instead. Because of this left-to-right shunt, the left atrium and ventricle become volume overloaded (they receive the shunted flow *plus* normal pulmonary venous return) and left ventricular failure may ensue. Also, the increased pulmonary blood flow can ultimately result in pulmonary hypertension and Eisenmenger's syndrome, with reversal of the shunt, such that blood flows from the pulmonary artery, through the ductus, into the descending aorta. In this case, the flow of desaturated blood to the lower extremities causes cyanosis of the feet; the upper extermities are not cyanotic, as they continue to receive normally saturated blood from the proximal aorta.

Symptoms

Children with a small patent ductus are generally asymptomatic. Those with a large left-to-right shunt gradually develop symptoms of congestive heart failure such as tachypnea, tachycardia, poor feeding, and slow growth.

Physical Examination

The most common finding in patients with left-to-right shunting through a PDA is a *continuous* murmur, heard best at the upper left sternal border (see Fig. 2.10). The murmur is heard throughout the cardiac cycle since there is a gradient between the aorta and lower pressure pulmonary artery in both systole and diastole. However, if pulmonary hypertension develops, the gradient between the aorta and the pulmonary artery decreases, leading to diminished flow through the ductus, and the murmur becomes shorter (the diastolic component may disappear) and softer.

Laboratory Studies

If the patent ductus arteriosus is small, the *chest radiograph* may be normal. With a large patent ductus, however, there is an enlarged cardiac silhouette (left atrial and left ventricular enlargement) with prominent pulmonary vascular markings. In adults, calcification of the patent ductus may be vi-

sualized. The *EKG* shows left atrial enlargement and left ventricular hypertrophy when a large shunt is present. The *echocardiogram* may visualize the PDA; flow through the ductus is usually readily apparent by Doppler flow imaging. Cardiac catheterization is usually not necessary to diagnose a patent ductus arteriosus. When performed in patients with a left-to-right shunt, it demonstrates a step-up in oxygen saturation in the pulmonary artery compared with the right ventricle, and angiography shows the flow of contrast from the aorta through the patent ductus arteriosus into the pulmonary artery.

Treatment

In the absence of other congenital cardiac abnormalities or severe pulmonary vascular disease, patent ductus arteriosus should be treated by surgical division or ligation of the abnormal connection. Experimental transcatheter techniques to close small and moderate-sized defects have shown great promise.

Congenital Aortic Stenosis

Congenital aortic stenosis (AS) is a narrowing of the aortic orifice due to abnormal development of the valve (Fig. 16.14). The abnormal valve usually has a unicuspid or bicuspid leaflet structure instead of the normal tricuspid configuration. Aortic stenosis accounts for 6% of congenital cardiac abnormalities, and is four times as common in males than females.

Pathophysiology

Because the valvular orifice is narrowed, left ventricular systolic pressure must increase in order to pump blood across the valve into the aorta. As a result, the left ventricle hypertrophies. The stenotic valve also creates a high-pressure jet of blood that continuously impacts on the proximal aortic wall and causes that vessel to dilate.

Symptoms

The clinical picture of aortic stenosis depends on the severity of the lesion. Most children with congenital aortic stenosis are asymptomatic and develop normally. When symptoms do occur, they usually include easy fatigueability, exertional dyspnea, angina pectoris, and syncope similar to adult aortic stenosis (see Chapter 8). However, the infant with a severely stenosed aortic valve may develop congestive heart failure with signs of tachycardia and tachypnea.

Physical Examination

Auscultation of the heart in congenital aortic stenosis reveals a systolic ejection murmur, loudest at the base of the heart and that radiates toward the neck. It is often preceded by a systolic ejection click, especially when mild stenosis is present (see Chapter 2). In more advanced disease, a palpable thrill may accompany the murmur, and the ejection time of the murmur becomes longer. In severe disease, the markedly prolonged ejection time causes a delay in closure of the aortic valve; in fact, the aortic valve may close *after* the pulmonary valve, the opposite of the normal

situation—a phenomenon known as reversed splitting of S_2 (see Chapter 2).

Laboratory Studies

The *chest radiograph* of an infant with AS may show an enlarged left ventricle and a dilated ascending aorta. Often, the *EKG* shows left ventricular hypertrophy. *Echocardiography* can identify the structure of the aortic valve and the degree of left ventricular hypertrophy; Doppler assessment accurately estimates the pressure gradient between the left ventricle and the aorta, and can estimate the reduced valve area. *Catheterization* findings include an elevated left ventricular systolic pressure and a diminished aortic systolic pressure, with a pressure gradient identified across the aortic valve.

Treatment

In its more mild forms, aortic stenosis does not need to be corrected, but endocarditis prophylaxis should be followed (see Chapter 8). Severe congenital obstruction of the valve may require that the child

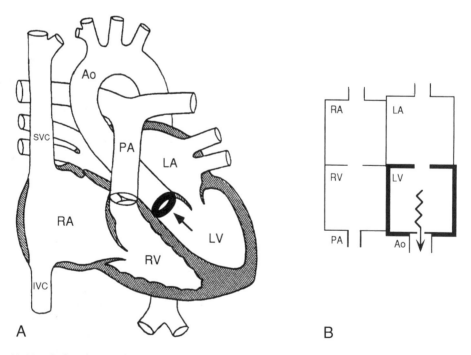

A   B

Figure 16.14. A. Congenital valvular aortic stenosis (arrow). **B.** Schematic representation of obstructed flow through the narrowed aortic valve (jagged arrow). Left ventricular (LV) hypertrophy results from the chronic increased pressure load. Poststenotic dilatation of the aorta (Ao) is common.

undergo balloon (via a catheter) or surgical valvuloplasty. If these procedures fail, the deformed aortic valve is surgically replaced.

Pulmonic Stenosis

Isolated pulmonic stenosis (Fig. 16.15) is the second most common type of congenital heart defect. It may occur at the level of the valve (e.g., from congenitally fused valve commisures), within the body of the right ventricle (due to obstructive cardiac muscle in the outflow tract), or in the pulmonary artery as a result of pulmonary artery hypoplasia. Valve stenosis is the most common form, making up greater than 90 percent of cases.

Pathophysiology

The result of pulmonic stenosis is obstruction to right ventricular systolic ejection, which leads to increased right ventricular pressure and chamber hypertrophy. In valvular pulmonic stenosis, blood is ejected with great force across the narrowed valve; as this force dissipates against the walls of the pulmonary artery, that vessel dilates. The clinical course is determined by the severity of the obstruction. In the setting of a normal cardiac output, a peak systolic transvalvular pressure gradient < 50 mmHg is considered *mild* pulmonic stenosis, between 50–80 mmHg is *moderate* stenosis, and *severe* stenosis is defined by a peak gradient > 80 mmHg.

Symptoms

Children with mild or moderate degrees of pulmonary stenosis are usually asymptomatic. These children are often first diagnosed when a systolic ejection murmur is heard on routine auscultation. Severe stenosis may produce dyspnea with exertion, exercise intolerance, and congestive heart failure.

Physical Examination

The physical findings in pulmonary stenosis depend on the severity of the obstruction. If the stenosis is severe, a loud murmur is heard at the upper left sternal border. The

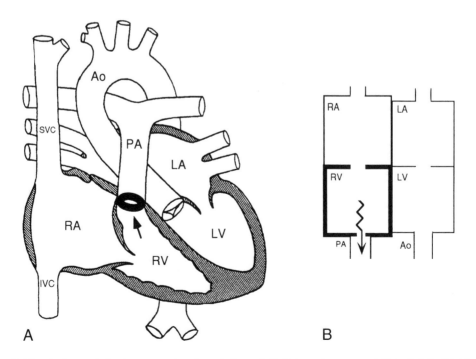

A   B

Figure 16.15. **A.** Congenital pulmonary valve stenosis (arrow). **B.** Schematic representation of obstructed flow through the narrowed pulmonary valve (jagged arrow). Right ventricular (RV) hypertrophy results from the chronically increased pressure load.

murmur is crescendo-decrescendo, begins with the first heart sound, and can obscure the aortic component of the second heart sound. A palpable thrill is often felt over the murmur. An increase in the splitting of the second heart sound is created by the delayed closure of the pulmonary valve.

In more moderate stenosis, an ejection click (a high-pitched sound associated with valve opening) follows the first heart sound, and precedes the crescendo-decrescendo systolic murmur. This murmur may end before a softer-than-normal pulmonary component of the second heart sound.

Laboratory Studies

In valvular pulmonary stenosis, the *chest radiograph* may demonstrate an enlarged right ventricle and poststenotic pulmonary artery dilation. The *EKG* shows right ventricular hypertrophy, in proportion to the degree of stenosis, usually accompanied by right axis deviation. Right atrial enlargement is usually evident in severe stenosis. *Echocardiography* with Doppler imaging is used to determine the pulmonary valve morphology, and to localize and measure the pressure gradient across the stenosis.

Treatment

Mild pulmonic stenosis usually does not progress, and does not require treatment. Moderate or severe valvular obstruction is treated in most cases by widening of the stenotic valve via transcatheter balloon valvuloplasty. Subvalvular or supravalvular obstruction requires open heart surgical correction. The associated right ventricular hypertrophy usually regresses following these interventions.

Coarctation of the Aorta

Coarctation is a pathologic narrowing of the aortic lumen that can occur anywhere along its length. It is most commonly observed distal to the origin of the left subclavian artery, in the region near the ductus arteriosus. This anomaly occurs approximately once in every 6000 live births, and is at least twice as common in males than females. Classically, two types of coarctation are distinguished according to the location of the aortic constriction in relation to the ductus arteriosus: preductal and postductal (Fig. 16.16). *Preductal* coarctation, in which narrowing occurs proximal to the ductus, occurs when an intracardiac anomaly during fetal life decreases blood flow through the left side of the heart and aortic isthmus, resulting in hypoplastic development of the aorta. The *postductal* type of coarctation develops postnatally, almost exclusively as an isolated lesion. It is most likely the result of muscular ductal tissue extending into the aorta during fetal life; when ductal tissue constricts following birth, the ectopic tissue within the aorta also constricts, creating a "napkin ringlike" obstruction. In distinction to the "preductal" type, no associated hypoplasia of the aorta occurs. In both types of coarctation, blood flow to the head and upper extremities is preserved, while flow to the descending aorta and lower extremities may be diminished. However, the clinical features of the two types of coarctation are quite distinct.

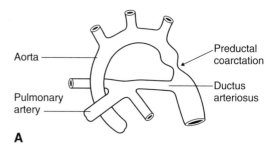

A

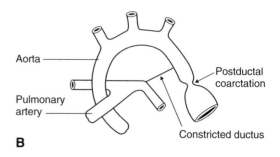

B

Figure 16.16.   Coarctation of the aorta. A. Preductal coarctation. **B.** Postductal coarctation.

Preductal Coarctation of the Aorta

In utero, the hypoplastic aorta is of no consequence, since the open ductus arteriosus allows blood to bypass the obstruction. It is only after birth when the ductus closes that the coarctation becomes clinically important. The aortic narrowing results in an increase in the left ventricular afterload and reduced blood flow to the descending aorta and lower body.

Patients with preductal coarctation usually present very shortly after birth with congestive heart failure (dyspnea, tachypnea, and tachycardia) and signs of low cardiac output (such as cool, mottled extremities). These infants may also exhibit **differential cyanosis** if the ductus arteriosus remains open: The upper half of the body, supplied by the left ventricle and the ascending aorta, is perfused with oxygenated blood; however, the lower half of the body appears cyanotic, as it is largely supplied by right-to-left flow (desaturated blood) from the pulmonary artery, across the still patent ductus arteriosus into the descending aorta. Hypertension is usually detected in the upper extremities supplied by arteries that branch from the aorta proximal to the obstruction, whereas the pressure is reduced in the lower extremities distal to the obstruction.

The *chest radiograph* shows cardiomegaly and pulmonary congestion. *Echocardiography* can demonstrate the severity of coarctation and other accompanying congenital heart defects.

The management of preductal coarctation begins with administration of prostaglandin E_1 to maintain ductal patency so as to increase flow to the lower half of the body, followed by surgical repair.

Postductal Coarctation of the Aorta

Severe postductal coarctation causes an increase in left ventricular afterload that may lead to congestive heart failure. If the coarctation is less severe, compensatory alterations may gradually develop and buffer the effects of the aortic narrowing. These include: 1) the development of left ventricular hypertrophy in the face of increased afterload, and 2), the formation of compensatory collateral blood vessels from the intercostal and internal mammary arteries that help perfuse the lower body. If the coarctation is not repaired in childhood, these collateral vessels can become very large and erode the undersurface of the ribs.

The clinical course of patients with postductal coarctation usually takes one of two routes. In the majority of newborns, the obstruction is not severe, and these patients grow and mature normally. However, some newborns with severe postductal coarctation develop congestive heart failure from pressure overload of the left ventricle. Within the first several weeks of life these infants present with tachypnea, dyspnea, tachycardia, and hepatomegaly.

On physical examination, this anomaly often presents as hypertension in the upper body (i.e., as measured in the right arm), but a significantly lower pressure when measured distal to the site of coarctation. That is, if the coarctation occurs distal to the takeoff of the left subclavian artery, the systolic pressure in the arms is greater than that in the legs. If the coarctation occurs *proximal* to the takeoff of the left subclavian artery, the systolic pressure in the right arm may exceed that in the left arm . A systolic pressure difference of 15–20 mmHg between the right arm and leg is sufficient to suspect coarctation. However, it is not unusual to see a pressure difference that exceeds 40 mmHg. A midsystolic ejection murmur (due to turbulence of flow through the narrowed coarctation) may be audible over the chest and/or back. A prominent dilated and tortuous collateral arterial circulation may create continuous murmurs over the chest.

Compensatory vessels that have eroded the undersurface of the ribs can be seen by *chest radiography* in the form of rib notching, although this is rarely seen before 5 years of age. Chest radiographs may also show an indented aorta at the site of coarctation. In patients with uncomplicated coarctation, the *EKG* shows left ventricular hypertrophy due to the pressure load placed on the left ventricle. *Echocardiography* can confirm the diagnosis of postductal coarctation and assess the pressure gradient across the lesion. Magnetic resonance imaging can demonstrate detailed images of the length and severity of coarctation; diagnostic catheterization and angiography are rarely necessary.

In severe postductal coarctation, transcatheter balloon dilation or surgery is performed to widen the stenotic segment. Even milder coarctation can lead to hypertensive heart disease, aortic dissection, and endocarditis, so that elective repair is usually recommended in childhood.

Cyanotic Lesions

Tetralogy of Fallot

The tetralogy of Fallot is characterized by a group of consistent cardiac malformations that result from a single defect: an abnormal anterosuperior and rightward displacement of the infundibular septum, resulting

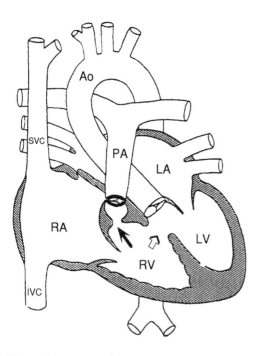

Figure 16.17. Tetralogy of Fallot is characterized by four associated anomalies: 1) a ventricular septal defect (hollow arrow), 2) obstruction to right ventricular outflow (solid arrow), 3) an overriding aorta that receives blood from both ventricles, and 4) right ventricular hypertrophy.

in an unequal division of the bulbus cordis into pulmonary and aortic outflow tracts. This unequal division directly results in the four anomalies associated with this condition (Fig. 16.17): 1) a ventricular septal defect due to septal malalignment, 2) subvalvular pulmonic stenosis because of obstruction from the infundibular septum, 3) an overriding (dextroposed) aorta that receives blood from both ventricles, and 4) right ventricular hypertrophy due to the high pressure load of the pulmonic stenosis. Tetralogy of Fallot is the most common form of cyanotic congenital heart disease seen after infancy.

Pathophysiology

Increased resistance by the pulmonary stenosis causes deoxygenated systemic venous return to be diverted from the right ventricle, through the VSD, to the overriding aorta and systemic circulation, resulting in systemic hypoxemia and cyanosis. The degree of shunting across the VSD is a function of the severity of the pulmonary stenosis, as well as the relative systemic and pulmonary vascular resistances.

Symptoms

Children with tetralogy of Fallot often experience dyspnea on exertion or when crying. In addition, "spells" may occur following exertion or feeding, characterized by irritability, cyanosis, hyperventilation, and sometimes syncope or convulsions due to cerebral hypoxemia. Children learn to alleviate their symptoms early in life through "squatting," which increases systemic resistance, thereby decreasing the right-to-left shunt and directing more blood to the lungs.

Physical Examination

Children with moderate pulmonary stenosis are often mildly cyanotic. Those with severe pulmonary stenosis may present with profound cyanosis in the first few days of life. Chronic hypoxemia caused by the right-to-left shunt commonly results in clubbing of the fingers and toes. The right ventricular hypertrophy characteristic of tetralogy of Fallot may be appreciated on physical examination as a palpable heave along the left sternal border. A systolic ejection murmur heard best at the left upper sternal border is created by turbulent blood flow through the stenotic right ventricular outflow tract and may sometimes be accompanied by a palpable thrill. The second heart sound is single and loud, composed of a normal aortic component; the pulmonary component is soft and usually inaudible.

Laboratory Studies

Chest radiography demonstrates prominence of the right ventricle and a decrease in the size of the main pulmonary artery segment giving the appearance of a "boot-shaped" heart. Pulmonary vascular markings are typically diminished. The *EKG* shows right ventricular hypertrophy and right axis deviation. *Echocardiography* displays and quantifies the extent of RV outflow tract obstruction and the malaligned ventricular septal defect can be visualized. *Cardiac catheterization* with right ventricular angiography demonstrates the morphology of the RV outflow tract and the size of the main branches of the pulmonary artery.

Treatment

The definitive treatment of tetralogy of Fallot is surgical correction, which consists of closure of the ventricular septal defect and enlargement of the subpulmonary infundibulum with the use of a pericardial patch. In the majority of cases, patients who have undergone successful surgical repair go on to become asymptomatic adults.

Transposition of the Great Arteries

Transposition of the great arteries (TGA) is present when the great vessels inappropriately arise from the opposite ventricle; that is, the aorta originates from the right ventricle and the pulmonary artery originates from the left ventricle (Fig. 16.18). This anomaly accounts for 7% of congenital heart defects and may occur in isolation, or may be accompanied by other congenital malformations, such as VSD or PDA.

The precise cause of transposition

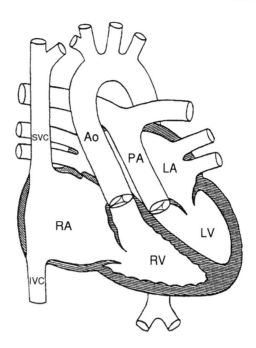

Figure 16.18.   Transposition of the great arteries. The aorta (Ao) and pulmonary artery (PA) arise abnormally from the right (RV) and left (LV) ventricles, respectively.

remains unknown. Historically, it was thought that it was the result of failure of the aorticopulmonary septum to spiral in a normal fashion during fetal development. Recently, it has been suggested that the defect may be the result of abnormal growth and absorption of the subpulmonary and subaortic infundibuli during the division of the truncus arteriosus. Normally, reabsorption of the subaortic infundibulum places the forming aortic valve posterior and inferior to the pulmonary valve and in continuity with the left ventricle. In TGA, the process of infundibular reabsorption possibly is reversed, placing the pulmonary valve over the left ventricle instead.

Pathophysiology

Transposition of the great arteries separates the pulmonary and systemic circulations by placing the two circulations in parallel rather than in series. This arrangement forces desaturated blood from the systemic venous system to pass through the right ventricle and then return to the systemic circulation through the aorta without undergoing oxygenation in the lungs. Similarly, oxygenated pulmonary venous return passes through the left ventricle and back through the pulmonary artery to the lungs without imparting oxygen to the systemic circulation. The end result is an extremely hypoxic, cyanotic neonate. Without intervention to create mixing between the two circulations, transposition of the great arteries is a lethal condition.

TGA is compatible with life *in utero* because flow through the ductus arteriosus and foramen ovale allow oxygen delivery to the peripheral tissues. Oxygenated fetal blood flows from the placenta through the umbilical vein to the right atrium, where the majority travels into the left atrium through the foramen ovale. The oxygenated blood in the left atrium then passes into the left ventricle and is pumped out the pulmonary artery. The majority of pulmonary artery flow traverses the ductus arteriosus into the aorta instead of the high resistance pulmonary vessels, whereupon oxygen is provided to the developing tissues.

After birth, normal physiologic closure of the ductus and the foramen ovale eliminates the shunt between the parallel circulations, and would result in acidosis and death, as oxygenated blood could not reach the systemic tissues. However, if the ductus arteriosus and foramen ovale remain patent, either normally or with exogenous prostaglandins and surgical procedures, communication between the parallel circuits is maintained and sufficiently oxygenated blood may be provided to the brain and other organs.

Symptoms and Physical Examination

Infants with transposition appear blue, with the intensity of the cyanosis dependent on the degree of intermixing between the parallel circuits. Generalized cyanosis is usually apparent on the first day of life, progressing rapidly as the ductus closes. Auscultation may reveal an intensified second heart sound, which reflects closure of the anteriorly placed aortic valve just under the chest wall. Prominent murmurs are uncommon and may signal an associated defect.

Laboratory Studies

Chest radiography is usually normal, although the base of the heart may be narrow due to the more anterior-posterior orientation of the aorta and pulmonary artery. The *EKG* demonstrates right ventricular hypertrophy, reflecting the fact that the RV is the systemic pumping chamber. The definitive diagnosis of transposition can be made by *echocardiography,* which demonstrates the abnormal orientation of the great vessels.

Treatment

Transposition of the great arteries is a medical emergency. Initial treatment includes maintenance of the ductus arteriosus by prostaglandin administration and creation of an interatrial communication (using a balloon catheter). These procedures allow mixing of the two circulations until definitive corrective surgery can be performed.

SUMMARY

1. The significance of congenital heart lesions can be predicted from an understanding of cardiovascular embryonic development and the necessary transition to the postnatal circulatory pathways.
2. Cardiac malformations occur in 0.8% of infants. Such lesions can be grouped into cyanotic or acyanotic defects, depending on whether the abnormality results in right-to-left heart shunting of blood.
3. Acyanotic defects often result in volume (atrial septal defect, ventricular septal defect, patent ductus arteriosus) or pressure (aortic stenosis, pulmonic stenosis, coarctation of the aorta) overload. Chronic volume overload due to a large left-to-right shunt can ultimately result in pulmonary hypertension and reversal of the shunt (Eisenmenger's syndrome).
4. Among the most common cyanotic defects are tetralogy of Fallot and transposition of the great arteries.

ADDITIONAL READING

Armstrong BE. Congenital cardiovascular disease and cardiac surgery in childhood. Curr Opin Cardiol 1995;10:58–67,68–77.

Emmanouilides GC, Riemanschneider TA, Allen HD, et al., eds. Moss and Adams' Heart Disease in Infants, Children and Adolescents. 5th ed. Baltimore: Williams & Wilkins, 1995.

Fyler DC, ed. Nadas' Pediatric Cardiology. Philadelphia: Hanley & Belfus, 1992.

Mahoney LT. Acyanotic congenital heart disease. Cardiol Clin 1993;11:603–616.

Moore KL, Persaud TVN. The Developing Human. 5th ed. Philadelphia: WB Saunders, 1993.

Mullins CE, Mayer DC. Congenital Heart Disease—A Diagrammatic Atlas. New York: Alan R. Liss, Inc., 1988.

Park MK. Pediatric Cardiology for Practitioners. 3rd ed. St. Louis: CV Mosby, 1996.

Perloff JK. The Clinical Recognition of Congenital Heart Disease. 4th ed. Philadelphia: WB Saunders, 1994.

Rosenkranz ER. Surgery for congenital heart disease. Curr Opin Cardiol 1994;9:200–215.

Van Praagh R, Et Al. Tetrology of Fallot: underdevelopment of the pulmonary infundibulum and its sequelae. Am J Cardiol 1970;26:25–33.

Acknowledgments The previous edition of this chapter was written by Lakshmi Halasyamani, MD, Andrew Karson, MD, and Michael Freed, MD.

Cardiovascular Drugs

Steven N. Kalkanis,
David Sloane, Gary R. Strichartz,
and Leonard S. Lilly

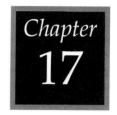

Chapter
17

This chapter reviews the physiologic basis and clinical use of cardiovascular drugs. Although a multitude of drugs is available to benefit cardiac disorders, these agents can fortunately be grouped by their pharmacologic actions into a small number of categories. Additionally, many drugs are useful in more than one form of heart disease.

INOTROPIC DRUGS

Inotropic drugs are used to increase the force of ventricular contraction when myocardial systolic function is impaired. The pharmacologic agents in this category include the cardiac glycosides, sympathomimetic amines, and phosphodiesterase inhibitors. Although they work through different mechanisms, they are all thought to improve cardiac contraction by increasing the intracellular calcium concentration, thus augmenting actin and myosin interactions. The hemodynamic effect is to shift a depressed ventricular performance curve (Frank-Starling curve) in an upward direc-

tion (Fig. 17.1), so that for a given ventricular filling pressure, stroke volume and cardiac output are increased.

Digitalis and Other Cardiac Glycosides

The cardiac glycosides are often called "digitalis" because commonly used drugs of this class are based on extracts of the foxglove plant, *Digitalis purpurea*. In this discussion, the term digitalis is used to describe the entire group of cardiac glycosides, including digoxin, digitoxin, and ouabain. These compounds are composed of an aglycone ring (steroid nucleus and lactone ring) that confers the pharmacologic activity, and a varying number of sugar residues that contribute to the drug's pharmacokinetics.

Mechanism of Action

There are two desired effects of digitalis: 1) to improve contractility of the failing

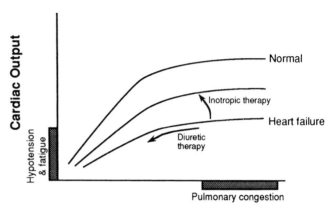

Figure 17.1. Ventricular performance (Frank-Starling) curve. In heart failure, the curve is displaced downward, so that at a given left ventricular end-diastolic pressure (LVEDP), the cardiac output is lower than in a normal individual. Diuretics reduce LVEDP, but do not change the position of the curve; thus pulmonary congestion improves, but cardiac output may fall. Inotropic drugs displace the curve upward, toward normal, so that at any LVEDP, the cardiac output is higher.

heart (mechanical effect), and 2) to prolong the refractory period of the AV node in patients with supraventricular arrhythmias (electrical effect).

Mechanical Effect

The action by which digitalis improves contractility appears to be inhibition of the sarcolemmal Na$^+$/K$^+$-ATPase pump, normally responsible for maintaining transmembrane Na$^+$ and K$^+$ gradients. By binding to and inhibiting this pump, digitalis causes the intracellular [Na$^+$] to rise. As shown in Figure 17.2, an increase in intracellular sodium content reduces Ca^{++} extrusion from the cell by the Na$^+$/Ca^{++} exchanger. Consequently, more Ca^{++} is pumped into the sarcoplasmic reticulum. As a result, when subsequent action potentials excite the cell, a greater than normal amount of Ca^{++} is released to the myofilaments, thereby enhancing the force of contraction. The magnitude of the positive inotropic effect correlates with the degree of Na$^+$/K$^+$-ATPase inhibition.

Electrical Effect

Digitalis affects the electrical properties of cardiac tissue directly. More important, it modifies autonomic nervous system activity by enhancing vagal tone and reducing sympathetic activity.

In the normal heart, the most important therapeutic electrical effect of digitalis occurs at the AV node (Table 17.1), where it

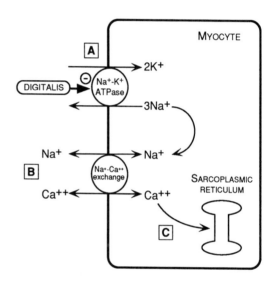

Figure 17.2. Mechanism of action of digitalis (inotropic effect). A. Digitalis inhibits the sarcolemmal Na$^+$-K$^+$ ATPase, causing intracellular [Na$^+$] to rise. *B.* Increased cytosolic [Na$^+$] reduces the transmembrane Na$^+$ gradient; thus, the Na$^+$/Ca^{++} exchanger drives less Ca^{++} out of the cell. **C.** The increased [Ca^{++}] is stored in the sarcoplasmic reticulum, such that with subsequent action potentials, greater than normal Ca^{++} is released to the contractile elements in the cytoplasm, intensifying the force of contraction.

slows conduction velocity and increases refractoriness, mostly via augmenting vagal activity. As a result, digitalis decreases the frequency of transmission of atrial impulses through the AV node to the ventricles. This is beneficial in reducing the rate of ventricular stimulation in patients with rapid supraventricular tachycardias such as atrial fibrillation or atrial flutter. In addition, by

TABLE 17.1. Electrophysiologic Effects of Digitalis

Region	Mechanism of Action	Effect
Therapeutic Effects		
AV node	Vagal effect: ↓ conduction velocity ↑ effective refractory period	1. ↓ rate of transmission of atrial impulses to the ventricles in supraventricular tachyarrhythmias 2. ↓ conduction velocity and ↑ refractory period may interrupt reentrant circuits passing through the AV node
Toxic Effects		
Sinoatrial node	↑ vagal and direct suppression	1. Sinus bradycardia 2. Sinoatrial block (impulse not transmitted from SA node to atrium)
Atrium	Delayed afterdepolarizations (triggered activity), ↑ slope of phase 4 depolarization (↑ automaticity)	1. Atrial premature beats 2. Nonreentrant SVT (ectopic rhythm)
	Variable effects on conduction velocity and ↑ refractory period (can fragment conduction and lead to reentry)	3. Reentrant PSVT
AV node	Direct and vagal-medicated conduction block	1. AV block (first, second or third degree)
AV junction (between AV node and His bundle)	Delayed afterdepolarizations (triggered activity), ↑ slope of phase 4 depolarization (↑ automaticity)	1. Accelerated junctional rhythm
Purkinje fibers and ventricular muscle	Delayed afterdepolarizations (triggered activity), ↓ conduction velocity and ↑ refractory period (can lead to reentry)	1. Ventricular premature beats
	↑ slope of phase 4 depolarization (↑ automaticity)	2. Ventricular tachycardia

PSVT = paroxysmal supraventricular tachycardia; AV = atrioventricular

enhancing the refractoriness of the AV node, digitalis may convert reentrant arrhythmias (e.g., PSVT) to a normal rhythm.

However, if digitalis concentrations rise into the toxic range, further enhancement of vagal tone and more extreme inhibition of the Na^+/K^+-ATPase pump can result in adverse electrophysiologic effects. For example, in atrial and ventricular Purkinje fibers, a high digitalis concentration has three important actions that may lead to dangerous arrhythmias (Fig. 17.3):

1. *Less negative resting potential.* Inhibition of the Na^+/K^+-ATPase causes the resting potential to become less negative. Recall from Chapter 1 that the Na^+/K^+-ATPase normally removes 3 Na^+ ions from the cell in exchange for 2 inwardly moving K^+ ions; inhibition of the pump results in a decrease of this pump-mediated outward current and a resulting depolarization of the cell. As a result, there is a voltage-dependent partial inactivation of the fast Na^+ channels, and subsequently a slower rise of phase 0 depolarization and reduction in conduction velocity (see Fig. 1.16). The slowed conduction, if present heterogeneously among neighboring cells, enhances the possibility of reentrant arrhythmias.

2. *Decreased action potential duration.* At high digitalis concentrations, the cardiac action potential shortens. This relates in part to the digitalis-induced elevated intracellular $[Ca^{++}]$, which increases the activity of a Ca^{++}-dependent K^+ channel. The opening of this channel promotes K^+ efflux and more rapid *repolarization*. In addition, high intracellular $[Ca^{++}]$ inactivates the Ca^{++} channels, decreasing the inward *depolarizing* Ca^{++} current. The decrease in action potential duration and the associated shortened

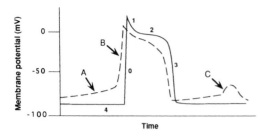

Figure 17.3. Direct effects of digitalis on the Purkinje cell action potential. The solid tracing represents depolarization and repolarization of a normal cell; the dashed tracing demonstrates the effects of digitalis: The maximum diastolic potential is less negative, and there is an increase in the slope of phase 4 depolarization (**A**), endowing the cell with intrinsic automaticity, and the potential for ectopic rhythms. Because depolarization of the cell occurs at a more positive voltage, the rate of rise of phase 0 is decreased (**B**), and conduction velocity is slowed, which, if present heterogeneously among neighboring cells, can produce conditions for reentry. Delayed afterdepolarizations may develop at high concentrations of digitalis (**C**) in association with an increased intracellular calcium concentration, and can result in triggered tachyarrhythmias.

refractory period increase the time during which cardiac fibers are responsive to external stimulation, allowing greater opportunity for propagation of arrhythmic impulses.

3. *Enhanced automaticity.* Digitalis enhances cellular automaticity and may generate ectopic rhythms by two mechanisms:

a. The less negative membrane resting potential may induce phase 4 gradual depolarization, even in nonpacemaker cells (see Chapter 11), and an action potential is triggered each time the threshold voltage is reached.

b. The digitalis-induced increase in intracellular $[Ca^{++}]$ may trigger delayed afterdepolarizations (Fig. 17.3). If an afterdepolarization reaches the threshold voltage, an action potential (ectopic beat) is generated. Ectopic beats may lead to additional afterdepolarizations and self-sustaining arrhythmias such as ventricular tachycardia.

Thus, digitalis in toxic concentrations may lead to several types of ectopic or reentrant rhythms (Table 17.1). In addition, the augmented direct and indirect vagal effects of toxic doses of digitalis slow conduction through the AV node, such that high degrees of AV block, including complete heart block, can occur.

Clinical Uses

The most common use of digitalis is as an inotropic agent to treat heart failure due to decreased ventricular contractility (see Chapter 9). Digitalis increases the force of contraction, augments cardiac output, and thereby improves left ventricular emptying, reduces LV size, and decreases the elevated diastolic ventricular filling pressures typical of patients with systolic dysfunction. Digitalis is *not* of benefit in forms of heart failure associated with normal ventricular contractility (e.g., high-output failure associated with thyrotoxicosis, pulmonary congestion due to mitral stenosis, or in the setting of pure *diastolic* dysfunction).

Once the mainstay of therapy in congestive heart failure (CHF), the use of digitalis has waned in the face of newer therapies, especially angiotensin-converting enzyme inhibitors (see Chapter 9 and below). Nonetheless, digitalis continues to be useful in treating patients with CHF complicated by atrial fibrillation (it has the added benefit of slowing the ventricular heart rate), or when symptoms do not respond adequately to ACE inhibitors and diuretics. Unlike ACE inhibitors, digitalis does not prolong life-expectancy in patients with chronic heart failure.

The second common use of digitalis is as an antiarrhythmic agent in the treatment of atrial fibrillation, atrial flutter, and paroxysmal supraventricular tachycardia (PSVT). In atrial fibrillation and flutter, digitalis reduces the number of impulses transmitted across the AV node, thereby slowing the ventricular rate. Digitalis may also be effective at terminating PSVT, likely because of enhanced vagal tone, which slows impulse conduction, prolongs the effective refractory period, and can therefore interrupt reentrant circuits that pass through the AV node.

The use of digitalis as an antiarrhythmic has also become less frequent in recent years, because other agents such as β-blockers, calcium channel blockers, and adenosine are more effective and work more rapidly. Nonetheless, in the treatment of supraventricular arrhythmias in the presence of congestive heart failure, digitalis remains an important option.

Pharmacokinetics

Digitalis has an oral availability ranging from 75% to 100%, and has a large volume of distribution. The major forms of digitalis, digoxin and digitoxin, differ in their excretion pathways: Digoxin is excreted unchanged by the kidney, whereas digitoxin is metabolized by the liver, is excreted into the bile, and undergoes enterohepatic cycling. The reabsorbed metabolites are cardioactive and contribute to the extended half-life of digitoxin (168 hours, as compared with 40 hours for digoxin). One might therefore consider using digitoxin in a patient with diminished renal function because it has little dependence on the kidneys for its excretion. Of the two drugs, digoxin is used much more commonly.

A series of loading doses of digitalis is administered to raise the drug's concentration into the therapeutic range. The maintenance dosage depends on the ability of the patient to excrete the drug (i.e., the patient's age, or renal function, in the case of digoxin). If a loading dose is not given, the steady-state concentrations of digoxin or digitoxin are established in four to five half-lives, or 7 days and 3 weeks, respectively. The maintenance dose of digitalis must be constantly reassessed in light of a patient's cardiac condition (and renal status, in the case of digoxin) in order to avoid toxicity.

Toxicity

The potential for digitalis toxicity is significant because of a low toxic-to-therapeutic drug concentration ratio. Although many side effects are minor, life-threatening arrhythmias may also result.

Extracardiac signs of acute digitalis toxicity are often gastrointestinal (nausea, vomiting, anorexia), thought to be mediated by the action of digoxin on the area postrema of the medulla. Cardiac toxicity includes a host of arrhythmias (Table 17.1) that may precede extracardiac warning symptoms. The most frequently encountered rhythm disturbance is the development of ventricular extrasystoles. In addition, various degrees of AV block may occur because of the direct and vagal effects on AV nodal conduction. Digitalis toxicity is the most common cause of nonreentrant supraventricular tachycardia (due to enhanced automaticity or delayed afterdepolarizations).

Many factors may contribute to digitalis intoxication, the most common of which is hypokalemia, often caused by the concurrent administration of diuretics. Hypokalemia exacerbates digitalis toxicity as it further inhibits the Na^+/K^+-ATPase pump. Other conditions that promote digitalis toxicity include hypomagnesemia and hypercalcemia. In addition, the concurrent administration of quinidine may raise the serum digoxin concentration by decreasing its excretion and reducing its volume of distribution. Thus, it is prudent to lower the digoxin dosage by one-half when quinidine is added to a patient's regimen to avoid this complication.

The treatment of digitalis-induced tachyarrhythmias includes administration of potassium (if hypokalemia is present) and often intravenous lidocaine (see below). High-grade AV block may require temporary pacemaker therapy. In patients with severe intoxication, administration of Fab fragments of antidigitalis antibodies may be life-saving.

Sympathomimetic Amines

Sympathomimetic amines are inotropic drugs that bind to cardiac $β_1$-receptors. Stimulation of these receptors increases the activity of adenylate cyclase, causing increased cAMP formation (Fig. 17.4). Increased cAMP activates protein kinases, which promote intracellular calcium influx

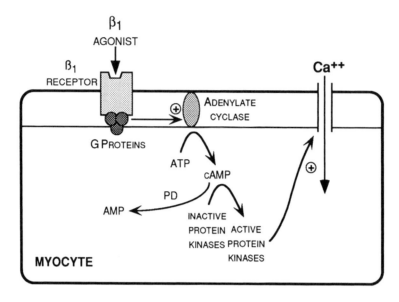

Figure 17.4. Mechanism by which β-adrenergic stimulation increases intracellular [Ca⁺⁺]. β_1-receptor stimulation acts through G proteins (guanine nucleotide regulatory proteins) to activate adenylate cyclase. The latter increases cAMP production, which mediates protein kinase phosphorylation of cellular proteins, including ion channels. Phosphorylation of the slow Ca^{++} channel increases calcium influx. cAMP is degraded by phosphodiesterase (PD).

by phosphorylating the slow calcium channels. The increased calcium entry triggers a corresponding rise in Ca^{++} release from the sarcoplasmic reticulum, which enhances the force of contraction. Intravenous dopamine and dobutamine are the most useful of the sympathomimetic amines in the treatment of acute heart failure. Norepinephrine, epinephrine, and isoproterenol are used in special circumstances as described below. Table 17.2 summarizes the receptor actions and major hemodynamic effects of these agents.

Dopamine is an endogenous catecholamine and the precursor of norepinephrine. It possesses an unusual combination of actions that make it attractive in the treatment of heart failure associated with hypotension and poor renal perfusion. There are several types of receptors with different affinities for dopamine. At low doses, < 2 μg/kg/min, dopamine interacts primarily with D_1-dopaminergic receptors that are distributed in the renal and mesenteric vascular beds. Stimulation of these receptors causes local vasodilation and increases renal blood flow and glomerular filtration, fa-

cilitating diuresis. Medium doses of dopamine, 2 to 10 μg/kg/min, increase inotropy by stimulation of cardiac β_1-receptors directly and indirectly by promoting release of norepinephrine (NE) from sympathetic nerve terminals. This action increases the heart rate, cardiac contractility, and stroke volume, all of which augment cardiac output.

At high doses, > 10 μg/kg/min, dopamine also stimulates systemic α-receptors, thereby causing vasoconstriction and elevating systemic resistance. High-dose dopamine is indicated in hypotensive states such as shock. However, such doses are inappropriate in most patients with cardiac failure because the peripheral vasoconstriction increases the resistance against which the heart must contract (i.e., higher afterload), further impairing left ventricular output.

The major toxicity of dopamine arises in patients who are treated with high-dose therapy. The most important side effects are acceleration of the heart rate (which increases oxygen consumption) and stimulation of tachyarrhythmias.

TABLE 17.2. Sympathomimetic Drug Effects

	Receptor Stimulation			
Drug	*D_1 (↑ renal perfusion)*	*α (vasoconstriction)*	*$β_1$ (↑ contractility)*	*$β_2$ (vasodilation)*
Dopamine	+ (low dose)	++++ (high dose)	++++ (mid or high dose)	++ (mid dose)
Dobutamine	0	+	++++	+
Norepinephrine	0	++++	++++	0
Epinephrine	0	++++	++++	++
Isoproterenol	0	0	++++	++++

Dobutamine is a synthetic analog of dopamine that stimulates $β_1$-, $β_2$- and α- receptors. It increases cardiac contractility by virtue of the $β_1$ effect but does not increase peripheral resistance because of the balance between α-mediated vasoconstriction and $β_2$-mediated vasodilation. Thus, it is useful in the treatment of CHF not accompanied by hypotension. Unlike dopamine, dobutamine does not stimulate dopaminergic receptors (i.e., no renal vasodilating effect), nor does it facilitate the release of NE from peripheral nerve endings. Like dopamine, it is useful for short-term therapy (less than 1 week), after which time it loses its efficacy, presumably because of down-regulation of adrenergic receptors. The major adverse effect is the development of tachyarrhythmias.

Norepinephrine is an endogenous catecholamine synthesized from dopamine in adrenergic postganglionic nerves and in adrenal medullary cells (where it is both a final product and the precursor of epinephrine). Via its $β_1$ activity, norepinephrine has positive inotropic and positive chronotropic effects. Acting at peripheral α receptors, norepinephrine is also a potent vasoconstrictor. The increase in total peripheral resistance causes the mean arterial blood pressure to rise.

With this combination of effects, norepinephrine is useful in patients suffering from "warm shock," in which the combination of cardiac contractile dysfunction and peripheral vasodilation lower the blood pressure. However, the intense vasoconstriction elicited by this drug make it less attractive than others in treating most cases of shock. Norepinephrine's side effects include precipitation of ischemia (due to the augmented afterload and force of contraction) and tachyarrhythmias.

Epinephrine, the predominant endogenous catecholamine produced in the adrenal medulla, is formed by the decarboxylation of norepinephrine. As indicated in Table 17.2, epinephrine is an agonist of α, $β_1$-, and $β_2$-receptors. Administered as an intravenous infusion at low doses (< .01 μg/kg/min) epinephrine's stimulation of the $β_1$-receptor increases ventricular contractility, shortens systole, and speeds impulse generation (e.g., by enhancing phase 4 depolarization in SA nodal cells). As a result, stroke volume, heart rate, and cardiac output all increase. However, at this dose range $β_2$-mediated vasodilation may reduce total peripheral resistance and blood pressure.

At higher doses, (> 0.2 μg/kg/min), epinephrine is a very potent vasopressor since α-mediated constriction dominates over $β_2$-mediated vasodilation. In this case, the effects of positive inotropy, positive chronotropy, and vasoconstriction act together to raise the arterial blood pressure.

Epinephrine is therefore used most often when the combination of inotropic and chronotropic stimulation are desired, such as in the setting of cardiac arrest. The α-associated vasoconstriction may also beneficially help support the blood pressure in that setting. The most common toxic effect is the precipitation of tachyarrhythmias. Epinephrine should be avoided in patients on beta-blocker therapy, since unopposed $α_1$ vasoconstriction could produce acute severe hypertension and its complications (see Chapter 13).

Isoproterenol is a synthetic epinephrine

analog. Unlike norepinephrine and epinephrine, it is a "pure" β agonist, having activity almost exclusively at β_1- and β_2-receptors, with almost no α receptor effect. In the heart, isoproterenol has positive inotropic and chronotropic effects, thereby increasing cardiac output. In peripheral vessels, stimulation of β_2-receptors results in vasodilation and reduced peripheral resistance, which may cause the blood pressure to fall.

Isoproterenol is sometimes used in emergency circumstances to increase the heart rate in patients with bradycardia or heart block (e.g., as a temporizing measure prior to pacemaker implantation). It may also be useful in patients with systolic dysfunction and slow heart rates with high systemic vascular resistance (a situation sometimes encountered after cardiac surgery in patients on prior beta-blocker therapy). Isoproterenol should be avoided in patients with myocardial ischemia in whom the increased heart rate and inotropic stimulation would further increase myocardial oxygen consumption.

Phosphodiesterase Inhibitors

Amrinone and **milrinone** are nondigitalis, noncatecholamine inotropic agents.

They exert their positive inotropic actions by inhibiting phosphodiesterase in cardiac myocytes (Fig. 17.4). This inhibition reduces the breakdown of intracellular cAMP, the ultimate result of which is enhanced $[Ca^{++}]$ entry into the cell and increased force of contraction. These agents also have vasodilating properties

Amrinone and milrinone are used in the treatment of CHF only if there has been insufficient improvement with conventional vasodilators, digitalis and diuretics. This is because of the high incidence of adverse effects, including serious ventricular arrhythmias. Amrinone has not been shown to improve the clinical state with chronic use in CHF patients, and chronic milrinone therapy has actually demonstrated an increase in mortality. Roles for these agents are currently limited to short-term therapy in hospitalized patients.

The most important effects of the inotropic drugs are summarized in Table 17.3.

VASODILATOR DRUGS

Vasodilator drugs play a central role in the treatment of heart failure and hypertension. As described in Chapter 9, the fall in

---

TABLE 17.3. Inotropic Drugs

Drug	Mechanism of Action	Major Adverse Effects
Cardiac glycosides • Digoxin • Digitoxin	Inhibition of sarcolemmal Na^+/K^+ ATPase	**GI:** nausea, vomiting **Cardiac:** atrial, nodal, and ventricular tachyarrhythmias; high-degree AV block
Sympathomimetic amines • Dopamine	Low dose (< 2 μg/kg/min): D_1 receptor stimulation results in mesenteric and renal arterial dilatation (facilitates diuresis) Medium dose (2–10 μg/kg/min): β_1 receptor stimulation and release of norepinephrine from sympathetic nerve terminals (inotropic effect) High dose (> 10μg/kg/min): α-receptor stimulation (peripheral vasoconstriction)	Tachycardia, arrhythmias, hypertension, drug tolerance
• Dobutamine	β_1, β_2, and α receptor stimulation.	Tachyarrhythmias, drug tolerance
Phosphodiesterase inhibitors • Amrinone • Milrinone	Increased intracellular cAMP due to inhibition of its breakdown by phosphodiesterase	**GI:** nausea, vomiting **Cardiac:** arrhythmias (Amrinone only): thrombocytopenia

cardiac output in CHF triggers two important compensatory pathways: the adrenergic nervous system, and, because of a reduction in renal blood flow, the renin-angiotensin system (see Fig. 9.9). As a result of these activations, two potent vasoconstrictors are released into the circulation: norepinephrine and angiotensin II. These hormones bind to receptors in arterioles and veins, where they incite vasoconstriction. Initially, vasoconstriction is beneficial in CHF because it maximizes left ventricular preload (through venous constriction) and maintains systemic blood pressure (by arterial constriction).

However, venous constriction may ultimately cause excessive venous return to the heart, with a rise in the pulmonary capillary hydrostatic pressure and development of pulmonary congestion. In addition, excessive arteriolar constriction increases the resistance against which the LV must contract, and therefore ultimately impedes forward cardiac output. Vasodilator therapy is directed at modulating the excessive constriction of veins and arterioles, so as to reduce pulmonary congestion and augment forward cardiac output (see Fig. 9.10).

Vasodilators are also useful antihypertensive drugs. Recall from Chapter 13 that blood pressure is the product of cardiac output and systemic vascular resistance. Vasodilator drugs decrease arteriolar resistance and therefore lower elevated blood pressure.

Individual vasodilator drug classes act at specific vascular sites (Fig. 17.5). Nitrates, for example, are primarily venodilators, whereas hydralazine is a pure arteriolar dilator. Some drugs, such as the ACE inhibitors, α-blockers, and sodium nitroprusside, are balanced vasodilators that act on both sides of the circulation.

Angiotensin-Converting Enzyme Inhibitors

The renin-angiotensin system plays an intricate role in cardiovascular homeostasis. The major effector of this pathway (Fig. 17.6) is angiotensin II (AII), which is formed by the cleavage of angiotensin I by angiotensin-converting enzyme (ACE). All of the actions of AII known to affect blood pressure control are mediated by its binding to angiotensin II receptors of the AT_1 subtype (see Fig. 13.6). Interaction with this receptor generates a series of intracellular reactions that cause, among other effects, vasoconstriction, and the adrenal release of aldosterone, which promotes Na^+ reabsorption from the distal nephron. As a result of these actions on vascular tone and sodium homeostasis, AII plays a major role in blood pressure and blood volume regulation. By blocking the formation of AII, ACE inhibitors decrease the systemic arterial pressure (decreased vasoconstriction) and facilitate natriuresis (e.g., decreased aldosterone and reduced Na^+ reabsorption from the distal nephron).

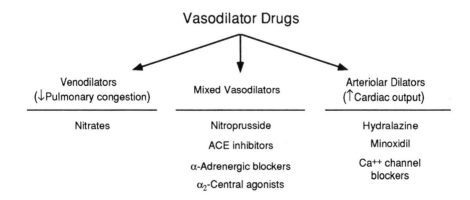

Figure 17.5. Examples of vasodilator drugs and their sites of action: the venous bed, the arteriolar bed, or both.

Another action of ACE inhibitors, which likely contributes to their hemodynamic effects, is related to bradykinin (BK) metabolism, as shown in Figure 17.6. The natural vasodilator BK is normally degraded to inactive metabolites by angiotensin-converting enzyme, such that ACE *inhibitors* prevent that degradation. As a result, BK accumulates and contributes to the antihypertensive effect, likely by stimulating the endothelial release of nitric oxide and the biosynthesis of vasodilating prostaglandins.

Clinical Uses

Hypertension

In hypertensive patients without CHF, ACE inhibitors lower blood pressure with little change in cardiac output or heart rate. One might assume that because this class of drug interferes with the renin-angiotensin system, it would be effective only in patients with "high-renin" hypertension, but

that is not the case. Rather, they are effective in most hypertensive patients, regardless of serum renin levels. The reason for this is not clear, but may relate to the additional antihypertensive effects of bradykinin and vasodilatory prostaglandins discussed above. In addition, several researchers have demonstrated the presence of renin-angiotensin activity within tissues outside of the circulation, including the walls of the vasculature, where ACE inhibitors may exert an effect regardless of circulating renin concentrations.

ACE inhibitors increase renal blood flow in hypertensive patients, usually without altering glomular filtration rate (GFR), because of dilation of both the afferent and efferent glomerular arterioles. Used alone in hypertension, ACE inhibitors show similar efficacy compared with diuretics and β-blockers, but are often better tolerated. They do not adversely affect serum glucose or lipid concentrations, and do not result in hypokalemia, as do diuretics. Studies have shown that ACE inhibitors are preferred

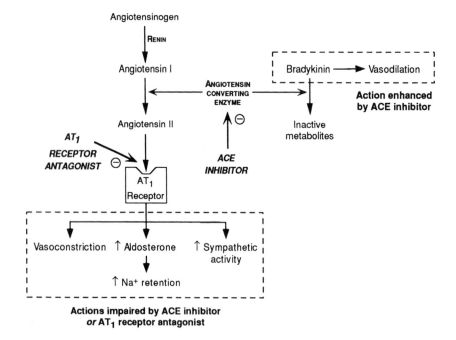

Figure 17.6. The renin-angiotensin system. Angiotensin converting enzyme (ACE) generates angiotensin II, which results in actions including vasoconstriction, sodium retention, and increased sympathetic activity. ACE inhibitors and angiotensin II type 1 (AT$_1$) receptor antagonists impair these effects. ACE also promotes the degradation of the natural vasodilator bradykinin; thus ACE inhibition, but not AT$_1$ receptor inhibition, results in accumulation of bradykinin, and enhanced vasodilation.

therapy in diabetic hypertensive patients, because they slow the development of diabetic nephropathy (a syndrome of progressive renal deterioration, proteinuria, and hypertension) through favorable effects on intraglomerular pressure.

Congestive Heart Failure

In CHF, ACE inhibitors reduce peripheral vascular resistance (decrease afterload) and cardiac filling pressures (decrease preload), and increase cardiac output. The rise in cardiac output usually matches the fall in peripheral resistance such that blood pressure tends not to fall (remember: BP = CO x TPR), except in those patients who are intravascular volume deplete, as might result from overvigorous diuretic therapy. The augmented cardiac output reduces the drive for neurohormonal stimulation in CHF (see Chapter 9), such that elevated levels of norepinephrine fall. In addition, survival in patients with symptomatic heart failure has been shown to increase significantly when treated with an ACE inhibitor, more so than with any other anti-CHF drug regimen.

Of the many oral ACE inhibitors available, three have been studied the most extensively: **captopril, enalapril,** and **lisinopril;** all of the available agents are listed in Table 17.4. The primary excretory pathway of most ACE inhibitors is via the urine, such

that dosage of these should generally be reduced in patients with renal dysfunction.

The important benefits of ACE inhibitor therapy on ventricular remodeling and survival following myocardial infarction are described in Chapter 7.

Toxicity

Side effects of the ACE inhibitors are potentially serious, but are not common.

Hypotension

This is a rare side effect when ACE inhibitors are used to treat hypertension. It is more likely to occur in heart failure patients in whom intravascular volume depletion has resulted from vigorous diuretic use. Such patients have marked activation of the renin-angiotensin system, and therefore the blood pressure is largely maintained by the vasoconstricting actions of circulating AII. The administration of an ACE inhibitor in that setting may result in hypotension due to the sudden reduction of AII levels. This side effect is avoided by temporarily reducing the diuretic regimen, and starting the ACE inhibitor at low dosage.

Hyperkalemia

Because ACE inhibitors indirectly reduce serum aldosterone concentrations, the serum potassium concentration may rise,

TABLE 17.4. Drugs That Interfere With the Renin-Angiotensin System

	Frequency of Administration	Metabolic Elimination Pathway
ACE Inhibitors		
Approved for hypertension and CHF		
Captopril	bid–tid	Renal
Enalapril	qd–bid	Renal
Fosinopril	qd	Renal/hepatic
Lisinopril	qd	Renal
Quinapril	qd–bid	Renal
Ramipril	qd–bid	Renal
Approved for hypertension only		
Benazepril	qd	Renal
Moexipril	qd	Hepatic/renal
Trandolapril	qd	Hepatic/renal
Angiotensin II Receptor Antagonists		
Losartan	qd	Hepatic/renal
Valsartan	qd	Hepatic/renal

but only rarely into the clinically important hyperkalemic range. Conditions that can further increase serum potassium levels and may result in dangerous hyperkalemia include renal insufficiency, diabetes (due to hyporeninemic hypoaldosteronism often present in elderly diabetics), and concomitant use of potassium-sparing diuretics. Therefore the latter, as well as potassium supplements, should generally be avoided during ACE inhibitor therapy.

Renal Insufficiency

As described above, administration of an ACE inhibitor to individuals with *intravascular volume depletion* may result in hypotension, as well as decreased renal perfusion and azotemia. Correction of the volume depletion or reduction of the ACE inhibitor dosage usually corrects this complication.

ACE inhibitor therapy can also precipitate renal failure in patients with *bilateral renal artery stenosis* because such patients rely on high efferent glomerular arteriolar resistance (which is highly dependent on AII) to maintain intraglomerular pressure and filtration. Administration of an ACE inhibitor abruptly decreases efferent arteriolar tone and glomerular hydrostatic pressure, and may therefore worsen GFR in this setting.

Cough

Irritation of the upper airways has been reported in up to 15% of patients on ACE inhibitor therapy, resulting in a dry cough. Its mechanism has not been established, but may relate to the increased bradykinin concentration. This side effect resolves after the drug is discontinued.

Other Effects

Very rare adverse reactions to the ACE inhibitors include angioedema and agranulocytosis.

Angiotensin II Type 1 Receptor Antagonists

Angiotensin II type 1 receptor antagonists (also termed AT_1 receptor antagonists) are the latest addition to the armamentar-

ium of oral antihypertensive agents. There are at least two distinct types of AII receptors: AT_1 and AT_2. All of the actions of AII known to affect blood pressure control are mediated by its binding to receptors of the AT_1 subtype (e.g., vasoconstriction, aldosterone release, renal Na^+ reabsorption, increased sympathetic nervous system activity). The AT_2 receptor subtype is abundant during fetal development and has been located in some adult tissues, but its actions are unknown.

AT_1 receptor antagonists are nonpeptide drugs that inhibit the effects of AII by competing with it for AT_1 receptors. As a result, AII-mediated effects, such as vasoconstriction, aldosterone secretion and renal sodium ion reabsorption, are inhibited (Fig. 17.6), resulting in a lowering of the blood pressure in hypertensive individuals. AT_1 receptor antagonists provide a somewhat more complete blockade of the renin-angiotensin system than ACE inhibitors, because the latter drugs do not completely block formation of AII (some AI is converted to AII by circulating enymes other than ACE). Unlike ACE inhibitors, serum bradykinin levels are not affected by the AT_1 receptor antagonists (Fig. 17.6). In clinical studies, AT_1 receptor antagonists have demonstrated antihypertensive effects comparable to ACE inhibitors or beta-blockers.

The prototype AT_1 receptor antagonist, **losartan,** is quickly absorbed from the GI tract and reaches a peak serum concentration within 1 hour. It is excreted primarily in the bile, but also in part in the urine. Its main metabolite is more active than the drug itself and has a longer half-life. Similar to ACE inhibitors, the blood pressure lowering effect of losartan is enhanced when concurrent thiazide diuretic therapy is administered. In contrast to ACE inhibitors, cough does not appear to be a side effect. Another potential advantage of losartan is that it reduces serum uric acid levels by an unknown mechanism, a characteristic that may prove useful in treating hypertensive patients who also have gout.

Clinical trials have demonstrated that losartan is well-tolerated. Hypotension and hyperkalemia (due to reduced aldosterone levels), predictable consequences of AII inhibition, are possible side effects.

Direct-Acting Vasodilators

Hydralazine, minoxidil, sodium nitroprusside, and diazoxide are examples of direct-acting vasodilators (Table 17.5). Hydralazine and minoxidil are primarily used as long-term oral vasodilators, while nitroprusside and diazoxide are administered intravenously in more acute settings.

Hydralazine acts as a potent and direct arteriolar dilator at the level of the precapillary arterioles, and has no effect on systemic veins. The exact cellular mechanism of its effect remains unknown. The fall in blood pressure following arteriolar dilation results in a baroreceptor-mediated increase in sympathetic outflow and cardiac stimulation (e.g., reflex tachycardia), which could precipitate myocardial ischemia in patients with underlying coronary artery disease. Therefore, hydralazine is often combined with a β-blocker to blunt this undesired response.

Hydralazine is used primarily as a second-line antihypertensive, in combination with other drugs, usually after ACE inhibitors, calcium channel blockers, betablockers and diuretics have failed to satisfactorily control a patient's blood pressure. Hydralazine is also sometimes used, in combination with the venodilator isosorbide dinitrate to treat heart failure in pa-

tients with systolic dysfunction. This combination improves symptoms in patients with mild-moderate heart failure, and has been shown to reduce long-term mortality in that setting, but not as effectively as ACE inhibitors.

Hydralazine possesses low bioavailability because of its extensive first-pass hepatic metabolism. However, its metabolism depends on whether the patient displays fast or slow acetylation; on average, 50% of Americans are fast and 50% are slow hepatic acetylators. Slow acetylators show less hepatic degradation, higher bioavailability, and increased antihypertensive effects, whereas fast acetylators demonstrate the opposite. Hydralazine has a short half-life (2 to 4 hours) in the circulation, but its effect persists as long as 12 hours because most of the drug is avidly bound to vascular tissue.

The most common side effects of hydralazine include headache (increased cerebral vasodilatation), palpitations (reflex tachycardia), flushing (increased systemic vasodilatation), nausea, and anorexia. As indicated above, tachycardia due to reflex adrenergic stimulation may precipitate anginal attacks in patients with coronary artery disease, if hydralazine is not jointly administered with a β-blocker. Finally, a systemic lupus–like syndrome, characterized by arthralgias, myalgia, skin rashes, and fever, may develop, especially in slow acetylators. This syndrome occurs in about 10% of slow acetylators, and is reversed by discontinuing the drug.

Minoxidil also results in arteriolar va-

TABLE 17.5. Direct Vasodilators

Drugs	Clinical Use	Route of Administration	Major Adverse Effects
Hydralazine	• Hypertension (chronic and acute therapy) • CHF	Oral, IV bolus, intramuscular	• Hypotension, tachycardia • Headache, flushing • Angina • Drug-induced lupus
Minoxidil	• Chronic therapy of hypertension	Oral	• Reflex tachycardia • Na$^+$ retention • Hypertrichosis
Nitroprusside	• Hypertensive emergencies • Acute CHF	Intravenous infusion	• Hypotension • Cyanide and thiocyanate toxicity
Diazoxide	• Hypertensive emergencies	Intravenous bolus	• Hypotension • Na$^+$ retension • Hyperglycemia

sodilation without significant venodilation, similar to hydralazine. Its mechanism of action may involve an increase in potassium channel permeability, which results in smooth muscle cell hyperpolarization and subsequent relaxation. Like other agents that selectively cause arteriolar dilation, reflex adrenergic stimulation leads to increased heart rate and contractility, an undesired effect which can be blunted by coadministration of a β-blocker. In addition, decreased renal perfusion often results in fluid retention, so that a diuretic must usually be administered concurrently.

Minoxidil's primary clinical indication is in the treatment of severe or intractable hypertension, and is especially useful in patients with renal failure who are often refractory to other antihypertensive regimens. It is well absorbed from the GI tract and is metabolized primarily by hepatic glucuronidation, but about one-fifth is excreted unchanged by the kidney. Although it has a short half-life, its pharmacologic effects persist even after serum drug concentration falls, probably because, like hydralazine, the drug is avidly bound to vascular tissue.

Side effects of minoxidil, in addition to reflex sympathetic stimulation and fluid retention, include hypertrichosis (excessive hair growth), and occasionally a pericardial effusion (mechanism unknown).

Sodium nitroprusside (SNP), a potent dilator of *both* arterioles and veins, is used to treat hypertensive emergencies, and in intensive care units for intravenous control of blood pressure. It is also used for preload and afterload modulation in severe CHF. SNP is a complex of iron, cyanide groups, and a nitroso moiety, and red blood cell me-

tabolism of the drug results in the liberation of nitric oxide (Fig. 17.7). Nitric oxide causes vasodilation through activation of guanylate cyclase in vascular smooth muscle (see Chapter 6 and below).

SNP's hemodynamic effects result from its ability to decrease arterial resistance and to increase venous capacitance. In patients with normal LV function, it can actually decrease cardiac output because of the reduction in venous return (see Fig. 9.10). However, in a patient with impaired LV contractile function, the decreased systemic resistance induced by SNP leads to an increase in the forward cardiac output, while venous dilation reduces preload and return of blood to the heart. The latter decreases pulmonary capillary hydrostatic pressure and improves symptoms of pulmonary congestion.

SNP is the treatment of choice for many hypertensive emergencies (see Chapter 13) because of its great potency and rapid action. Often, a sympatholytic drug such as a β-blocker must be administered concurrently to counteract the baroreceptor-mediated reflex increase in sympathetic outflow that may accompany the use of this drug.

SNP must be given by continuous intravenous infusion. Its onset of action is 30 sec after administration; the peak effect is achieved in 2 minutes and dissipates within minutes of its discontinuation. After red blood cells metabolize SNP into nitric oxide and cyanide, the liver, in the presence of a sulfhydryl donor, transforms cyanide into thiocyanate; the thiocyanate, in turn, is excreted by the kidney. *Thiocyanate accumulation and toxicity,* manifested by blurred vision, tinnitus, disorientation and/or nausea, may occur with continued use, espe-

Figure 17.7. Sodium nitroprusside is a complex of iron, cyanide (CN), and a nitroso group. RBC metabolism liberates CN and the active vasodilator nitric oxide. The CN is metabolized in the liver to thiocyanate, which is eliminated by the kidneys.

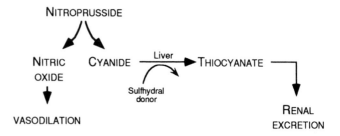

cially in the setting of renal impairment. Thus it is important to monitor serum levels of thiocyanate if SNP is administered for more than 24 hours. In addition, excessive infusion rates of SNP, or a deficiency in hepatic thiosulfate stores, can result in lethal *cyanide toxicity,* the early signs of which include metabolic acidosis, headache, and nausea, followed by loss of consciousness.

Diazoxide is another potent *arteriolar* dilator. Its mechanism of action involves activation of ATP-sensitive potassium channels, leading to arteriolar smooth muscle hyperpolarization and vasodilation. As with other vasodilators, the fall in resistance leads to a reflex activation of the adrenergic nervous system with tachycardia, and to fluid retention associated with activation of the renin-angiotensin system. This drug has been used primarily for hypertensive emergencies; however, its use has declined in favor of newer and better-tolerated agents.

Diazoxide is available only for intravenous administration, and it has a rapid onset of action. Excessive hypotension and reflex sympathetic stimulation represent its main toxicities. In addition, diazoxide inhibits insulin release from the pancreatic islet cells and can lead to hyperglycemia.

Calcium Channel Blockers (CCBs)

The CCBs are discussed here as a group, but many differences exist among the drugs of this class. The common property of Ca^{++} channel blockers is their ability to impede the influx of Ca^{++} through membrane channels in cardiac and smooth muscle cells. Two principal types of voltage-gated Ca^{++} channels have been identified in cardiac tissue, termed L and T. The L-type channel is responsible for the Ca^{++} entry that maintains phase 2 of the action potential (the "plateau" in Fig. 1.13). The T-type Ca^{++} channel likely plays a role in the initial depolarization of nodal tissues. It is the L-channel that is antagonized by current CCBs.

The cellular mechanism of calcium channel antagonists has been partly delineated. Increased concentrations of intracellular

Ca^{++} lead to augmented contractile force in both myocardium and vascular smooth muscle. In both cases, the net effect of Ca^{++} channel blockade is to decrease the amount of Ca^{++} available to the contractile proteins within these cells, which translates into vasodilation of vascular smooth muscle and a negative inotropic effect in cardiac muscle.

Vascular Smooth Muscle

Contraction of vascular smooth muscle depends on the cytoplasmic Ca^{++} concentration, which is regulated by the transmembrane flow of Ca^{++} through voltage-gated channels during depolarization. Intracellular Ca^{++} interacts with calmodulin to form a Ca^{++}-calmodulin complex. This complex stimulates myosin light chain kinase (MLCK), which phosphorylates myosin light chains, and allows myosin and actin to interact and cause contraction. CCBs promote relaxation of vascular smooth muscle by inhibiting Ca^{++} entry through the voltage-gated channels. Other organs possessing smooth muscle are also susceptible to this relaxing effect, including gastrointestinal, uterine, and bronchiolar tissues.

Cardiac Cells

Cardiac muscle also depends on Ca^{++} influx during depolarization for contractile protein interactions, but by a different mechanism than that in vascular smooth muscle. Ca^{++} entry into the cardiac cell upon depolarization triggers additional intracellular Ca^{++} release from the sarcoplasmic reticulum, leading to contraction (see Chapter 1). By blocking Ca^{++} entry, CCBs therefore interfere with excitation-contraction coupling and cause decreased force of contraction. Because the pacemaker tissues of the heart (e.g., SA and AV node) are the most dependent on the inward Ca^{++} current for their depolarization, one would expect that CCBs reduce the rate of sinus firing and AV nodal conduction. Some but not all CCBs have this property (Table 17.6). The effect on cardiac conduction appears to depend not only on whether the specific CCB reduces the inward Ca^{++} current, but

TABLE 17.6. Calcium Channel Blockers

Drug	Vasodilation	Negative Inotropic Effect	Suppress AV Node Conduction	Major Adverse Effects
Verapamil	+	+++	+++	• Hypotension • Bradycardia, AV block • CHF • Constipation
Diltiazem	++	++	++	• Hypotension • Peripheral edema • Bradycardia
Dihydropyridines: Amlodipine Felodipine Isradipine Nicardipine Nifedipine Nisoldipine	+++	0 to +	0	• Hypotension • Headache, flushing • Peripheral edema

also whether it delays recovery of the Ca^{++} channel to its preactivated state. **Verapamil** and **diltiazem** have this property, whereas **nifedipine** and the other dihydropyridines do not (see below).

Clinical Uses

As a result of their actions on vascular smooth muscle and cardiac cells, CCBs are useful in several cardiovascular disorders through the mechanisms summarized in Table 17.7. In angina pectoris, they exert beneficial effects by reducing myocardial oxygen consumption, as well as by potentially increasing oxygen supply through coronary dilatation. The latter effect is also useful in the treatment of coronary artery vasospasm.

CCBs are often used to treat hypertension, and unlike β-blockers or ACE inhibitors, they are particularly effective in elderly patients. Nifedipine and the other dihydropyridines are the most potent vasodilators of this class, but diltiazem and verapamil are also effective.

CCBs are usually administered orally, and once-a-day formulations are available for each of these agents. Routes of excretion vary. For example, nifedipine and verapamil are eliminated primarily in the urine, whereas diltiazem is excreted via the liver.

Common side effects (Table 17.6) include the development of hypotension due to excessive vasodilation, and ankle edema, presumably because of local vasodilation of peripheral vascular beds. Verapamil and diltiazem may result in bradyarrhythmias, and should be used with caution (or not at all) in patients already on β-blocker therapy.

The safety of *short-acting* calcium channel blockers has been called into question in recent years. In some studies, a higher incidence of myocardial infarction or mortality has been reported in patients with hypertension or coronary disease taking such agents. Although more data from randomized controlled trials are needed to clarify this risk, it is recommended that the long-acting (i.e., once-a-day) formulations of CCBs be prescribed, rather than the short-acting preparations. In patients with coronary artery disease, beta-blockers and/or nitrates are preferred over CCBs for initial therapy, as described in Chapter 6.

Organic Nitrates

The nitrates constitute one of the oldest treatments of angina pectoris; they are also used in other ischemic syndromes, as well as in heart failure. The main physiologic action of the nitrates is vasodilatation, particularly of the systemic veins.

TABLE 17.7. Clinical Effects of Calcium Channel Blockers

Condition	Mechanism

1. Angina pectoris	↓Myocardial oxygen consumption
	  ↓ blood pressure
	  ↓ contractility
	  ↓ heart rate (verapamil and diltiazem)
	  ↑ Myocardial oxygen supply
	  ↑ coronary dilatation

2. Coronary artery spasm	Coronary artery vasodilatation
3. Hypertension	Arteriolar smooth muscle relaxation
4. Supraventricular arrhythmias	(Verapamil and diltiazem): Decrease conduction velocity and increase refractoriness of AV node via blockade of slow inward Ca^{++} current

Mechanism of Action

Nitrates produce vascular smooth muscle relaxation. The proposed mechanism involves the conversion of the administered drug to nitric oxide (NO) at or near the plasma membrane of vascular smooth muscle cells (Fig. 17.8). Nitric oxide, in turn, activates guanylate cyclase to produce cyclic GMP (cGMP). The intracellular accumulation of cGMP leads to smooth muscle relaxation. This mechansim of vascular smooth muscle relaxation is similar to that associated with nitroprusside and endogenous endothelial-derived nitric oxide.

Hemodynamic and Antianginal Effects

At low doses, nitroglycerin, the prototypical organic nitrate, produces greater dilation of *veins* than arterioles. The resulting venodilation causes venous pooling, diminished venous return, and hence decreased right and left ventricular preload. Systemic arterial resistance is generally unaffected, but cardiac output may fall because of the diminished preload, especially in patients with intravascular volume depletion (see Fig. 9.10). *Arterial* dilation occurs to some extent in the coronary arteries, and may also occur in the facial vessels and the meningeal arterioles, giving rise to the side effects of flushing and headache, respectively.

At *high* doses, nitrates result in widespread arteriolar dilation, as well as venodilation. Arteriolar dilation may result in systemic hypotension and reflex tachycardia. However, the reflex sympathetic effect is not manifest in patients with heart failure, because decreasing afterload in that situa-

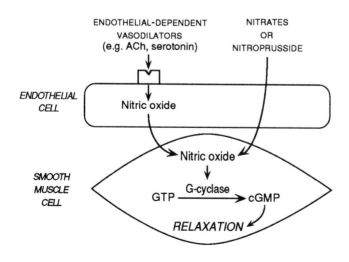

Figure 17.8. Organic nitrates incite vascular smooth muscle (SM) relaxation by conversion to nitric oxide (NO) at or near the cell membrane. Nitroprusside and endothelial-dependent vasodilators also promote NO delivery to vascular smooth muscle and cause relaxation. In the SM, NO stimulates formation of cyclic GMP (cGMP), which mediates relaxation.

tion actually improves cardiac output and reduces the sympathetic drive.

The major use of nitrates is in the treatment of angina pectoris. The main therapeutic action in this condition is the nitrate-induced reduction of preload, secondary to venodilation and reduced LV filling. The reduced preload lowers ventricular wall stress and myocardial oxygen consumption, which alleviates the oxygen imbalance in ischemic states. Nitrates are also useful in patients with coronary artery spasm (Prinzmetal's variant angina) because of nitrate-induced dilatation of the coronary arterioles.

Agents and Pharmacokinetics

There are many available formulations of nitrates. When the relief of acute angina is the objective, rapid onset of action is essential. On the other hand, in the long-term prevention of anginal attacks in a patient with chronic coronary artery disease, duration of action and predictability of effect are more crucial than the speed of drug effect.

Sublingual **nitroglycerin tablets** or **spray** is valuable in the treatment of acute angina. The peak action of these agents occurs within 3 minutes, because they are rapidly absorbed into the bloodstream via the oral mucosa; their effect, however, diminishes rapidly, falling off within 15 to 30 minutes, as the drug is deactivated in the liver. These forms of nitroglycerin are also effective when taken prophylactically, immediately before situations known by the patient to produce angina (e.g., walking up a hill or a flight of stairs).

The "long-acting" nitrates are used to prevent chest pain in the chronic management of angina pectoris. Low doses of oral nitroglycerin are ineffective because of rapid hepatic degradation; therefore, the long-term preventive agents must be given in sufficient dosage to saturate the liver's deactivating capacity. In this situation, high oral doses of **sustained-release nitroglycerin, isosorbide dinitrate,** or **isosorbide mononitrate** are routinely used. These agents have a duration of action of 2 to 14 hours. Transdermal patches or nitroglycerin paste applied to the skin also deliver a sustained release of nitroglycerin. However, the efficacy of long-acting nitrate therapy is attenuated by the rapid development of drug tolerance with continuous use. For this reason, it is important that the dosing regimens allow a drug-free interval of several hours each day to maintain drug efficacy.

Intravenous nitroglycerin is administered and titrated by continuous infusion. This route is most useful in the treatment of hospitalized patients with unstable angina or acute heart failure.

Adverse Effects

The most common adverse effects of the nitrates include hypotension, reflex tachycardia, headache, and flushing.

ANTIADRENERGIC DRUGS

Drugs that interfere with the sympathetic nervous system are used widely in the treatment of cardiovascular disorders. Such agents act at many different loci within the central and peripheral nerve pathways. Figure 17.9 demonstrates these sites of action, which include the central nervous system (CNS), postganglionic sympathetic nerve endings, and peripheral α- and β-receptors.

Normally, when a sympathetic nerve is stimulated, norepinephrine (NE) is released, traverses the synapse, and stimulates postsynaptic α- and β-receptors. The consequences of receptor stimulation depends on the organ involved (Table 17.8). The effect of α-receptor stimulation on vascular smooth muscle is vasoconstriction, whereas β_2 stimulation causes vasodilation. In the CNS, α_2 stimulation *inhibits* sympathetic outflow to the periphery, thereby contributing to vasodilatation.

In addition, NE within the synapse can bind to *presynaptic* β- and α_2-receptors, which provides a feedback mechanism that modulates further release of the hormone.

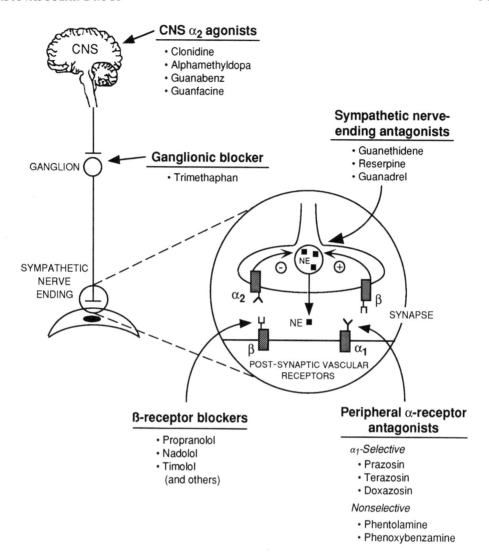

Figure 17.9. Sites of action of the antiadrenergic drugs. Note that receptors at the sympathetic nerve ending bind norepinephrine (NE) and provide feedback: The β-receptor stimulates, and the α₂-receptor inhibits, further NE release. CNS, central nervous system.

The β-receptor increases, and the α_2 inhibits, further NE release.

Central Adrenergic Inhibitors

α_2-receptors are located in the presynaptic neurons of the CNS, and when *stimulated* by an α_2-agonist, lead to diminished sympathetic outflow from the medulla. This translates into diminished peripheral vascular resistance and decreased cardiac stimulation, resulting in a fall in blood pressure and heart rate. Thus the central adrenergic *inhibitors* are actually centrally acting α_2-receptor *agonists*. The α_2 agonists are used as second-line agents in the treatment of hypertension. They are not sufficiently potent to serve as vasodilators in the treatment of heart failure.

The common α_2 agonists are shown in Figure 17.9. They are all available as oral preparations, and clonidine can also be prescribed as a skin patch that is applied and left in place for 1 week at a time, facilitating drug compliance. Side effects of α_2 agonists

TABLE 17.8. Responses to Adrenergic Receptor Stimulation

Receptor Type	Distribution	Response
α_1	Vascular smooth muscle (arterioles and veins)	Vasoconstriction
α_2	Presynaptic adrenergic nerve terminals	Inhibition of NE release
	Vascular smooth muscle (coronary and renal arterioles)	Vasoconstriction
β_1	Heart	Increase heart rate
		Increase contractility
		Speed AV node conduction
	Kidney (JG cells)	Increase renin release
	Presynaptic adrenergic nerve terminals	Increase NE release
	Adipose tissue	Stimulates lipolysis
β_2	Vascular smooth muscle (arterioles, except skin and cerebral)	Vasodilation
	Bronchial smooth muscle	Bronchodilation
	Liver	Stimulates glycogenolysis

include sedation, dry mouth, bradycardia, and if the drug is stopped suddenly, the possibility of a sudden, paradoxical rise in blood pressure.

Sympathetic Nerve-Ending Antagonists

This group includes guanethidine, reserpine, and guanadrel. **Guanethidine** and **guanadrel** are actively transported into the postganglionic neuron via the NE reuptake pump, and once inside bind to NE vesicles, preventing the release of NE upon nerve stimulation. Gradually, this depletes the vesicles of their contents, and as NE is released into the cytoplasm, it is degraded.

Early in the course of therapy, guanethidine decreases BP and cardiac output by slowing the heart rate and increasing venous capacitance, via the reduction of NE. There is no compensatory rise in peripheral resistance, because the drug effectively blocks sympathetically mediated reflex vasoconstriction. Guanethidine was used extensively in the early 1970s as an antihypertensive, but its side effects (primarily postural hypotension) and the development of better agents have demoted it to the "rarely used" status. Guanadrel has a shorter duration of action, and may have fewer side effects.

Reserpine was the first drug found to interfere with the sympathetic nervous system, and its use ushered in many of the concepts employed today in hypertension

management. It binds to storage vesicles in postganglionic and central neurons, leading to the destruction of those vesicles and the release and degradation of NE. The antihypertensive effect is due to the depletion of catecholamines, which causes the force of myocardial contraction and total peripheral resistance to decrease.

Reserpine's CNS toxicity represents its chief drawback as an antihypertensive. It often produces sedation and can impair concentration. The most serious potential toxicity is psychotic depression, and patients with a history of depression should not receive this drug. Newer, better-tolerated antihypertensive agents have largely supplanted the use of reserpine.

Peripheral α-Receptor Antagonists

Peripheral α antagonists (Table 17.9) are divided into those that act on both α_1- and α_2-receptors, and those that inhibit α_1 alone. α_1-selective receptor antagonists (**prazosin, terazosin, doxazosin**) are used in the treatment of hypertension. Their selectivity for the α_1-receptor explains their ability to produce less reflex tachycardia than nonselective agents: Normally, drug-induced vasodilation results in baroreceptor-mediated stimulation of the sympathetic nervous system and an undesired increase in heart rate. This effect is amplified by drugs that block the presynaptic α_2-receptor, as feedback inhibition of NE release is prevented. However, α_1 selective agents do not block the

TABLE 17.9 Alpha-Receptor Blockers

Mechanism/Drug	Indications	Major Adverse Effects
Selective peripheral α_1 blockade Prazosin Terazosin Doxazosin	• Hypertension • Benign prostatic hyperplasia	• Postural hypotension • Headache, dizziness • [No reflex tachycardia]
Nonselective α blockade Phentolamine Phenoxybenzamine	• Pheochromocytoma	• Postural hypotension • Reflex tachycardia • Arrhythmias

negative feedback on the α_2-receptor. Thus, further NE release and reflex sympathetic side effects are blunted.

The principal indication for α_1 antagonists is the treatment of hypertension. One of their advantages is that they do not adversely affect the serum concentrations of cholesterol and triglycerides as do other antihypertensives such as diuretics and β-blockers. They have been evaluated for use in the treatment of heart failure, but appear to lose their effectiveness over time (drug tolerance), and unlike other vasodilator regimens (ACE inhibitors or hydralazine plus nitrates), do not reduce mortality in chronic CHF. Terazosin and doxazosin are also indicated to treat the symptoms of benign prostatic hyperplasia, as they beneficially relax prostatic smooth muscle tone.

Phentolamine and **phenoxybenzamine** are nonselective α-blockers. They are used primarily in the treatment of pheochromocytoma, a tumor that abnormally secretes catecholamines into the circulation. Otherwise, these drugs are rarely used, as the α_2 blockade impairs normal feedback inhibition of NE release, an undesired effect, as indicated above.

β-Adrenergic Receptor Antagonists

The β-adrenergic antagonists are used for a number of cardiovascular conditions, including ischemic heart disease, hypertension, and tachyarrhythmias.

Because catecholamines increase inotropy, chronotropy, and conduction velocity of the heart, it follows that β-receptor antagonists decrease inotropy, slow the heart rate, and decrease conduction velocity. When stimulation of the β-receptors is low, as in a normal resting individual, the effect of blocking agents is likewise mild. However, when the sympathetic nervous system is activated (e.g., during exercise), these antagonists can substantially diminish catecholamine-mediated effects.

The β-blockers can be distinguished from one another by specific properties (Table 17.10): 1) the relative affinity of the drug for β_1- and β_2-receptors, 2) whether partial β-*agonist* activity is present, 3) whether α_1-receptors are also blocked, and 4) differences in pharmacokinetic properties. The goal of β_1-*selective* agents is to achieve myocardial receptor blockade, with less effect on bronchial and vascular smooth muscle (tissues that exhibit β_2-receptors), so as to produce less bronchospasm and vasoconstriction in susceptible individuals.

During short-term use, nonselective β antagonists tend to reduce cardiac output because of the decrease in heart rate and contractility, and they slightly increase peripheral resistance because of β_2-receptor

TABLE 17.10. β-adrenergic Blockers

	Nonselective β-blockers	β_1-selective β-blockers
No β-agonist activity	Propranolol Nadolol Timolol Labetalol*	Atenolol Betaxolol Esmolol[†] Metoprolol
β-agonist activity	Carteolol Penbutolol Pindolol	Acebutolol

*Also has α_1-adrenergic blocking properties.
[†]Administered intravenously only.

blockade. β antagonists that have partial agonist activity (such as pindolol), or those that possess some α-blocking activity (such as labetolol), can actually lower peripheral resistance by interacting with their respective β₂- and α-receptors.

Clinical Uses

Ischemic Heart Disease

The beneficial effects of β-blockers in the management of angina is related to their ability to decrease myocardial oxygen demand (see Chapter 6): They reduce the heart rate, blood pressure (afterload), and contractility. The negative inotropic effect is directly related to blockade of the cardiac β-receptor (Fig. 17.4), which results in decreased calcium influx into the myocyte. β-blockers have also been shown to improve survival and reduce the rate of reinfarction following acute MI. The exact mechanism by which mortality is reduced is unknown, but may relate in part to the antiarrhythmic activity of β-blockers (described below).

Hypertension

β-blocking agents reduce the blood pressure in hypertensives but often do not display this effect in normotensive individuals. In fact, despite their widespread use as antihypertensives, the mechanisms responsible for this effect are not well understood. With initial use, the antihypertensive effect is thought to result from the decrease in cardiac output, in association with slowing of the heart rate and mild decrease in contractility. However, with chronic administration, other mechanisms are likely at work, including reduced secretion of renin and possible CNS actions.

Other conditions that benefit from beta-blocker therapy include tachyarrhythmias (see below) and hypertrophic cardiomyopathy (see Chapter 10).

Toxicity

Fatigue may occur during the course of β-blocker therapy, and is most likely a CNS side effect. β-blockers with less lipid solubility (e.g., nadolol) do not penetrate the blood-brain barrier and have fewer CNS adverse effects than more lipid-soluble drugs, such as propranolol. Other potential adverse effects relate to the predictable consequences of β blockade:

1. β_2 blockade associated with use of nonselective agents (or large doses of β_1-selective blockers) can exacerbate *bronchospasm*, worsening preexisting asthma or chronic obstructive lung disease.
2. The impairment of AV nodal conduction by β_1 blockade can precipitate conduction blocks.
3. The negative chronotropic and inotropic effects associated with β_1 blockade can precipitate *heart failure* in patients with impaired LV systolic function.
4. β_2 blockade can precipitate arterial *vasospasm*. This can precipitate Raynaud's phenomenon or worsen peripheral vascular disease, potentially resulting in claudication or gangrene (see Chapter 15).
5. Abrupt withdrawal of a β-antagonist after chronic use can theoretically precipitate angina or myocardial infarction in patients with CAD ("rebound ischemia") because of "up-regulation" of the number of β-receptors during the period of adrenergic blockade, rendering the heart more susceptible to circulating catecholamines after the drug is stopped.
6. Undesirable reduction of HDL cholesterol and elevation of triglycerides can occur through an unknown mechanism. This effect appears to be less pronounced with those blockers that have partial β-agonist activity, or combined β- and α-blocking properties (see Table 17.10).
7. β_2 blockade may impair recovery from hypoglycemia in diabetics suffering an insulin reaction. In addition, β-blockers may mask the sympathetic warning signs of hypoglycemia, such as tachycardia. If β-blockers are used in diabetics, β_1-selective agents are generally preferable.

Finally, β-antagonists should be used with caution in combination with verapamil (or diltiazem) because each can impair myocardial contractility and AV nodal conduction, and could therefore precipitate heart failure or AV conduction blocks.

ANTIARRHYTHMIC DRUGS

Drug therapy is a common approach to the treatment of cardiac tachyarrhythmias. However, despite their benefits, antiarrhythmic drugs are among the most dangerous pharmacologic agents because of their frequent serious adverse effects. Therefore, a thorough understanding of their mechanisms of action, indications, and toxicities is of particular importance.

Although a number of classification systems for these agents exist, antiarrhythmic drugs are commonly separated into four groups, based on their general mechanisms of action (Table 17.11):

1. *Class I* drugs block the fast sodium channel responsible for phase 0 depolarization of the action potential. They are further divided into three subtypes based on the magnitude of sodium channel blockade and the effect of the drug on the duration of the cellular refractory period.

2. *Class II* drugs are β-adrenergic receptor blockers.

3. *Class III* drugs are those that markedly prolong the action potential with little effect on the rise of phase 0 depolarization. The mechanism of action of some of these drugs appears to be blockade of the repolarizing K^+ current (during phases 2 and 3 of the action potential).

4. *Class IV* drugs block the slow L-type calcium channel.

Drugs that do not conveniently fit into these classes include adenosine and the digitalis glycosides.

Regardless of the class, the goal of the antiarrhythmic therapies discussed in this section is to abolish the mechanisms by which tachyarrhythmias occur. These mechanisms (as descibed in Chapter 11) are: 1) increased automaticity of pacemaker or nonpacemaker cells, 2) reentrant pathways, and 3) triggered activity.

In the case of arrhythmias due to *increased automaticity,* treatment is aimed at: 1) reducing the slope of spontaneous phase 4 diastolic depolarization, and/or 2) raising the threshold potential. These actions reduce or extinguish the excess rate of cell firing.

Antiarrhythmic drugs inhibit *reentrant* rhythms by a different mechanism. Recall

TABLE 17.11. Classification of Antiarrhythmic Drugs

Class		General Mechanism		Examples
I		**Na⁺ channel blockade**		
	IA	Moderate block:	↓↓ phase 0 upstroke rate Prolong repolarization	Quinidine Procainamide Disopyramide
	IB	Mild block:	↓ phase 0 upstroke rate Shorten repolarization	Lidocaine Tocainide Mexiletine Phenytoin (DPH)
	IC	Marked block:	↓↓↓ phase 0 upstroke rate No change in repolarization	Flecainide Propafenone
II		**β-blockers**		Propranolol Esmolol Metoprolol and many others
III		**Marked prolongation of repolarization**		Amiodarone Sotalol Bretylium Ibutilide
IV		**Ca⁺⁺ channel blockers**		Verapamil Diltiazem

that the initiation of a reentrant circuit relies on a region of unidirectional block and slowed retrograde conduction (Fig. 17.10). For a reentrant rhythm to sustain itself, the length of time it takes for an impulse to propagate around the circuit must exceed the effective refractory period of the tissue. If an impulse returns to an area of myocardium that was depolarized moments earlier but has not yet recovered excitability, it cannot restimulate that tissue. Thus, one strategy to stop reentry is to lengthen the tissue's refractory period. When the refractory period is pharmacologically prolonged, a propagating impulse confronts inactive sodium channels, cannot conduct further, and is extinguished.

A second means to interrupt reentrant circuits is to *additionally impair* impulse propagation within the already slowed retrograde limb. This is accomplished via pharmacologic blockade of the Na^+ channels responsible for phase 0 depolarization. Such blockade fully abolishes the compromised impulse conduction within the retrograde limb and breaks the self-sustaining loop.

The elimination of the third type of tachyarrhythmia, *triggered activity*, requires suppression of early and delayed afterdepolarizations (as described in Chapter 11).

An ideal pharmacologic agent would suppress ectopic foci and interrupt reentrant loops without affecting normal conduction pathways. Unfortunately, when the concentrations of antiarrhythmic drugs exceed their narrow therapeutic ranges, even

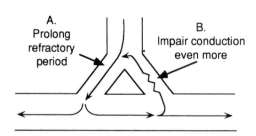

Figure 17.10. Two strategies to interrupt reentry are (A) to prolong the tissue refractory period, so that returning impulses find the tissue unexcitable, or (B) to further reduce conduction, so that the impulse "dies out" in the slow retrograde limb of the circuit.

normal electrical activity may become suppressed. In addition, most antiarrhythmic drugs have the potential to aggravate rhythm disturbances (termed a *"proarrhythmic effect"*). For example, this may occur when an antiarrhythmic drug prolongs the action potential, and induces early afterdepolarizations, resulting in a triggered-type of arrhythmia (see Chapter 11). Drug-induced proarrhythmia, which may result in ventricular tachycardia or ventricular fibrillation, occurs most often in patients with reduced left ventricular function or in those with an increased QT interval (a sign that the action potential is prolonged).

Class IA Antiarrhythmics

Mechanisms of Action

Effect on Arrhythmias Due to Increased Automaticity

Class IA agents produce moderate blockade of the fast sodium channels. Because fewer channels are available to conduct sodium into the cell, these drugs raise the threshold potential and slow the upstroke of the action potential (phase 0). In addition, perhaps by inhibition of pacemaker channels, the slope of phase 4 depolarization is depressed (Fig. 17.11) so that it takes longer to reach threshold and fire the action potential. These effects are most pronounced at Purkinje fibers and abnormal ectopic pacemakers. Because IA agents have little effect on the automaticity of the SA node, it can resume its function as the cardiac pacemaker after ectopic foci are suppressed.

Effect on Reentrant Arrhythmias

Because sodium channel blockade slows the rate of phase 0 depolarization by reducing the magnitude of the inward current, it reduces cellular and tissue conduction velocities. If impaired sufficiently within a reentrant circuit, the impulse will die out within the already slowed retrograde limb, aborting the rhythm. In addition, lengthening of the action potential by these drugs and their relatively slow dissociation from

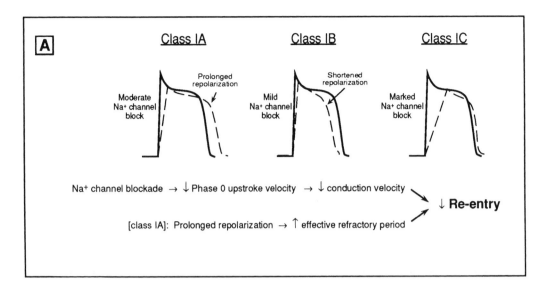

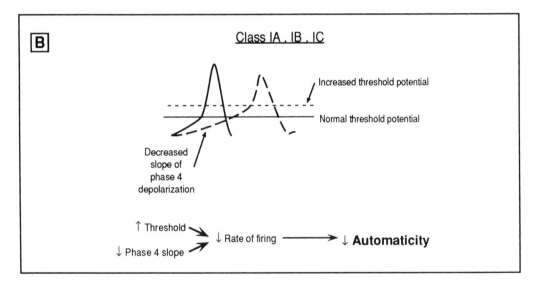

Figure 17.11.   Electrophysiologic effects of the class I antiarrhythmic drugs on the (A) Purkinje cell action potential and (B) pacemaker cell action potential.

Na$^+$ channels after repolarization both prolong the cell's refractory period (Fig. 17.11) such that an impulse traveling in the reentrant loop encounters unexcitable tissue and is extinguished.

Effect on the Electrocardiogram

Because the conduction velocity is decreased and the action potential duration and repolarization are prolonged, the effect of class IA agents is to mildly prolong the QRS and QT intervals (Table 17.12). At higher dosage, these intervals may become substantially lengthened, potentially setting the stage for afterdepolarizations and drug-induced arrhythmias.

Clinical Uses

Class IA drugs are used to treat a wide variety of reentrant and ectopic supraventricular and ventricular tachycardias (Table

TABLE 17.12. Effect of Antiarrhythmic Drugs on Electrocardiographic Intervals

Class	PR	QRS	QT
IA	0	↑	↑
IB	0	0	0 or ↓
IC	↑	↑	0 or ↑
II	0 or ↑	0	0 or ↓
III	0 or ↑	↑	↑
IV	↑	0	0

TABLE 17.13. Common Clinical Uses of the Antiarrhythmic Drugs

Class	Use
IA	• Atrial fibrillation & flutter • Paroxysmal SVT • Ventricular tachycardia
IB	• Ventricular tachycardia • Digitalis-induced arrhythmias
IC	• Ventricular tachycardia • (Sometimes): atrial fibrillation and paroxysmal SVT
II	• Atrial or ventricular premature beats • Paroxysmal SVT • Atrial fibrillation and flutter • Ventricular tachycardia (Ischemia-related)
III	• Ventricular tachycardia *(Amiodarone and sotalol, but not bretylium):* • Atrial fibrillation and flutter • Bypass-tract mediated PSVT
IV	• PSVT • Atrial fibrillation and flutter (↓ VR) • Multifocal atrial tachycardia (↓ VR)

PSVT, Paroxysmal supraventricular tachycardia; VR, Ventricular rate

17.13). The most common uses are for the conversion of atrial flutter or fibrillation to normal sinus rhythm, and as chronic treatment for reentrant supraventricular tachycardias, ventricular ectopic beats, and ventricular tachycardia.

Specific Class IA Drugs

Quinidine is the most commonly used oral antiarrhythmic drug. In addition to the electrophysiologic effects inherent to class IA agents, it also has an anticholinergic action that may *augment* conduction at the AV node, antagonizing its direct suppressant effect. Quinidine also displays an α-adrenergic blocking action that may cause hypotension, especially with parenteral intravenous administration. Therefore, it is generally administered only by the oral route. Because quinidine is metabolized primarily by the liver, its dosage must be reduced in patients with hepatic dysfunction.

Cardiac and noncardiac side effects occur frequently during quinidine therapy. The most common are related to the gastrointestinal tract, including diarrhea in one-third of patients. Cardiac toxicities are serious and potentially fatal. For example, excessive prolongation of the QT interval (usually > 0.5 sec) is associated with a form of life-threatening ventricular tachycardia known as torsades de pointes ("twisting of the points"), described in Chapter 12.

Quinidine also raises blood digoxin levels by decreasing the body's clearance and volume of distribution of the drug; digitalis-associated arrhythmias may therefore be precipitated. Thus, it is important to re-

duce the digoxin dosage by one-half when quinidine is initiated.

Finally, the anticholinergic effect of quinidine may actually *speed* AV nodal conduction, in contrast to its direct effect on tissue excitability, and cause an *acceleration* of the ventricular rate in patients with atrial fibrillation or flutter. This response is avoided by combining quinidine with a negative chronotropic agent such as digitalis, a β-blocker, verapamil or diltiazem.

The electrophysiologic effects of **procainamide** are similar to those of quinidine. They both depress phase 0 depolarization in the atria and ventricles, slow conduction, prolong the action potential duration and refractory period. However, there are several important differences between these two drugs. First, procainamide does not prolong the action potential (and QT interval) as much as quinidine, although toxic arrhythmias such as torsades de pointes can occur. Second, procainamide has less-pronounced anticholinergic effects than quinidine, so that facilitation of AV nodal conduction is less marked. Furthermore, procainamide does not produce α blockade, but does have mild ganglionic blocking effects that may cause peripheral vasodilatation and a negative cardiac inotropic effect, particularly when the drug is administered intravenously. However, because hypotension associated with intravenous procainamide is much less common than with quinidine, the former is used when an intravenous form of administration is required.

Procainamide can be administered by mouth, intramuscularly, or intravenously. More than 50% of procainamide is excreted unchanged in the urine; the remainder undergoes acetylation by the liver to form N-acetyl procainamide (NAPA), which is subsequently excreted by the kidneys. In renal failure, or in "rapid acetylators," high serum levels of NAPA may accumulate. NAPA shares procainamide's ability to prolong the action potential and refractory period, but it does not alter the rate of phase 4 depolarization or the slope of phase 0 upstroke of the action potential.

Early cardiac side effects of procainamide are similar to those of quinidine: In patients with atrial fibrillation or flutter, the ventricular rate may paradoxically increase, because of the anticholinergic properties of the drug. Proarrhythmic effects, such as torsades de pointes, appear to be dose-related.

Noncardiac side effects are common. Although GI symptoms are less often seen than with quinidine, fever and rash are frequent. Approximately one-third of patients develop a systemic lupus–like syndrome after 6 months of therapy, manifested by arthralgias, rash, and connective tissue inflammation. It most often occurs among slow acetylators, and is reversible upon cessation of the drug.

Disopyramide's electrophysiologic and antiarrhythmic effects are similar to those of quinidine. However, the two drugs have four main differences:

1. GI side effects are much less common with disopyramide.
2. Disopyramide does not increase serum digoxin levels.
3. Disopyramide has a much greater anticholinergic effect, so that common side effects include constipation, urinary re-

tention (bladder sphincter tone is ACh-dependent), and exacerbation of glaucoma (intraocular pressure is increased by the anticholinergic action).
4. Disopyramide, more so than quinidine or procainamide, has a pronounced negative inotropic effect and must be used with caution in patients with left ventricular contractile dysfunction.

Disopyramide is administered orally. The primary excretory pathway is via the kidneys, and toxic levels may accumulate in patients with renal insufficiency.

The most important side effects of disopyramide include precipitation of congestive heart failure and the anticholinergic side effects listed above. In addition, because of its negative inotropic effect, disopyramide should be administered cautiously, or not at all, in conjunction with other drugs that reduce ventricular contraction such as β-blockers or verapamil. Other cardiac side effects include QT prolongation and precipitation of ventricular arrhythmias (including torsades de pointes), similar to other type IA agents.

Class IB Antiarrhythmics

Class IB drugs inhibit the fast sodium channel and typically *shorten* the action potential duration and the refractory period. The shortening of the action potential is attributed to blockade of small sodium currents that normally continue through phase 2 of the action potential.

Class IB drugs at therapeutic concentrations do not substantially alter the electrical activity of normal tissue; rather, they preferentially act on diseased or ischemic cells. Conditions present during ischemia such as acidosis, faster rates of cell stimulation, increased extracellular potassium concentration, and less negative diastolic membrane potential all increase the ability of class IB drugs to block the sodium channel. These drugs promote conduction block in ischemic cells because of a reduction in the slope of phase 0 depolarization with slowing of the conduction velocity, thus inhibiting certain reentrant arrhythmias (Fig. 17.11). Similar to other class I drugs, the automaticity of ectopic pacemakers is also suppressed by decreasing phase 4 spontaneous depolarization and (in the case of some drugs of this class) by raising the threshold potential. In addition, intravenous lidocaine is useful in suppressing delayed afterdepolarizations.

Type IB agents have little effect on *atrial* tissue at therapeutic concentrations, due to the shorter atrial action potential (especially during tachycardia) allowing less time for the drug to bind to and block the Na^+ channel. Thus, these drugs are ineffective in atrial fibrillation, atrial flutter, and supraventricular tachycardias. Their most common use is in the suppression of ventricular arrhythmias, especially in association with ischemia or digitalis toxicity.

Because the QT interval is not prolonged by this group, early afterdepolarizations do not occur, and torsades de pointes is not an expected complication.

Specific Class IB Drugs

Lidocaine is the antiarrhythmic drug most commonly used acutely to suppress ventricular arrhythmias in hospitalized patients. It is administered intravenously only, because oral administration results in unpredictable plasma levels. As a result of rapid distribution and hepatic metabolism, lidocaine must be administered as a continuous infusion following two or three loading boluses. The half-life of the drug depends greatly on hepatic blood flow: Reduced flow (as in heart failure or in older individuals) or intrinsic liver disease can greatly increase serum lidocaine concentrations and toxic effects, and therefore the infusion rate must be lowered in such patients.

The most common side effects of lidocaine are not cardiac; rather, they are related to the central nervous system and include confusion, dizziness, and seizures. These effects are dose-related and can be prevented by following serum levels or re-ducing the infusion rate when liver disease or decreased hepatic blood flow is present.

Tocainide is an analog of lidocaine whose structure protects it from first-pass hepatic metabolism, so that it can be administered orally. Its electrophysiologic effects are similar to those of lidocaine. Toxic effects are common, and include those related to the CNS (dizziness, tremor, numbness) and to the GI tract (nausea, diarrhea). The potential for serious blood disorders, such as a decreased white blood cell count, have limited the usefulness of this drug. Approximately one-half of the dose of tocainide is excreted unchanged in the urine, so that administration must be reduced in patients with renal dysfunction.

Mexiletine is structurally similar to lidocaine and shares its electrophysiologic properties. Unlike lidocaine, but similar to tocainide, it is administered orally. Ninety percent of mexiletine is metabolized in the liver to inactive products, and the dosage of the drug should be reduced in patients with hepatic dysfunction.

Dose-related side effects of mexiletine are common, especially of the CNS (dizziness, tremor, slurred speech) and the GI tract (nausea, vomiting). The toxic hematologic effects of tocainide do not occur with mexiletine.

Diphenylhydantoin (DPH) is an antiseizure medication that is occasionally also used as an antiarrhythmic. Its role is generally limited to the treatment of digitalis-induced arrhythmias, because it inhibits triggered automaticity (digitalis-induced delayed afterdepolarizations) without worsening digitalis-induced AV block.

DPH can be administered by the intravenous or oral routes. It is primarily metabolized in the liver. Its degradation is slowed by hepatic disease and drugs that compete for hepatic enzymes, such as the phenothiazines and isoniazid. Serious adverse effects of DPH occur related to the CNS (ataxia, drowsiness, nystagmus) and GI tract (nausea, anorexia), and protracted use may cause hyperplasia of the gums and lymph nodes.

Class IC Antiarrhythmics

The class IC drugs are the most potent sodium channel blockers. They markedly decrease the upstroke of the action potential and conduction velocity in atrial, ventricular, and Purkinje fibers (Fig. 17.11). Although they have little effect on the duration of the action potential, repolarization, or refractory period of Purkinje fibers, the refractory period within the AV node and accessory bypass tracts is markedly prolonged.

The group IC agents are potent drugs that most commonly have been prescribed to treat ventricular arrhythmias. However, their use has come into question, as these drugs have significant proarrhythmic qualities. Studies have shown an *increased* mortality in patients taking members of this class (flecainide, encainide (no longer marketed) or moricizine) for asymptomatic ventricular ectopy following myocardial infarction. In addition, long-term treatment with the class IC drug propafenone *increased* mortality in patients surviving sudden cardiac arrest. Thus, drugs of this subclass are used only occasionally in the treatment of ventricular arrhythmias in patients who have other underlying heart abnormalities, such as coronary artery disease or heart failure. Recently, class IC drugs have been shown to be effective (and reasonably safe) in preventing supraventricular arrhythmias in patients who have otherwise healthy hearts.

In addition to its electrophysiologic effects, **flecainide** is a negative inotrope that can precipitate congestive heart failure in patients with reduced left ventricular function. Thus at present, its use is limited to the treatment of life-threatening ventricular arrhythmias and certain supraventricular arrhythmias (Table 17.13) in patients without other underlying structural heart disease.

Flecainide is well absorbed after oral administration. Approximately 40% of the drug is excreted unchanged in the urine, and the remainder is converted to inactive metabolites by the liver. As indicated above, cardiac toxicities include the aggravation of ventricular arrhythmias, and precipitation of congestive heart failure in patients with underlying left ventricular dysfunction. Noncardiac side effects are referable to the central nervous system and include confusion, dizziness, and blurred vision.

The electrophysiologic properties of **propafenone** are similar to those of flecainide, but in addition it has a weak β-adrenergic blocking action. It is metabolized by the liver, but there is much genetic variation, such that an individual's dosage must be carefully titrated by observing the drug's effect. It is not yet known whether propafenone shares the same proarrhythmic properties as the other IC agents. Extracardiac side effects are not common; they include dizziness and disturbances of taste.

Moricizine has both IB and IC properties. CNS-mediated side effects occur and include dizziness, vertigo, and agitation.

Class II Antiarrhythmics

The class II drugs are the β-adrenergic blockers, which are used in the management of both supraventricular and ventricular arrhythmias (Table 17.13). Most of the antiarrhythmic properties of this group can be attributed to inhibition of cardiac sympathetic activity. Additional actions of some β-blockers, such as β1 cardioselectivity or a "membrane stabilizing effect," seem to have little influence on antiarrhythmic activity.

Chapter 11 described how β-adrenergic stimulation results in an increased slope of phase 4 depolarization and an increased firing rate of the SA node. β-adrenergic blockers inhibit these effects, thus reducing automaticity (Fig. 17.12). This action extends to the cardiac Purkinje fibers, where arrhythmias due to *enhanced automaticity* are inhibited. In addition, because afterdepolarizations may be caused by excessive catecholamines, β-blockers may prevent *triggered arrhythmias* induced by that mechanism. All β-blockers increase the effective refractory period of the AV node, and there-

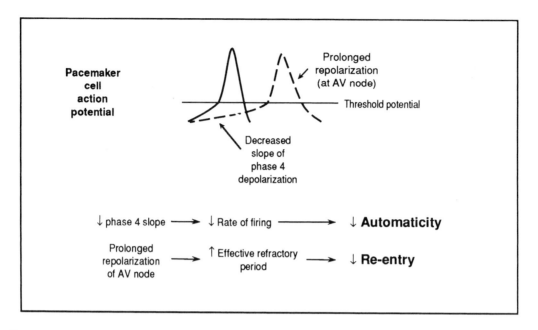

Figure 17.12. Electrophysiologic effects of the class II antiarrhythmic drugs on the pacemaker cell action potential.

fore, these drugs are effective at interrupting *reentrant rhythms* that pass through it. β-blockers may also have a beneficial antiarrhythmic effect by decreasing myocardial oxygen demand and reducing myocardial ischemia. Several drugs from this group have been shown to reduce mortality following myocardial infarction (see Chapter 7), which may in part relate to their antiarrhythmic effect.

β-blockers affect the EKG by prolonging the AV nodal conduction time so that the PR interval may become prolonged (Table 17.12). The QRS and QT intervals are usually unaffected.

Clinical Uses

β-blockers are most useful in suppressing tachyarrhythmias induced by excessive catecholamines (e.g., during exercise, emotional stimulation). They are also frequently used to slow the ventricular rate in atrial flutter and fibrillation by reducing conduction and increasing the refractoriness of the AV node. In addition, β-blockers may terminate reentrant supraventricular arrhythmias (e.g., PSVT) in which the AV node constitutes one limb of the reentrant pathway.

β-blockers are effective in suppressing ventricular premature beats and other ventricular arrhythmias, especially when induced by exercise, and in the treatment of coronary disease by reducing ischemia. They are also effective in treating ventricular arrhythmias in the setting of a prolonged QT interval because, unlike group IA agents, they do not prolong that interval.

The toxicities of β-blockers were presented earlier in this chapter.

Class III Antiarrhythmics

Class III drugs are structurally dissimilar from one another, but share the property of markedly prolonging the action potential and refractoriness of Purkinje and ventricular muscle fibers (Fig. 17.13). As opposed to class I agents, they generally have little effect on phase 0 depolarization or conduction velocity.

Amiodarone is a powerful antiarrhythmic with many potential adverse reactions. Its major therapeutic effect is to prolong the

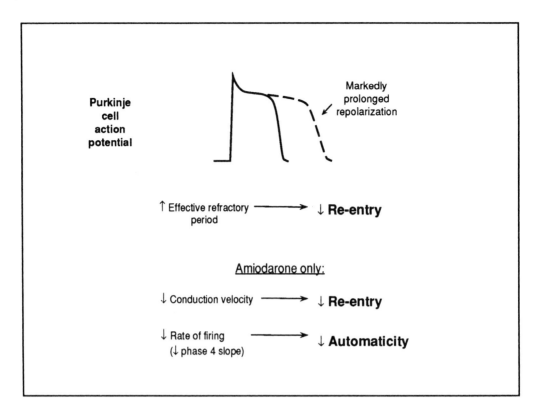

Figure 17.13.   Electrophysiologic effects of the class III antiarrhythmic drugs on the Purkinje cell action potential.

action potential duration and refractoriness of all cardiac fibers. However, it also shares actions with each of the other antiarrhythmic classes: The slope of phase 0 depolarization may be depressed through sodium channel blockade (class I effect), it exerts a β-blocking effect (class II), and also demonstrates weak calcium channel blockade (class IV). As a result, the electrophysiologic effects of amiodarone are to decrease the sinus node firing rate, suppress automaticity, interrupt reentrant circuits, and prolong the PR, QRS, and QT intervals on the EKG (Table 17.12).

In addition, amiodarone is a vasodilator (because of α-receptor and calcium channel blocking effects), and a negative inotrope (β-blocker and calcium channel blocker effects). The vasodilation is more prominent than the negative inotropic effect, so that cardiac output does not usually suffer in patients treated with this drug.

Although the use of amiodarone is sometimes limited by its potential toxicities and

very long half-life, it is more effective than most other antiarrhythmic drugs in preventing and treating a wide spectrum of ventricular and supraventricular tachyarrhythmias. These include atrial fibrillation, atrial flutter, ventricular tachycardia, ventricular flutter, and paroxysmal supraventricular tachycardias, including those involving bypass tracts. As a result, its use is expanding, particularly among patients with underlying ventricular dysfunction, who often develop proarrhythmic adverse events on other antiarrhythmic agents. In addition, *low-dose* regimens of amiodarone are generally effective and well-tolerated for long-term suppression of atrial fibrillation and flutter.

Amiodarone is absorbed slowly from the GI tract, requiring 5 to 6 hours to reach peak plasma concentrations. It is highly lipophilic, and thus extensively sequestered in tissues and undergoes very slow hepatic metabolism. Its elimination half-life is long and quite variable, averaging 25 to 60 *days*. The drug is excreted by the biliary tract, lacrimal glands, and skin, but not the kidney, so that its dosage need not be adjusted in patients with renal failure. However, the delayed onset of action and very long duration of action make amiodarone a difficult drug to regulate if side effects ensue.

There are numerous potential side effects associated with amiodarone's use. The most serious is pulmonary toxicity, manifested as a pneumonitis leading to pulmonary fibrosis. Its origin is unclear, but may represent a hypersensitivity reaction and, if recognized early, is reversible.

The other life-threatening side effects of amiodarone relate to cardiac toxicity: Symptomatic bradycardia and aggravation of ventricular arrhythmia each occur in approximately 2% of treated patients. As amiodarone significantly prolongs the QT interval, early afterdepolarizations and torsades de pointes can occur. In addition, because of amiodarone's negative inotropic effect, congestive heart failure can rarely be precipitated with intravenous use.

Gastrointestinal side effects include anorexia, nausea, and elevation of liver function tests, all of which improve with lower dosages of the drug. Abnormalities of thyroid function studies are also common, because amiodarone inhibits the peripheral conversion of T_4 to T_3; the serum T_4 rises and serum T_3 falls. Approximately 10% of patients will have changes in thyroid function without signs or symptoms, but frank hyperthyroidism or hypothyroidism occurs in 3%–5% of patients. Neurologic side effects include proximal muscle weakness, peripheral neuropathy, ataxia, tremors, headache, and sleep disturbances. Another common adverse effect is the development of corneal microdeposits that can be detected in almost all patients on amiodarone therapy, but these rarely affect vision.

As a result of these potential adverse effects, routine electrocardiograms, chest radiographs, and thyroid and liver function tests are performed in patients on chronic therapy. Amiodarone interacts with and increases the activity of certain drugs, including warfarin and digoxin, such that the dosages of these must be decreased. Be-

cause amiodarone prolongs the QT interval, other drugs that do the same should not be used concurrently, such as class IA antiarrhythmics. Other drugs that share negative chronotropic or negative inotropic effects (β-blockers, verapamil, diltiazem) should also generally be avoided.

Sotalol is a nonselective beta-blocker with additional antiarrhythmic properties. It prolongs the duration of the action potential, increases the refractory period of atrial and ventricular tissue, and inhibits conduction in accessory bypass tracts. The phase 0 upstroke velocity is not altered in the usual dosage range. Sotalol is effective against both supraventricular and ventricular arrhythmias. It is as effective as quinidine at preventing recurrent atrial fibrillation after cardioversion, but is better tolerated. It appears to be more potent than class I agents in the treatment of serious ventricular arrhythmias.

Sotalol is excreted exclusively by the kidneys, and its dosage must be adjusted in the presence of renal disease. Possible side effects include those of beta-blockers in general (see above). Like all drugs that prolong the QT interval, the most serious potential adverse effect is the triggering of the ventricular arrhythmia torsades de pointes.

Bretylium tosylate is a drug administered intravenously to treat life-threatening ventricular tachycardia or fibrillation. It is used when intravenous lidocaine and/or procainamide have failed, often in the setting of acute myocardial infarction. Its mechanism of action is different from all of the other antiarrhythmic agents in that it acts at postganglionic adrenergic nerve terminals, where it initially releases norepinephrine but then inhibits subsequent release. Thus, after initial stimulation, sympathetic activity of the heart decreases. The initial catecholamine release can transiently aggravate arrhythmias, but continued therapy lengthens the action potential duration and refractoriness of atrial, ventricular, and Purkinje fibers, and the threshold for ventricular fibrillation is substantially raised.

Immediately after bretylium administration, the blood pressure may rise because of the catecholamine release. However, significant orthostatic *hypotension* may follow because of the drug's antiadrenergic actions.

Ibutilide is an intravenous antiarrhythmic agent used for the acute conversion of atrial fibrillation or atrial flutter of recent onset. This agent prolongs the action potential duration and increases atrial and ventricular refractoriness. The mechanism relates to activation of a slow inward current that prolongs the plateau (phase 2) of the action potential, rather than by blocking outward potassium currents that is typical of other class III drugs. In clinical trials, the success rate for conversion of atrial flutter is approximately 60%, but only 30% for those in atrial fibrillation.

Since ibutilide prolongs the QT interval, the potentially fatal arrhythmia torsades de pointes can be precipitated, and the drug should be administered with careful electrocardiographic monitoring.

Class IV Antiarrhythmics

Class IV drugs exert their electrophysiologic effects by selective blockade of the slow L-type cardiac calcium channels, and include **verapamil** and **diltiazem,** but not nifedipine or the other dihydropyridines. They are most potent in tissues where the action potential depends on calcium currents, such as the sinoatrial and atrioventricular nodes. Within nodal tissue, calcium channel blockade decreases phase 4 spontaneous depolarization (resulting in decreased automaticity), elevates threshold, decreases the rate of rise of phase 0 depolarization and conduction velocity, and lengthens the refractory period of the AV node (Fig. 17.14). These electrophysiologic actions translate into their clinical effects:

1. The heart rate slows.
2. Transmission of rapid atrial impulses through the AV node to the ventricles decreases, thus slowing the ventricular rate in atrial fibrillation and atrial flutter.
3. Reentrant rhythms traveling through the AV node may terminate.

The primary antiarrhythmic use of class IV drugs, especially verapamil, is in the treatment of reentrant paroxysmal supraventricular tachycardia. Formerly, intravenous verapamil was the treatment of choice for acute episodes of this rhythm, but intravenous adenosine (see below) has now assumed that role. The class IV antiarrhythmics are also useful in slowing the ventricular rate in atrial fibrillation and flutter.

The pharmacology and toxicities of calcium channel blockers were presented earlier in this chapter. The most important side effect of verapamil or diltiazem, administered intravenously as an antiarrhythmic, is hypotension. In addition, these agents should be avoided in patients on β-blocker therapy, because of the additive negative inotropic and chronotropic effects.

Adenosine

Adenosine is an endogenous nucleoside with a very short half-life. Administered intravenously, it is currently the most useful drug for the termination of paroxysmal supraventricular tachycardia.

Adenosine has substantial electrophysiologic effects on specialized conduction tissues, especially the sinoatrial and atrioventricular nodes. By binding to myocyte surface receptors, it activates specific potassium channels (Fig. 17.15). The resultant increase in the outward potassium current hyperpolarizes the membrane potential, and therefore decreases spontaneous depolarization of the sinoatrial node.

In addition, adenosine decreases intracellular cyclic AMP (cAMP) concentrations by inhibiting adenylate cyclase, the result of which is a decrease in the inward pacemaker current (I_f), as well as a decreased calcium inward current (Fig. 17.15). The net effect of adenosine, then, is to slow the SA node firing rate and to decrease AV nodal conduction. Ventricular myocytes are relatively immune to these effects, at least in part because the specific potassium channels responsive to adenosine are not present in those cells.

Transient AV block induced by adenosine terminates reentrant pathways that include the AV node as part of the circuit.

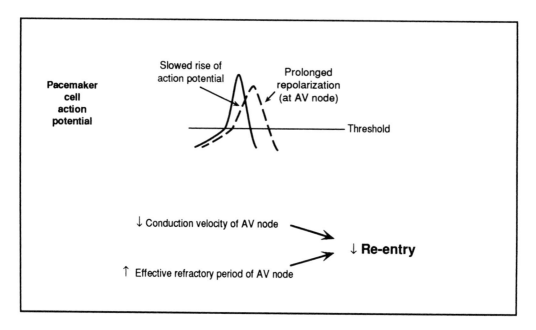

Figure 17.14. Electrophysiologic effects of the class IV antiarrhythmic drugs on the pacemaker cell action potential.

Since the half-life of adenosine is only 10 sec, side effects (headache, chest pain, flushing, bronchoconstriction) are very transient. Because methylxanthines (caffeine, theophylline) competitively antagonize the adenosine receptor, higher doses of adenosine may be necessary in patients using those substances. Conversely, dipyridamole inhibits the breakdown of adenosine, and amplifies its effect.

In summary, the antiarrhythmic drugs have complex actions with multiple cardiac and noncardiac toxicities. The potential of inducing dangerous arrhythmias exists with most agents.

Although symptomatic or life-threatening rhythm disturbances may warrant antiarrhythmic drug therapy, there is a trend away from treating asymptomatic arrhythmias, no matter how dangerous they appear, because of the potential adverse drug effects. For example, there is thus far no evidence that treating asymptomatic ventricular arrhythmias following myocardial infarction prolongs survival, and drugs of antiarrhythmic class IC have been shown to increase mortality in that setting, as indicated above. Concerns about the long-term

effects and safety of antiarrhythmic drugs have prompted the development of non-pharmacologic means of treatment, such as surgical or catheter ablation of aberrant pathways and ectopic tissue, and implantation of electrical defibrillators.

Whenever antiarrhythmic drugs are used, patients must be followed closely, the effectiveness of the drug demonstrated, and surveillance for toxicity continued over the long term through repeated examination, measurement of drug levels, electrocardiographic monitoring, and sometimes invasive electrophysiologic testing.

DIURETICS

Diuretics increase the renal excretion of Na^+ and H_2O, and are most often used in the treatment of heart failure and hypertension. In heart failure, enhanced renal reabsorption of sodium and water, with subsequent expansion of the extracellular volume, contributes greatly to peripheral edema and pulmonary congestion. Diuretics eliminate excess sodium and water, and are therefore the cornerstone of therapy to

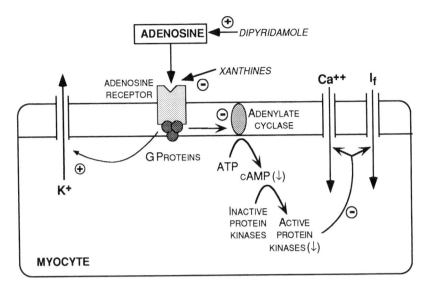

Figure 17.15.   Mechanism of antiarrhythmic action of adenosine. Stimulation of the myocyte adenosine receptor activates potassium channels, and the resultant outward K^+ current hyperpolarizes the membrane (resulting in decreased automaticity). Adenosine also inhibits membrane adenylate cyclase activity; the subsequent reduction in active protein kinases decreases the inward pacemaker (I_f) and Ca^{++} currents (resulting in decreased automaticity and decreased conduction through the AV node). Xanthines compete for the adenosine receptor, blocking these effects. Dipyridamole interferes with cellular uptake and degradation of adenosine, and therefore amplifies its effect.

relieve congestive symptomatology (see Chapter 9). In the treatment of hypertension, diuretics act in part by elimination of intravascular volume, and in some cases through vascular dilatation.

In the kidney, the rate of glomerular filtration typically averages 135 to 180 L/day in normal adults. Most of the filtered Na^+ is reabsorbed by the renal tubules, leaving only a small quantity in the final urine (Fig. 17.16). Approximately 65% to 70% of the filtered Na^+ is reabsorbed isoosmotically in the proximal tubule by active transport. In the thick ascending limb of the loop of Henle (LOH), an additional 25% of the filtered sodium is reabsorbed, through a Na^+/K^+ cotransport system coupled to the uptake of two Cl^- ions. Because this region is impermeable to the reabsorption of water, hypotonic tubular fluid is formed here, and the surrounding interstitium becomes hypertonic. In the distal convoluted tubule, an additional small fraction of NaCl is reabsorbed (approximately 5%). In the cortical collecting duct, Na^+ permeability is modulated by an aldosterone-sensitive mecha-

nism, such that Na^+ is reabsorbed into the tubular cells in the presence of aldosterone, creating a lumen negative potential difference that enhances K^+ and H^+ excretion. Approximately 1%–2% of sodium reabsorption takes place at this location.

All but the terminal segment of the distal tubule is impermeable to water. In the cortical collecting tubule, however, water permeability and reabsorption is promoted by antidiuretic hormone (ADH) and driven by the osmotic gradient between the tubule and the hypertonic interstitium. Substances that interfere with ADH, such as ethanol consumption, therefore have diuretic actions.

The three most commonly used groups of diuretics are the loop diuretics, thiazide diuretics, and potassium-sparing diuretics (Table 17.14 and Fig. 17.16). These three classes are generally distinguished by the site of the kidney tubule where they act, and the potency by which they do so. Loop diuretics impair absorption in the thick ascending limb of the loop of Henle, thiazide diuretics act on the distal tubule

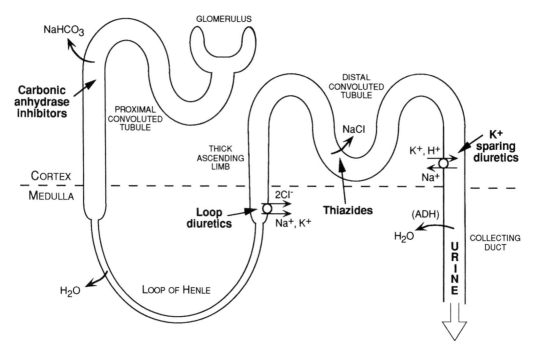

Figure 17.16. Schematic diagram of the renal tubules. Approximately 70% of filtered sodium is reabsorbed in the proximal convoluted tubule (PCT), 25% in the thick ascending limb of the loop of Henle, 5% in the distal convoluted tubule (DCT), and 1% to 2% in the cortical collecting tubule (mediated by the action of aldosterone). Antidiuretic hormone (ADH) increases the permeability of the distal nephron for water. Diuretics are secreted into the PCT and act at the sites shown.

and collecting segment, and potassium-sparing diuretics act on the aldosterone-sensitive region of the cortical collecting tubule. A fourth group, the carbonic anhydrase inhibitors, are weak diuretics rarely used in the treatment of hypertension or heart failure. They act at the proximal convoluted tubule, resulting in a loss of bicarbonate (and sodium) in the urine.

Diuretics, as the active pharmacologic agents, are secreted into the proximal renal tubule, and their major sites of action are shown schematically in Figure 17.16.

Loop Diuretics

These agents are so named because they act principally on the thick ascending limb of the loop of Henle (LOH). They are powerful diuretics that result in the excretion of 20% to 25% of the filtered Na^+ load through inhibition of the $Na^+/2Cl^-/K^+$ cotransport system. Because inhibition at this site im-

pairs the generation of a hypertonic interstitium, the gradient for passive water movement out of the collecting duct is diminished and water diuresis results.

Loop diuretics are of great importance in the acute management of pulmonary edema (administered intravenously) and in the management of chronic congestive heart failure or peripheral edema (given orally). Unlike most other diuretics, they tend to be effective even in the setting of impaired renal function. In addition to the diuretic effect, and even preceding it, drugs of this class may induce venodilatation, which is also of benefit in reducing venous return and pulmonary congestion (see Chapter 9). The mechanism of venodilatation appears to involve drug-induced prostaglandin generation, which acts to relax vascular smooth muscle.

Among the most common side effects of the loop diuretics are intravascular volume depletion, hypokalemia, and metabolic alkalosis. *Hypokalemia* arises because: 1) these

TABLE 17.14. Commonly Used Diuretics

Diuretic		Onset of Action (hours)	Duration of Action (hours)	Potential Adverse Effects
Thiazides				Hypokalemia, hypomagnesemia,
Chlorothiazide	PO:	1	6–12	hyponatremia, hypercalcemia,
	IV:	0.25	2	hyperglycemia, hyperuricemia,
Hydrochlorothiazide	PO:	2	12	hypercholesterolemia,
Chlorthalidone	PO:	2	24	hypertriglyceridemia, metabolic
Metolazone	PO:	1	12–24	alkalosis
Indapamide	PO:	1–2	16–36	
Loop Diuretics				Hypotension, hypokalemia,
Furosemide	PO:	1	6	hypomagnesemia,
	IV:	5 min	2	hyperglycemia, hyperuricemia,
Bumetanide	PO:	0.5–1	4–6	metabolic alkalosis
	IV:	0.25	0.5–1	
Torsemide	PO:	< 1	6–8	
	IV:	10 min	6–8	
Ethacrynic acid	IV:	0.25	3	
Potassium-Sparing Diuretics				Hyperkalemia, GI disturbances
Spironolactone	PO:	1–2 days	2–3 days	(spironolactone only): gynecomastia
Triamterene	PO:	2	12–16	
Amiloride	PO:	2	24	

agents impair the reabsorption of sodium in the loop of Henle, such that an increased amount of Na^+ is delivered to the distal tubule, where it prompts greater-than-usual exchange for potassium (and therefore more K^+ excretion into the urine); and 2) diuretic-induced intravascular volume depletion activates the renin-angiotensin system. The subsequent rise in aldosterone promotes additional Na^+/K^+ exchange, and hence hypokalemia. Administration of K^+ supplements, or a potassium-sparing diuretic, can offset the development of hypokalemia.

Metabolic alkalosis during loop diuretic therapy results from two mechanisms: 1) increased H^+ secretion into the distal tubule (and therefore into the urine) due to the secondary hyperaldosteronism described above, and 2) contraction alkalosis—increased sodium bicarbonate reabsorption by the proximal tubule (Fig. 17.16) is promoted by the reduced intravascular volume.

Additional side effects may also occur during loop diuretic therapy. *Hypomagnesemia* may result, because magnesium reabsorption depends on NaCl transport in the thick ascending limb of the LOH, the action blocked by these drugs. *Ototoxicity* (eighth

cranial nerve toxicity) can occasionally develop, impairing hearing and vestibular function. It is thought to arise from electrolyte disturbances of the endolymphatic system, most likely because of $Na^+/2Cl^-/K^+$ cotransport inhibition by the loop diuretic at that site.

The most commonly used loop diuretic is **furosemide,** the oral form of which demonstrates reliable gastrointestinal absorption but a short duration of action (4 to 6 hours), which limits its usefulness in the treatment of chronic hypertension. **Bumetanide** is a congener of furosemide, and shares its actions and adverse effects, but has greater potency and bioavailability. It also appears to have a lower incidence of ototoxcitity than the other drugs of this class. Bumetanide is sometimes useful in CHF when edema is refractory to other agents, and in individuals allergic to furosemide. **Torsemide** is a recently introduced loop diuretic that is effective in the treatment of hypertension at low dosage (with minimal diuretic effect), while at higher dosage, its diuretic action is similar to furosemide. **Ethacrynic acid** is the only nonsulfonamide loop diuretic and thus can be prescribed to patients who cannot tolerate sulfonamide compounds. However, ethacrynic acid is not widely used because of its relatively high incidence of ototoxicity.

Thiazide Diuretics

Thiazides and related compounds (chlorthalidone, indapamide, and metolazone) are commonly used diuretics because they demonstrate excellent GI absorption when administered orally, and are usually well tolerated. They are less potent than the loop diuretics, but, because of their sustained actions, they are useful in chronic conditions such as essential hypertension and mild congestive heart failure.

This class of drugs acts at the distal tubule, where they block the reabsorption of approximately 3% to 5% of the filtered sodium (Fig. 17.16). Na^+ reabsorption at this site is mediated through a Na^+/Cl^- cotransporter on the luminal membrane. The thiazides inhibit this carrier by a mechanism that has not been elucidated, but may involve competition for the Cl^- site. The antihypertensive effect is initially associated with a decrease in cardiac output, due to reduced intravascular volume, and unchanged peripheral resistance. With long-term thiazide use, however, cardiac output often returns to normal as total peripheral resistance becomes reduced by an unexplained vascular dilatation. **Indapamide** is unique among this class in that it displays a particularly prominent vasodilating effect.

Thiazides are most often administered orally. Diuresis occurs after 1 to 2 hours, but the full antihypertensive effect of continued therapy may not become manifest for up to 12 weeks (possibly related to the vasodilator mechanism alluded to above). **Chlorothiazide,** the parent compound, has a low lipid solubility and hence low bioavailability: Higher doses are therefore required to achieve therapeutic levels compared with the more commonly used **hydrochlorothiazide**. **Chlorthalidone** is slowly absorbed and hence has a long duration of action. **Metolazone,** unlike other drugs of this class, is sometimes effective in patients with reduced renal function.

Clinically, the thiazides differ from the loop diuretics in that they are less potent, have a longer duration of action, and (with the exception of metolazone) demonstrate poor diuretic efficacy in the setting of impaired renal function: They are generally not effective when the glomerular filtration rate is < 25 ml/min.

Thiazides have traditionally served as the cornerstone of antihypertensive therapy because of their low cost and general effectiveness. They are particularly effective in individuals with "volume-dependent" hypertension such as blacks and patients of advanced age (see Chapter 13). Because of potential adverse effects, however, other agents, including ACE inhibitors and Ca^{++} channel blockers, have risen to compete with diuretics as first-line antihypertensive therapy.

Thiazides are sometimes used in heart failure, generally for patients with mild chronic congestive symptoms. In addition, they can be combined with a loop diuretic for heart failure patients who have become refractory to the diuretic effect of the latter. The combination of the two classes lowers the dose-dependent adverse effects that accompany each drug, and because they act on sequential segments of the renal tubule, a more profound natriuretic effect ensues than with either agent used alone.

Among the most important potential adverse effects of thiazides are: 1) *hypokalemia* and *metabolic alkalosis,* which result in part from increased Na^+ delivery to the distal tubule, where exchange for K^+ and H^+ takes place, and partly from volume contraction and secondary hyperaldosteronism, as described for the loop diuretics above; 2) *hyponatremia,* which may occur during prolonged treatment because of continued Na^+ excretion in the setting of chronic free water consumption; 3) *hyperuricemia* (and possible precipitation of gout), which results from decreased clearance of uric acid; 4) *hyperglycemia,* which may occur because of either impaired pancreatic insulin release, or decreased peripheral glucose utilization; 5) *dyslipidemia,* which is characterized by increased LDL and triglycerides; and 6) *weakness, fatigability,* and *paresthesias,* which can occur with long-term use because of volume depletion and hypokalemia. Serum calcium levels often rise slightly during thiazide therapy, but this is uncommonly of clinical significance.

In past decades, the standard thiazide dosage was excessive compared with current practice. By using lower dosages, it is possible to accrue the benefits of this class of diuretics, while minimizing the adverse effects listed above.

Potassium-Sparing Diuretics

These agents are relatively weak diuretics that antagonize physiologic Na^+ reabsorption at the distal convoluted tubule and cortical collecting tubule. Potassium-sparing diuretics reduce K^+ excretion, and thus lessen the risk of hypokalemia. They are used when maintenance of serum potassium levels is crucial, and in states characterized by aldosterone excess (primary or secondary hyperaldosteronism). Two types of drugs make up this group: 1) aldosterone antagonists (e.g., spironolactone) and 2) direct inhibitors of Na^+ permeability in the collecting duct, which act independently of aldosterone (e.g., triamterene and amiloride).

Na^+ and K^+ exchange in the collecting tubules accounts for only a small percentage of sodium reuptake, so that a clinically important diuresis does not occur with these agents when used alone. Rather, they are often used in combination with the loop or thiazide classes for additive diuretic effect, and to prevent clinically important hypokalemia.

Spironolactone is a synthetic steroid that competes for the cytoplasmic aldosterone receptor, thereby inhibiting the aldosterone-sensitive Na^+ channel. Because Na^+ reabsorption through that channel is inhibited, no lumen-negative potential exists to drive K^+ and H^+ ion excretion at the distal nephron sites; thus, K^+ and H^+ ions are retained in the circulation.

The most serious complication of spironolactone treatment is the development of hyperkalemia, resulting from its im-

paired excretion. Thus, one should *avoid routine administration of K^+ supplements or ACE inhibitors (which also decrease serum aldosterone concentration) when potassium-sparing diuretics are used*, as they could contribute to this complication. Spironolactone also displays antiandrogenic activity that may produce gynecomastia in men and menstrual irregularities in women.

Triamterene and **amiloride** are structurally related potassium-sparing diuretics, possessing similar pharmacodynamic actions, that act *independently* of spironolactone. At the distal tubules, they inhibit the Na^+ channel, and therefore the excretion of K^+ and H^+ is diminished. Triamterene is metabolized by the liver, and its active product is secreted into the proximal tubule by the organic cation transport system. Amiloride is secreted directly into the proximal tubule, and appears unchanged in the urine. As with spironolactone, the most important potential adverse effect of these drugs is the development of hyperkalemia.

ANTITHROMBOTIC DRUGS

Platelets and the coagulation proteins play a key role in the pathogenesis of many cardiovascular disorders, including the acute coronary syndromes (unstable angina, acute myocardial infarction), deep venous thrombosus, and thrombi that may complicate atrial fibrillation, dilated cardiomyopathy, or mechanical prosthetic heart valves. Therefore, the modulation of platelet function and of the coagulation pathway is often critically important in cardiovascular therapeutics.

The formation of a thrombus, whether in normal hemostasis or in pathological clot formation, requires three events: 1) exposure of circulating blood elements to thrombogenic material (e.g., unmasking of subendothelial collagen after atherosclerotic plaque rupture), 2) activation of platelets, and 3) triggering of the coagulation cascade, ultimately resulting in a fibrin clot. Hemostasis effected by platelets and the coagulation system are closely interlinked — activated platelets accelerate the coagulation pathway, and certain coagulation proteins (e.g., thrombin) contribute to platelet aggregation.

In this section, we focus first on drugs that interfere with platelet function, then those that inhibit the coagulation cascade. Thrombolytic (also termed fibrinolytic) agents, which dissolve clots that have already formed, are described in Chapter 7.

Platelet Inhibitors

Platelets are responsible for primary hemostasis by a three part activation process: 1) adhesion to the site of injury, 2) release reaction (secretion of platelet products and activation of key surface receptors), and 3)

aggregation. For example, following blood vessel injury, platelets quickly *adhere* to exposed subendothelial elements (e.g., collagen) by means of membrane glycoprotein receptors, a process that is dependent on von Willebrand factor. Following adhesion to the vessel wall, platelets *release* the preformed contents of their granules (including calcium, ADP, serotonin, and thrombin). Platelet activation and granule secretion are stimulated by the binding of agonists (e.g., collagen and thrombin). During this process, platelet activation promotes *de novo* synthesis and secretion of thromboxane A_2 (TXA_2), a powerful vasoconstrictor and promoter of platelet aggregation (Fig. 17.17). ADP, thrombin and TXA_2 cause platelets to *aggregate* and

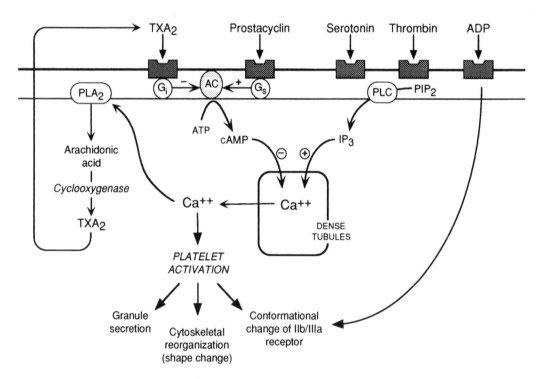

Figure 17.17. Platelet activation is mediated by intracytosolic [Ca^{++}]. Factors that promote and inhibit calcium release from the platelet dense tubules are shown. Thrombin and serotonin, acting at their specific receptors, stimulate the formation of inositol triphosphate (IP$_3$) from phosphatidylinositol diphosphosphate (PIP$_2$) by phospholipase C (PLC). IP$_3$ subsequently enhances the intracellular release of calcium. Thromboxane A$_2$ (TXA$_2$) also facilitates calcium release: It inhibits adenyl cyclase (AC) and reduces cyclic AMP (cAMP) formation. Since cAMP normally *prevents* Ca^{++} release from the ER, the reduction of this effect by TXA$_2$ *increases* Ca^{++} release into the cytosol. Conversely, endothelial-derived prostacyclin has the opposite effect: It reduces intraplatelet calcium release because it *stimulates* AC activity and cAMP formation. Calcium promotes the action of phospholopase A$_2$ (PLA$_2$), which generates the precursors of TXA$_2$ from the cell membrane. Platelet activation modulated by [Ca^{++}] ultimately results in granule secretion, cytoskeletal reorganization, and the critical conformational change in glycoprotein IIb/IIIa receptors that is necessary for platelet aggregation. ADP also contributes to the later action, through intermediaries that have not yet been defined.

thereby contribute to the formation of the primary hemostatic plug. During activation, there is also a critical conformational change in platelet membrane glycoprotein IIb/IIIa receptors. This alteration allows the previously inactive IIb/IIIa receptor to bind fibrinogen molecules, an act that tightly links platelets to one another, mediating the aggregation process.

Platelet activation is regulated to a great extent by release of stored Ca^{++} from the platelet dense tubular system. This action results in an increase in the intracytosolic calcium concentration, activation of protein kinases and ultimate phosphorylation of intraplatelet regulatory proteins. The increase in intracytosolic $[Ca^{++}]$ also stimulates phospholipase A_2, causing the release of arachidonic acid, the precursor of TXA_2 (Fig. 17.17). Calcium release is modulated by several factors. Acting at their respective platelet membrane receptors, thrombin and other agonists generate intermediaries that *stimulate* the release of calcium from the dense tubules (Fig. 17.17). TXA_2 increases the intracellular $[Ca^{++}]$ by binding to its platelet receptor, which *inhibits* the activity of adenylate cylase and thereby reduces cAMP formation and release of Ca^{++} from the dense tubules (Fig. 17.17). Converesely, endothelial cell-derived prostacyclin (PGI_2) *stimulates* adenylate cyclase activity, increases platelet cAMP concentration, and *inhibits* Ca^{++} release from the dense tubular system.

Current antiplatelet drugs interfere with platelet function at various points along the sequence of activation and aggregation. The most commonly used antiplatelet drug is aspirin. Other agents in clinical use include dipyridamole and ticlopidine. Potent new drugs that block the platelet IIb/IIIa receptor are under active study, and their roles in cardiovascular therapeutics are currently being defined.

Aspirin

As described in the previous section, TXA_2, an arachidonic acid metabolite, is an important mediator of platelet activation and clot formation. Aspirin (acetylsalicylic acid) acts by irreversibly acetylating (and thus blocking the action of) cyclooxygenase, an enzyme essential to prostaglandin and thromboxane synthesis from arachidonic acid (Fig. 17.17). Because platelets lack a nucleus and are therefore unable to synthesize new proteins, aspirin *permanently* disables TXA_2 production in exposed cells.

PGI_2, a major antagonist of TXA_2 that is produced by endothelial cells, shares a dependency upon cyclooxygenase activity for its formation, and aspirin, at high dosage, can impair its synthesis as well. Unlike platelets, however, endothelial cells *are* able to generate new cyclooxygenase to replace what has been deactivated by acetylation. Thus, when used in low dosage, aspirin effectively inhibits platelet TXA_2 synthesis without significantly interfering with the presence and beneficial actions of PGI_2.

Since the antiplatelet effect of aspirin is limited to inhibition of TXA_2 formation, platelet aggregation induced by other factors (e.g., ADP, collagen) is not significantly impeded. Thus, aspirin is not a "complete" antithrombotic agent.

Clinical Uses

Aspirin therapy has many proven clinical benefits in patients with cardiovascular disease (Table 17.15). In individuals with unstable angina, acute myocardial infarction, or a history of MI, aspirin conclusively reduces the incidence of future fatal and nonfatal coronary events. Similarly, in patients with chronic stable angina *without* a history of MI, aspirin successfully lessens the occurrence of subsequent myocardial infarction and mortality. In patients who have suffered a minor stroke or transient cerebral ischemic attacks, aspirin reduces the rate of future stroke and of cardiovascular events. And in patients who have undergone coronary artery bypass surgery, aspirin lessens the likelihood of graft occlusion.

The use of aspirin in patients for *primary* prevention (i.e., individuals without a history of cardiovascular events or symptoms) is of less clear benefit. When tested in a large

TABLE 17.15. Current Uses of Antithrombotic Drugs

Drug	Chronic angina	Unstable angina	Acute MI	Post-MI	Post-CABG	Transient ischemic attack	Proximal vein DVT	Mechanical heart valve	Atrial fibrillation
Platelet inhibitors									
Aspirin	+	+	+	+	+	+		(1)	(2)
Dipyridamole								(3)	
Ticlopidine						+			
Abciximab (4)									
Anticoagulants									
Heparin		+	(5)				+	(6)	(6)
LMWH							(7)		
Warfarin				(8)		(9)	+	+	+

(1) Sometimes used in combination with warfarin
(2) If patient at low risk of stroke, or if warfarin contraindicated
(3) Sometimes used in combination with warfarin for recurrent embolism, but combination of ASA + warfarin is better
(4) This platelet glycoprotein IIb/IIIa inhibitor is currently approved for use only in high-risk angioplasties
(5) After thrombolytic therapy with tPA, or if large akinetic segment present
(6) For hospitalized patients unable to take wafarin
(7) For prophylaxis after hip or knee replacement or abdominal surgery
(8) For 3–6 months if large akinetic segment present
(9) If an embolic source is identified
LMWH, Low molecular weight heparin; DVT, Deep venous thrombosis

cohort of healthy American middle-aged men, aspirin was associated with a reduced incidence of nonfatal MI, but an *increased* rate of nonfatal hemorrhagic stroke and gastrointestinal bleeding; there was no effect on total vascular mortality. Thus, while aspirin displays an extremely important role in patients with known cardiovascular disease, it is not evident that otherwise healthy people should routinely take aspirin for cardiovascular "protection." Large scale studies are in progress that are designed to shed more light on this issue.

At present, it is recommended that aspirin (in a low dosage of 75–325 mg/d) be administered to patients with clinical manifestations of coronary disease, in the absence of contraindications (i.e., aspirin allergy or complications described below). It should not be prescribed routinely for primary prevention purposes in healthy individuals. Pending the results of ongoing research, many physicians believe it appropriate to *consider* aspirin use in men > age 50 with multiple cardiac risk factors (i.e., a high likelihood of developing coronary disease, as described in Chapter 5). Finally, aspirin is not as beneficial as warfarin (described below) for the prevention of stroke in high-risk patients with atrial fibrillation,

and should only be used in that setting when warfarin cannot be safely administered.

Side effects

The most common adverse effects of aspirin are related to the gastrointestinal system, including dyspepsia and nausea, which often can be ameliorated by lowering the dosage and/or using enteric coated or buffered tablets. More serious potential side effects include gastrointestinal bleeding and hemorrhagic strokes. Since aspirin is excreted by the kidneys and competes with uric acid for the renal proximal tubule organic anion transporter, it may occasionally exacerbate gout.

Other Antiplatelet Drugs

Dipyridamole is sometimes used in patients who are intolerant to aspirin, but it is not as effective. It interferes with platelet adhesion to sites of vascular injury, it may potentiate the antiplatelet effect of PGI_2, and in high dosage, it enhances platelet cAMP levels, which lower cytosolic $[Ca^{++}]$ and inhibit platelet aggregation (Fig. 17.17).

By itself, dipyridamole has no proven

benefits, and should not be substituted for aspirin unless a patient is intolerant of the latter. It is used occasionally in combination with warfarin for an augmented anti-thrombotic effect in patients with recurrent thromboembolism from prosthetic heart valves, but the combination of aspirin plus warfarin is more effective. A more common contemporary use for dipyridamole is as a pharmacologic stress testing agent (see Chapters 3 and 6), in which it is administered intravenously to block cellular disposal of adenosine, thereby enhancing the coronary vasodilating actions of the latter.

Side effects of dipyridamole include gastrointestinal irritation, headache, dizziness, flushing, and sometimes angina pectoris secondary to excessive coronary vasodilation.

Platelet aggregation and contraction require a conformational change of the platelet membrane glycoprotein (GP) IIb/IIIa receptor that binds fibrinogen. **Ticlopidine,** or possibly one of its metabolites, inhibits this aspect of platelet function by irreversibly blocking the activation of the GP IIb/IIIa receptor, such that fibrinogen cannot bind and aggregation and contraction are prevented.

Ticlopidine is beneficial for the prevention of thrombotic stroke in patients who have suffered a prior stroke or transient cerebral ischemic attacks. However, its use has been limited out of concern for its most serious side effect, agranulocytosis, which can be life-threatening. Thus it is generally prescribed only for patients who are intolerant of aspirin. The short-term use of ticlopidine appears promising for the prevention of occlusion following placement of intracoronary stents.

A critical common pathway in platelet aggregation is the binding of fibrinogen molecules to exposed GP IIb/IIIa receptors, causing platelets to link together. Monoclonal antibodies have been manufactured that bind to this platelet receptor and inhibit aggregation. The first of these agents, **abciximab**, effectively prevents the binding of fibrinogen, von Willebrand factor, and other adhesive molecules to the IIb/IIIa receptor, and has been shown to reduce the

incidence of cardiac ischemic complications following coronary angioplasty. These agents are under active study for other possible benefits in ischemic syndromes.

Anticoagulant Drugs

Anticoagulant drugs interfere with the coagulation cascade, so as to impair secondary hemostasis. Since the final step in both the intrinsic and extrinsic coagulation pathways is the formation of a fibrin clot by the action of thrombin, major goals of anticoagulant therapy are to inhibit the activity of thrombin (e.g., heparin and similar compounds) or to decrease the production of functional prothrombin (e.g., warfarin).

Heparin

Heparin is a highly charged mucopolysaccharide polymer with multiple effects on coagulation. Although it has little anticoagulant effect by itself, it associates with antithrombin III (AT III) in the circulation, greatly increasing its anticoagulant properties. AT III is a natural protein that inhibits the action of thrombin, as well as other clotting factors. When heparin complexes with AT III, the affinity of the latter for thrombin increases 1000-fold, greatly interfering with thrombin's ability to generate fibrin from fibrinogen. The heparin-AT III complex also inhibits activated factor X, additionally contributing to the anticoagulant action. Furthermore, heparin demonstrates antiplatelet properties by binding to, and blocking the action of, von Willebrand factor.

Heparin is administered parenterally, as it is not absorbed from the GI tract. For most acute indications, an intravenous bolus injection is followed by a continuous infusion of the drug. The bioavailability of heparin varies from patient to patient because it is manufactured as a heterogeneous collection of molecules that bind to plasma proteins, macrophages and endothelial cells. Since some of these neutralize heparin's effect, the individual dose-effect relationship is often not predictable, and proper control of the drug's infusion rate requires frequent monitoring of blood studies for the anticoagulant effect (most commonly, the activated partial thromboplastin time).

The usual cardiovascular settings in which intravenous heparin is indicated include: 1) *unstable angina* (Chapter 6), 2) *acute MI* after thrombolytic therapy with tPA or if an extensive wall motion abnormality results (Chapter 7), 3) *pulmonary embolism* or *deep venous thrombosis (DVT)* of proximal veins (Chapter 15), and 4) when a patient on chronic anticoagulant therapy is unable to ingest the oral drug (e.g., perioperatively in a patient who has a mechanical prosthetic heart valve). Among hospitalized or bedridden patients not on intravenous heparin, fixed low dosages of *subcutaneous* heparin are often administered to prevent DVT.

The most important side effect of heparin is *bleeding*, including the possibility of intracranial hemorrhage with excessive anticoagulation. Heparin-induced *thrombocytopenia* occurs in approximately 2.5% of patients. It is asymptomatic in milder forms (in which thrombocytopenia is thought to result from direct heparin-induced platelet aggregation), but in more severe cases can lead to bleeding or *thrombosis* (due to the development of antiplatelet antibodies that result in platelet aggregation). Patients on long-term heparin therapy may develop a form of osteoporosis (decreased bone formation and increased rate of bone resorption) by a mechanism that has not yet been elucidated.

An overdose of heparin, or a life-threatening bleeding complication during its administration, can be treated with intravenous protamine sulfate, which forms a stable complex with heparin and immediately reverses the anticoagulation effect.

Low Molecular Weight Heparin

Some of the shortcomings of standard heparin (e.g., short half-life, unpredictable bioavailability) have been addressed by the development of low molecular weight heparin (LMWH), a recent entry into the clinical arena. LMWH is produced by depolymerization of standard heparin, yielding fragments approximately one-third the size. LMWH interacts with AT III, and this complex preferentially inhibits coagulation factor Xa. Theoretical advantages of LMWH over standard heparin are: 1) it can inhibit platelet-bound factor Xa, and thus may be a more effective anticoagulant, 2) it demonstrates less binding to plasma proteins and endothelial cells, so that it has more predictable bioavailability and a longer half-life, and 3) it has less of an effect on platelet function, so may be subject to fewer bleeding complications. From a practical standpoint, the major advantage is that LMWH is much easier to use: It can be administered as a subcutaneous injection once a day in a fixed dose, without laboratory monitoring.

In clinical studies, LMWH is at least as effective and safe as standard heparin in the prevention of DVT. Furthermore, the incidence of thrombocytopenia is much lower with LMWH. At the time of this writing, LMWH is approved for DVT prevention following hip, knee, or abdominal surgery, but it is likely that its clinical indications will continue to expand.

Direct Thrombin Inhibitors

The anticoagulation effect of heparin is limited because of its dependence upon AT III for its activity, and because it only inhibits *circulating* thrombin. Thrombin already bound to fibrin *within* a clot is resistant to the anticoagulant effect by the large heparin-AT III complex. Direct thrombin inhibitors are investigational agents that inhibit thrombin activity independently of AT III, are effective against both circulating thrombin and clot-bound thrombin, and may therefore be more effective anticoagulants. Unlike heparin, they do not result in thrombocytopenia.

Warfarin

Warfarin is an *oral* agent prescribed for long-term anticoagulation. It inhibits coag-

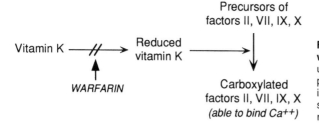

Figure 17.18. **Mechanism of action of warfarin.** Normally, factors II, VII, IX and X undergo carboxylation in the liver, in the presence of reduced vitamin K. Warfarin inhibits the formation of reduced vitamin K, such that nonfunctional coagulation factors result.

ulation by antagonizing the normal hepatic synthesis of vitamin K-dependent coagulation factors (factors II (prothrombin), VII, IX and X). Normally, the reduced form of vitamin K promotes the carboxylation of a glutamic acid residue within these coagulation factors, an action that is necessary for the factors to subsequently bind calcium and participate in coagulation (Fig. 17.18). By interfering with the formation of reduced vitamin K, warfarin indirectly inhibits carboxylation of the coagulation factors, rendering them inactive. Since certain natural coagulation inhibitors (protein C and protein S) are also vitamin K dependent, warfarin impairs their functions as well, which in some cases may counteract the drug's anticoagulant effect.

Warfarin's anticoagulation action has a delayed onset of 2–7 days, so that if an immediate effect is needed, intravenous heparin must be used concurrently for the first few days. The half-life of warfarin is 37 hours, and the drug's dosage must be individualized to achieve a therapeutic effect while minimizing the risk of bleeding complications. The extent of anticoagulation is monitored by measuring the prothrombin time, reported as an International Normalized Ratio (INR), for universal standardization. There are two "target" ranges of anticoagulant intensity. For patients at greatest risk of pathological thrombosis (e.g., mechanical heart valve), the desired INR is 2.5–3.5. In less thrombogenic circumstances (e.g., atrial fibrillation), the target INR is 2.0–3.0.

Many factors can influence the anticoagulation effect of warfarin and require alterations in its dosage. For example, liver disease or heart failure reduces the warfarin requirement, whereas a high dietary inges-

TABLE 17.16. Drugs That Alter the Anticoagulation Effect of Warfarin

Reduced anticoagulant effect	Increased anticoagulant effect
Barbiturates	Amiodarone
Rifampin	Cephalosporin antibiotics
Carbamazepine	Cimetidine
Cholestyramine	Erythromycin
Nafcillin	Fluconazole
Sucralfate	Isoniazid
	Ketoconazole
	Metronidazole
	Phenytoin
	Propafenone
	Trimethoprim-sulfamethoxazole

tion of vitamin K-containing foods (e.g., green leafy vegetables) increases the dosage need. Similarly, many pharmaceuticals alter warfarin's anticoagualtion effect, examples of which are shown in Table 17.16. Finally, the combined use of warfarin with aspirin or other antiplatelet agents increases the risk of a bleeding complication.

If serious bleeding arises during warfarin therapy, the drug's effect can be reversed within hours by the administration of vitamin K_1. However, in patients with mechanical heart valves, this antidote should be avoided unless a life-threatening bleed occurs, because of the possibility of rebound valve thrombosis.

Warfarin is teratogenic and should not be taken during pregnancy, especially in the first trimester.

SUMMARY

This chapter has presented an overview of the most commonly used cardiovascular drugs. These agents are covered in greater detail in the following references, but we hope that the tables, figures and brief explanations presented here will be useful to you now, and again as you consider the basic pathophysiology of heart disease while caring for patients on the wards.

ADDITIONAL READING

Abrams J. The role of nitrates in coronary heart disease. Arch Intern Med 1995;155:357–364.

Bauer JH, Reams GP. The angiotensin II type 1 receptor antagonists: a new class of antihypertensive drugs. Arch Intern Med 1995;155:1361–1368.

Camm AJ, Garratt CJ. Adenosine and supraventricular tachycardia. N Engl J Med 1991;325:1621–1628.

Cardiac Arrhythmia Suppression Trial (CAST) Investigators: Preliminary report. Effect of encainide and flecainide on mortality in a randomized trial of arrhythmia suppression after myocardial infarction. N Engl J Med 1989;321:406.

Collins R, Peto R, Baigent C, et al. Aspirin, heparin and fibrinolytic therapy in suspected acute myocardial infarction. N Engl J Med 1997;336:847–860.

Digitalis Investigation Group. The effect of digoxin on mortality and morbidity in patients with heart failure. New Engl J Med 1997;336:525–533.

Ferguson JJ, Waly HM, Wilson JM. Mechanism and role of platelets in Ischemic events: action of therapeutic agents. J Invas Cardiol 1996;8(Suppl B):1B–7B.

Goldstein S. β-blockers in hypertensive and coronary heart disease. Arch Intern Med 1996;156:1267–1276.

Goodfriend TL, Elliott ME, Catt KJ. Angiotensin receptors and their antagonists. N Engl J Med 1996;334:1649–1653.

Hirsh J, Fuster V. Guide to anticoagulant therapy. Part 2: Oral anticoagulants. Circulation 1994;89:1469–1480.

Hohnloser SH. Sotalol. N Engl J Med 1994;331:31–38.

Lefkovits J, Plow EF, Topol EJ. Platelet glycoprotein IIb/IIIa receptors in cardiovascular medicine. N Engl J Med 1995;332:1553–1559.

Messerli FH. Cardiovascular Drug Therapy. Philadelphia: WB Saunders, 1996.

Opie LH, Chatterjee K, Frishman W, et al. Drugs for the Heart. 4th ed. Philadelphia: WB Saunders, 1995.

Opie LH. Angiotensin-converting Enzyme Inhibitors. Scientific Basis for Clinical Use. New York: Wiley-Liss, 1994.

Parmley WW, Chatterjee K. Cardiovascular Pharmacology. London: Mosby-Year Book Europe, Ltd., 1994.

Patrano C. Aspirin as an antiplatelet drug. N Engl J Med 1994;330:1287–1294.

Roden DM. Risks and benefits of antiarrhythmic therapy. N Engl J Med 1994;331:785–791.

Schafer AI. Low-molecular-weight heparin for venous thromboembolism. Hosp Pract 1997; (January 15); 99–106.

Shen WK, Kurachi Y. Mechanisms of adenosine-mediated actions on cellular and clinical cardiac electrophysiology. Mayo Clin Proc 1995;70:274–291.

Shipley JB, Hess ML. Inotropic therapy for the failing myocardium. Clin Cardiol 1995;18:615–619.

Smith TW. Digoxin in heart failure. N Engl J Med 1993;329:51–53.

Smith TW, ed. Cardiovascular Therapeutics. Philadelphia: WB Saunders, 1996.

Task Force of the Working Group on Arrhythmias of the European Society of Cardiology. The Sicilian gambit: a new approach to the classification of antiarrhythmic drugs based on their actions on arrhythmogenic mechanisms. Circulation 1991;84:1831–1851.

Acknowledgments The previous edition of this chapter was written by Andrew C. Hecht, MD, Steven P. Leon, MD, Ralph A. Kelly, MD, and Leonard S. Lilly, MD. The authors wish to thank Drs. Bruce Ewenstein and Robert Handin for their helpful suggestions.

Index

Page numbers in italic represent figures; page numbers followed by a "t" represent tables.